A Complete Guide to Veterinary Medicine

A Complete Guide to Veterinary Medicine

Editor: Gerardo Bailey

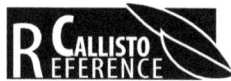

RCALLISTO REFERENCE

www.callistoreference.com

Callisto Reference,
118-35 Queens Blvd., Suite 400,
Forest Hills, NY 11375, USA

Visit us on the World Wide Web at:
www.callistoreference.com

ISBN: 978-1-63239-972-4 (Hardback)

Trademark Notice: Registered trademark of products or corporate names are used only for explanation and identification without intent to infringe.

Cataloging-in-Publication Data

A complete guide to veterinary medicine / edited by Gerardo Bailey.
    p. cm.
Includes bibliographical references and index.
ISBN 978-1-63239-972-4
1. Veterinary medicine. 2. Animals--Diseases. 3. Animal health. I. Bailey, Gerardo.
SF745 .C66 2018
636.089--dc23

Table of Contents

Preface

Veterinary medicine deals with the study and practice of treating, diagnosing, and preventing various diseases and disorders in animals. The field includes treating both domestic and wild animals with effective medication. This book provides significant information of this discipline to help develop a good understanding of veterinary medicine and related fields. It explains in detail the different studies conducted relating to this area. The text is compiled in such a manner, that it will provide in-depth knowledge about the theory and practice of veterinary medicine. It aims to serve as a resource guide for students and experts alike and contribute to the growth of the discipline.

The researches compiled throughout the book are authentic and of high quality, combining several disciplines and from very diverse regions from around the world. Drawing on the contributions of many researchers from diverse countries, the book's objective is to provide the readers with the latest achievements in the area of research. This book will surely be a source of knowledge to all interested and researching the field.

In the end, I would like to express my deep sense of gratitude to all the authors for meeting the set deadlines in completing and submitting their research chapters. I would also like to thank the publisher for the support offered to us throughout the course of the book. Finally, I extend my sincere thanks to my family for being a constant source of inspiration and encouragement.

Editor

Histomorphometric Evaluation of Superovulation Effect on Follicular Development after Autologous Ovarian Transplantation in Mice

Amin Tamadon,[1] Alireza Raayat Jahromi,[2] Farhad Rahmanifar,[3] Mohammad Ayaseh,[2] Omid Koohi-Hosseinabadi,[4] and Reza Moghiminasr[5]

[1]Transgenic Technology Research Center, Shiraz University of Medical Sciences, Shiraz, Iran
[2]Department of Clinical Sciences, School of Veterinary Medicine, Shiraz University, P.O. Box 1731-71345, Shiraz, Iran
[3]Department of Basic Sciences, School of Veterinary Medicine, Shiraz University, P.O. Box 1731-71345, Shiraz, Iran
[4]Laboratory Animal Center, Shiraz University of Medical Sciences, Shiraz, Iran
[5]Department of Stem Cells and Developmental Biology, Cell Science Research Center,
 Royan Institute for Stem Cell Biology and Technology, ACECR, Tehran, Iran

Correspondence should be addressed to Alireza Raayat Jahromi; raayat@shirazu.ac.ir
and Farhad Rahmanifar; rahmanifar@shirazu.ac.ir

Academic Editor: Sumanta Nandi

The effect of superovulation by pregnant mare serum gonadotropin (PMSG) on autologous transplanted ovaries in the lumbar muscles of mice was histomorphometrically evaluated using the indices of number and volume of different kind of follicles and volume of corpora lutea, ovary, and stroma. Angiogenesis was observed after mouse ovarian transplantation on days 14 and 21 after ovarian grafting. After transplantation, the total number and volume of primary and secondary follicles reduced, while PMSG superovulation increased the total number and total volume of tertiary follicles and also the ovarian volume after transplantation. Transplantation increased the average size of primary, secondary, and tertiary follicles. Therefore, primary and secondary follicles can survive after autologous transplantation but their reservations diminished by increasing the time of transplantation. However, number of tertiary follicles and their response to superovulation increased over time after transplantation.

1. Introduction

Ovary transplantation is a method for preservation of endangered and valuable species [1]. On the other hand, ovarian transplantation has the potential application for maintaining the fertility after chemotherapy and radiotherapy in women [2]. As a result of the ovarian transplantation, the possible depletion of follicle reserve and limitation of fertility restoration exist [3]. The major concern in grafting is that the graft survival is completely dependent on the establishment of neovascularization [4]. A number of follicles may be lost because of hypoxia and ischemia. For evaluation of the effect of ischemia after ovarian transplantation, whole or piece of small ovaries of laboratory rodents can be used [5]. To prevent ischemia and increase the rate of angiogenesis, surgery must

be rapid and the ovarian tissue should be placed in a highly vascular tissue [6]. It is shown that ischemia may cause disappearance of 50% or even greater percentage of primary follicles and almost all of the growing follicles 3 to 7 days after transplantation and before development of angiogenesis [7].

Steroidogenesis, proliferation, and differentiation of follicular granulosa cells of growing preovulatory stages of ovarian follicles are induced by follicle-stimulating hormone (FSH). However, primordial follicles' initial development is FSH independent [8], but FSH acts as survival factor in serum-free ovarian cortical tissue culture and during primordial follicular transition to primary and secondary follicles [9]. In addition, coordination of germ line and somatic compartments of follicle development in mouse is done by FSH [10]. FSH action in adult mouse can be induced using

TABLE 1: Groups and procedures for evaluation of superovulation effect on follicular development after autologous ovarian transplantation in mice.

Groups	Transplantation	PMSG injection and time	Day of sampling
Negative control	−	−	In the estrus phase
PMSG	−	+ (In the diestrus phase)	2 d after injection
Graft (14 d)	+	−	14 d after transplantation
Graft (21 d)	+	−	21 d after transplantation
Graft + PMSG (14 d)	+	+ (12 d after transplantation)	14 d after transplantation
Graft + PMSG (21 d)	+	+ (19 d after transplantation)	21 d after transplantation

pregnant mare serum gonadotropin (PMSG), a chorionic gonadotropin hormone of pregnant mare. PMSG superovulation can serve as a good model to understand the probable mechanism of FSH action in follicular development [11].

With that in mind that harvesting of mature oocytes for in vitro fertilization process increases the chances of reproductive success, PMSG is currently used for production of mature superovulated oocytes for in vitro fertilization of valuable species including endangered ones. In addition, it is not known if the transplanted preserved ovaries can respond to the superovulation to achieve this goal of harvesting higher number of matured oocytes. The aim of the present study was to (1) assess superovulation with PMSG on transplanted ovary as an indicator of posttransplantation normal activity of antral follicles, (2) evaluate histomorphometrically the effect of posttransplantation ischemia on different follicular stages, and (3) evaluate the effect of recovery time on follicular growth after autologous transplantation of murine ovaries by the induction of superovulation using PMSG.

2. Materials and Methods

2.1. Animals. The experimental study was approved by Ethics Committee of School of Veterinary Medicine, Shiraz University. Thirty-six female adult Balb/c mice weighing approximately 25–30 g were provided from Laboratory Animal Center, Shiraz University of Medical Sciences. The animals were kept at $23 \pm 1°C$ and $55 \pm 5\%$ relative humidity with 12 h light/dark cycle. They were given standard pellet and water *ad libitum* during experimental period.

The mice were randomly divided into 6 equal groups ($n = 6$), four transplantation groups and two control groups (Table 1). The transplantation groups included two transplantation (14 and 21 d) groups and two PMSG/transplantation (14 and 21 d) groups. The control groups were subdivided to a positive control PMSG group and a negative control group. The mice were entered into study on day of diestrus using vaginal smears. In PMSG positive control group, the mice received single intraperitoneal injection of PMSG (5 IU, Pregnecol, Bioniche Animal Health (A/Asia) Pty Ltd., Armidale, NSW, Australia) and 48 h later the animals were euthanized with ether and cervical dislocation. In the transplantation groups (14 and 21 d), the ovarian autotransplantation was done on both sides of spinal cord during the diestrus phase. After 14 d and 21 d, the mice of transplantation groups were sacrificed. In the PMSG/transplantation groups (14 and 21 d),

the same autotransplantation procedure was performed and after 12 d in the first group and 19 d in the second one PMSG (5 IU) was intraperitoneally injected and 48 h later the mice were euthanized. In the negative control group, surgery was not performed and the mice were sacrificed in the estrus phase. Stages of estrus cycle were determined based on vaginal smear method [12].

2.2. Ovarian Autotransplantation Surgical Method. Surgical procedures were performed under sterile conditions and in a 24°C temperature operating room. The diestrus mice were weighed and anesthetized with an IP injection of ketamine (100 mg/kg, Alfasan, Woerden, Netherland) and xylazine (10 mg/kg, Alfasan, Woerden, Netherland). Surgical area of abdomen and lateral lumbar region of the mice were surgically prepared. Both ovaries of the mice were removed from a midline abdominal incision and transferred to a sterile dish filled with prewarmed (39°C) sterile saline. Adipose and connective tissues were carefully removed from ovary using a stereomicroscope (SZM, Optika, Italy). The abdominal muscles and skin were sutured with a standard two-layer closure using a simple continuous suture pattern. Then, paralumbar incisions were made on both sides, parallel to the lumbar spinal cord. The ovaries were then grafted into the dorsal lumbar muscles and skin was routinely closed. Oxytetracycline spray was applied on the incision site. Animals were placed in individual controlled 25°C temperature recovery cages.

2.3. Histological Evaluation of Ovaries. On the day of sampling, animals were euthanized with ether and ovaries of control and PMSG groups and the transplanted ovarian tissues with their surrounding muscles of transplanting groups were removed. The tissues were fixed in fresh 10% buffered formalin solution in room temperature. After that they were implanted in paraffin. Ethanol and xylene were used for dehydration step. Samples were embedded in paraffin wax and serial sections at thicknesses of 20 μm were performed. During the block sectioning, serial sections were checked until the ovarian tissues appeared in the paraffin section. That was selected as the first section of ovary and the 10th section of every 10 consecutive slices were selected until the observation of the last section with ovarian tissue in the paraffin block. Selected sections were deparaffinized at 60°C and dehydrated in graded concentrations of xylene and ethanol rehydrated in room temperature and stained with hematoxylin and eosin stain.

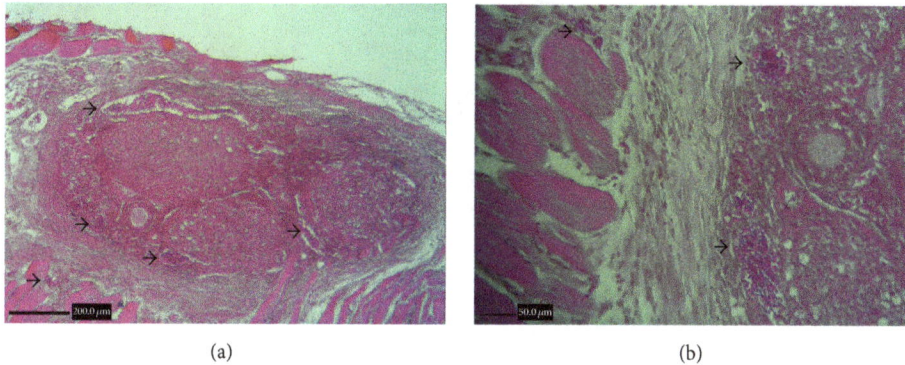

(a)

(b)

FIGURE 1: (a) Corpora lutea and secondary follicle in the section confirm ovarian function and folliculogenesis after 21 days' autologous ovarian transplantation in lateral lumbar muscles of mice without superovulation. (b) Angiogenesis, arrows show presence of blood cells in vessels of transplanted ovary and surrounding skeletal muscles. H&E staining.

2.4. Histomorphometric Analysis. Follicle types in ovarian sections were defined as previously explained [13] and the numbers of primary, secondary, and tertiary follicles were counted on light microscope (CX21, Olympus, Japan). Sections were also microscopically photographed with an adjusted digital camera (AM423U Eyepiece Camera, Dino-Eye, Taiwan) and Dino Capture 2.0 software (AnMo Electronics Corporation, New Taipei City, Taiwan). The area of total ovary, corpora lutea, and total follicles of each section were measured by drawing their scope using Digimizer software (MedCalc Software bvba; Mariakerke, Belgium).

Moreover, the volume of the ovary, developing follicles of all stages, and corpora lutea of all groups (V) were calculated according to the elliptical cone volume formula: $V = \pi D^2 h/6$, where π is equivalent to 3.14, D indicates the larger diameter, and h indicates the smaller diameter of the ovary, follicles, and corpora lutea. The mean follicle volume (v) was measured by taking the average of volume of ovarian tertiary follicles of all stages, according to the following formula: $v = V/N$, where N indicates the numbers of ovarian developing follicles of all stages. Furthermore, stromal volume (V_S) was calculated according to the following formula: $V_S = V_O - V_F$, where V_O is the volume of the ovary and V_F is the volume of the follicles.

2.5. Statistical Analysis. The data of histological indices of ovary were subjected to Kolmogorov-Smirnov test of normality and analyzed by one-way ANOVA and LSD post hoc test (SPSS for Windows, version 22, SPSS Inc., Chicago, Illinois). The P value of less than 0.05 was considered to be statistically significant. Group means and their standard error were reported in the text and graphs (GraphPad Prism version 5.01 for Windows, GraphPad software Inc., San Diego, CA, USA).

3. Results

Histological evaluation showed angiogenesis and folliculogenesis after grafting in ovaries in the transplantation and PMSG/transplantation groups (Figure 1). Moreover, in microscopic evaluation of ovaries in the PMSG group and the PMSG/transplantation (14 and 21 d) groups numerous large tertiary follicles were observed, but in the transplantation (14 and 21 d) groups and the control group the number and the size of tertiary follicles were smaller (Figure 2).

Histomorphometric analysis showed that there was a significant reduction in the number and total volume of primary follicles in the transplantation (14 and 21 d) and PMSG/transplantation (14 and 21 d) groups compared with the control and PMSG groups ($P < 0.05$, Figures 3(a) and 3(b)). The mean primary follicle volume in the transplantation (14 d) group was more than that in the other groups except for the PMSG/transplantation (14 d) group ($P < 0.05$, Figure 3(c)). Also there was a significant decrease in the mean primary follicle volume in the PMSG group in comparison with the other groups ($P < 0.05$).

Same as primary follicles, there was a significant reduction in the number of secondary follicles in the transplantation (14 and 21 d) and PMSG/transplantation (14 and 21 d) groups compared with the control and PMSG groups ($P < 0.05$, Figure 4(a)). Moreover, the total volume of secondary follicles in the PMSG group was more than the PMSG/transplantation (21 d) group ($P < 0.05$, Figure 4(b)). The mean secondary follicle volume in the transplantation (14 d) group was significantly more than the control, PMSG, and PMSG/transplantation (21 d) groups ($P < 0.05$, Figure 4(c)).

The number of tertiary follicles in the transplantation (21 d) and PMSG/transplantation (21 d) groups was significantly more than the control group ($P < 0.05$, Figure 5(a)). The total volume of tertiary follicles in the PMSG/transplantation (21 d) group was significantly greater than the control, PMSG, and transplantation (14 d) groups ($P < 0.05$, Figure 5(b)). The mean tertiary follicle volume in the PMSG/transplantation (14 and 21 d) group was more than the control and PMSG groups ($P < 0.05$, Figure 5(c)).

Ovary volume in the PMSG/transplantation (21 d) group was more than the control and transplantation (14 d) groups ($P < 0.05$, Figure 6(a)). Ovarian stromal volume in the PMSG group was more than the transplantation (14 and 21 d) groups ($P < 0.05$, Figure 6(b)).

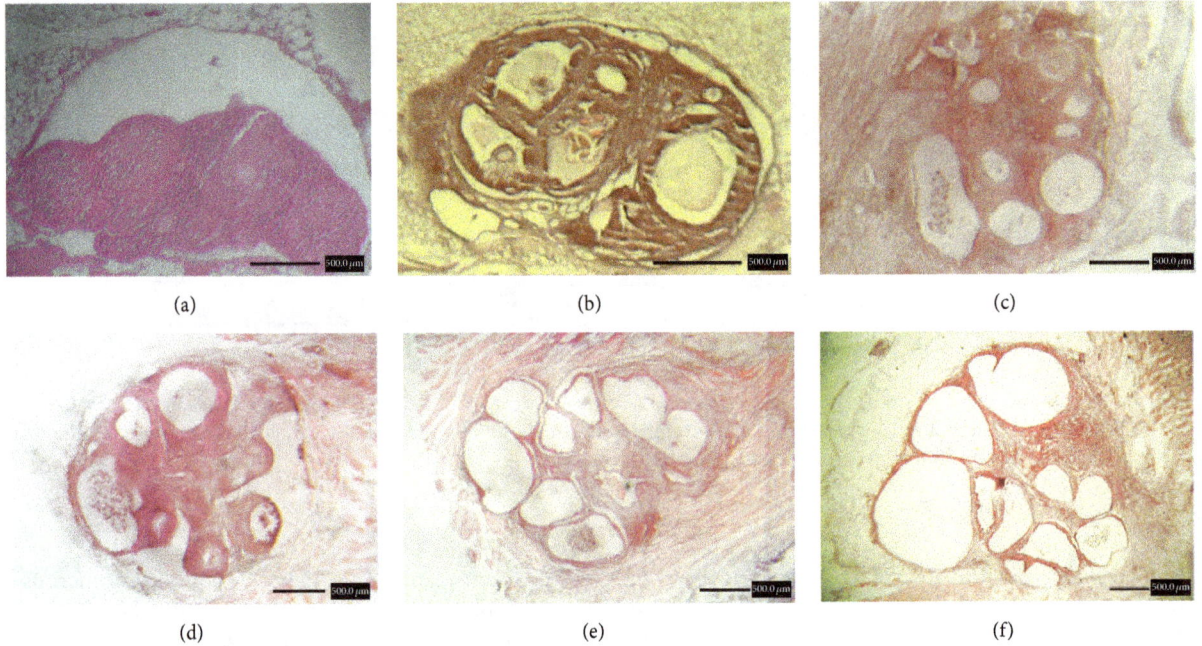

FIGURE 2: Comparison of the superovulatory effect of pregnant mare serum gonadotropin (PMSG) after autologous ovarian transplantation in mice. Ovaries of groups of (a) control, (b) PMSG, (c) transplantation (14 d), (d) transplantation (21 d), (e) PMSG/transplantation (14 d), and (f) PMSG/transplantation (21 d). H&E staining.

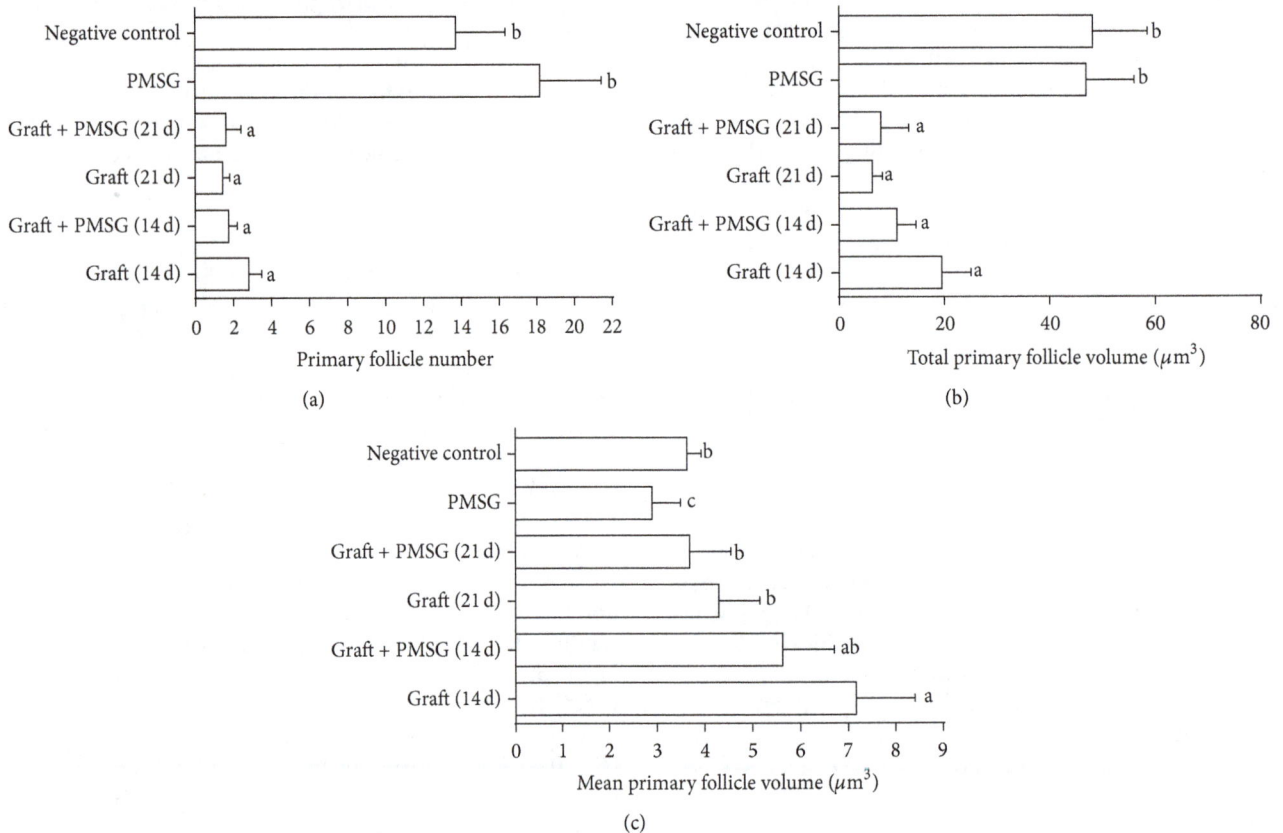

FIGURE 3: Mean and standard error of histomorphometric analysis of primary follicles (a) total number, (b) total volume, and (c) mean follicle volume in control group, pregnant mare serum gonadotropin (PMSG) group, transplantation (14 and 21 d), and PMSG/transplantation (14 and 21 d) groups after autologous ovarian transplantation and superovulatory effect of PMSG. [a, b, c] Different superscript letters show significant difference between different groups ($P < 0.05$).

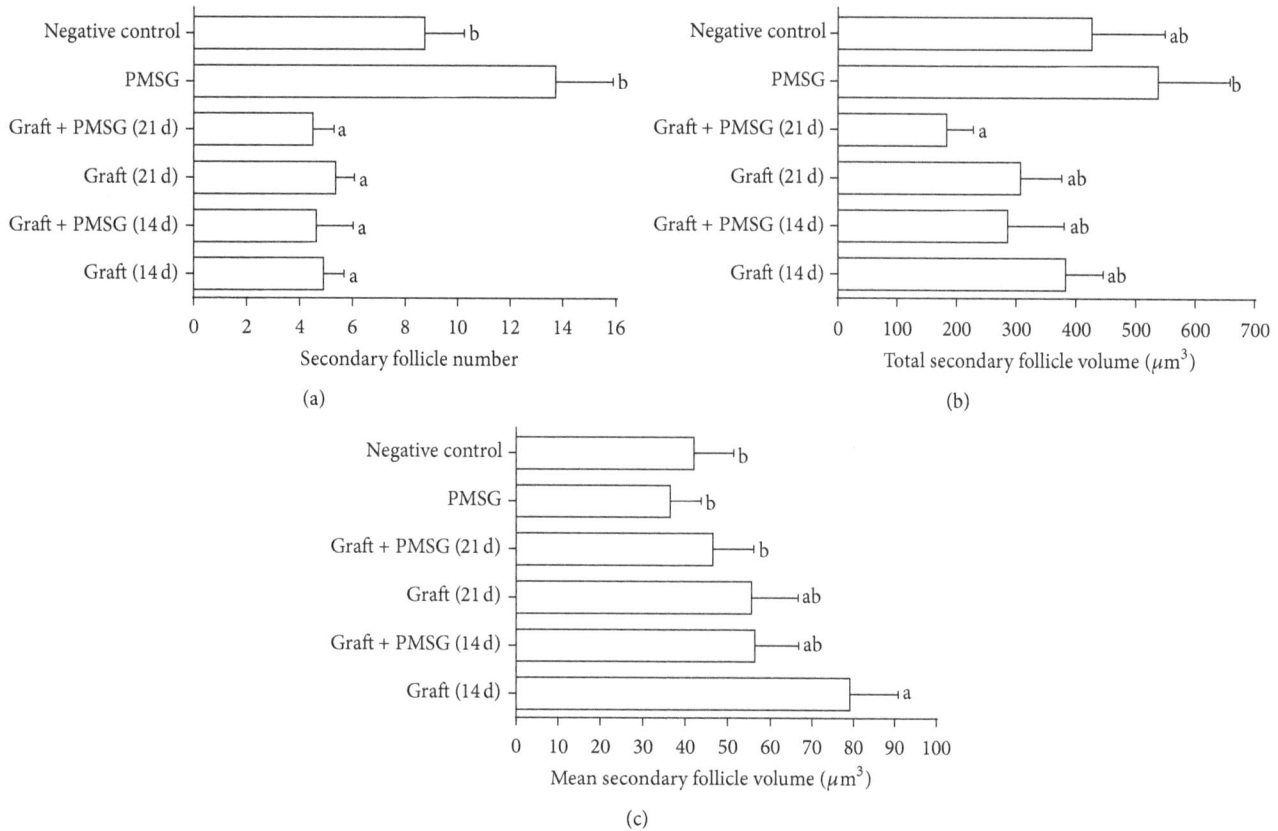

FIGURE 4: Mean and standard error of histomorphometric analysis of secondary follicles (a) total number, (b) total volume, and (c) mean follicle volume in control group, pregnant mare serum gonadotropin (PMSG) group, transplantation (14 and 21 d), and PMSG/transplantation (14 and 21 d) groups after autologous ovarian transplantation and superovulatory effect of PMSG. [a,b] Different superscript letters show significant difference between different groups ($P < 0.05$).

4. Discussion

In the present study, the impact of transplantation ischemia on survival and development of different follicular stages following whole ovary heterotopic autotransplantation were histomorphometrically evaluated after 14 and 21 d. The results indicated that survival and development of different follicular types were influenced by ischemia. Reduction in the number of primary and secondary follicles in the transplantation and PMSG/transplantation groups after 14 and 21 d showed the effect of ischemia on these follicular stages. However, the number and volume of these follicles decreased after grafting but estimated individual size of both types was increased after 14 days and again was decreased on day 21. Simultaneously, during the same period, increase of the number and volume of tertiary follicles showed follicular growth continued and was enhanced after heterotopic transplantation. Consistent with our findings, Xie et al. [3] recently showed that healthy rate of follicles and the number of follicles with positive proliferating cell nuclear antigen in primary follicles decreased 1 month after orthotopic autografting of the rabbit ovaries. Early follicular development is regulated by ovarian autocrine/paracrine regulators and interactions between oocyte-granulosa cells, ovarian stromal cells, and theca cells affect this process [14]. Grafting could induce deactivation

of primordial follicles [15]. Therefore, decrease in number of primary follicles can be affected by cessation of primordial follicle growth. Our findings indirectly and directly may indicate that follicular growth and development in early stage (primordial and primary follicles) were more influenced by ischemia in comparison with late stages (secondary and tertiary follicles), and follicle reservoirs in primordial and primary stages cannot be well replaced after transplantation ischemia.

In this study, we observed that ovarian tissue survived and follicles grew in muscular spaces of back muscle. A rapid blood supply can prevent loss of follicular pool and cessation of folliculogenesis after ovarian transplantation may reduce the follicular quality and response to hormonal alterations. Therefore, in this study the effect of intraperitoneal injection of PMSG on follicular growth after ovarian transplantation was evaluated as an index of presence of ovarian blood supply, angiogenesis, and folliculogenesis especially after primordial follicular stage. Significant differences in the primary, secondary, and tertiary follicle number and volume after transplantation and superovulation, which indicated the time despite the positive role in follicular survival and better angiogenesis, have a significant impact on follicular growth and maturation in response to superovulation. Anatomically, primary follicles in rodents are small and located very close

(a)

(b)

(c)

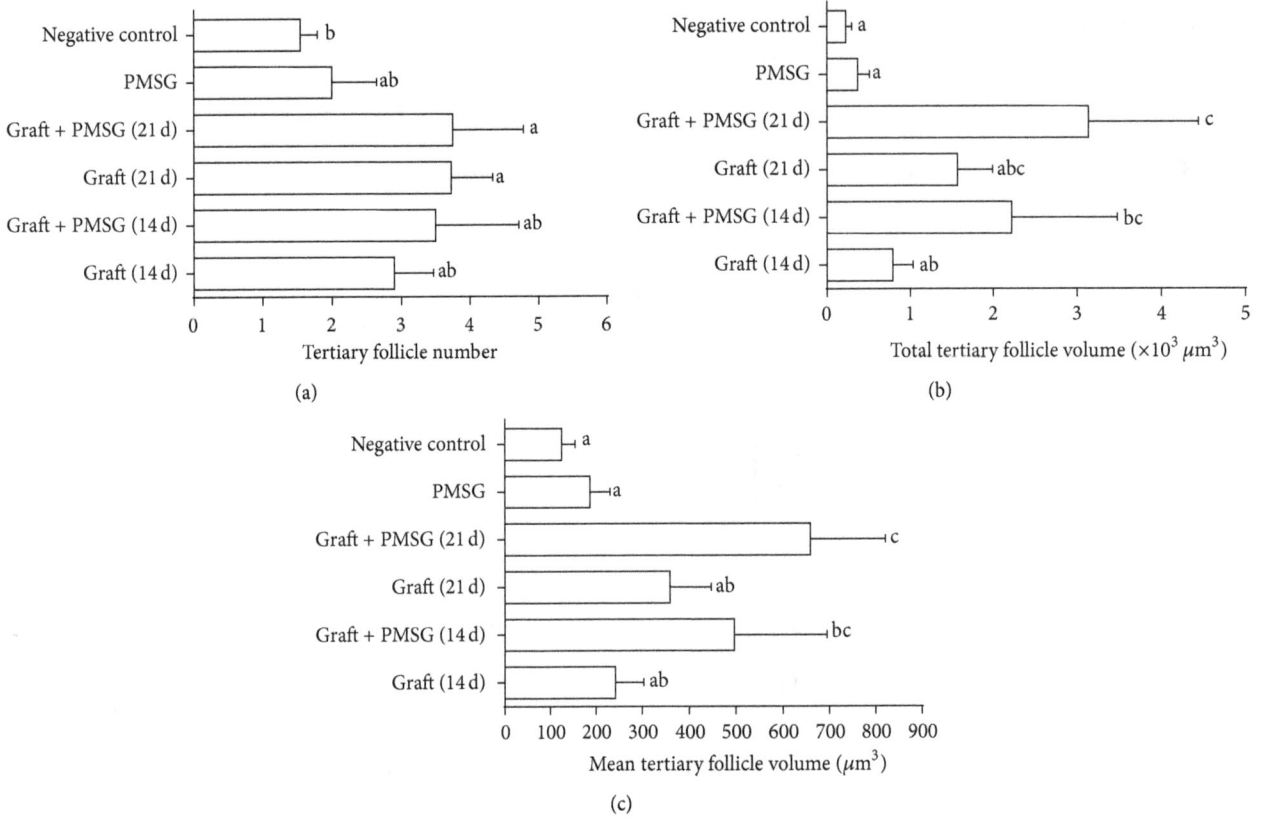

FIGURE 5: Mean and standard error of histomorphometric analysis of tertiary follicles (a) total number, (b) total volume, and (c) mean follicle volume in control group, pregnant mare serum gonadotropin (PMSG) group, transplantation (14 and 21 d), and PMSG/transplantation (14 and 21 d) groups after autologous ovarian transplantation and superovulatory effect of PMSG. [a,b,c]Different superscript letters show significant difference between different groups ($P < 0.05$).

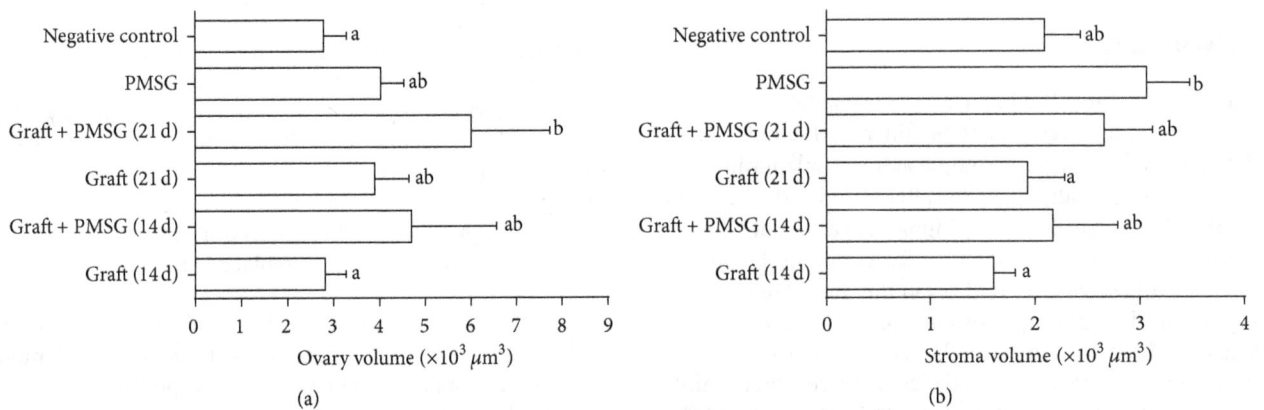

(a)

(b)

FIGURE 6: Mean and standard error of histomorphometric analysis of (a) ovarian volume and (b) stroma volume in control group, pregnant mare serum gonadotropin (PMSG) group, transplantation (14 and 21 d), and PMSG/transplantation (14 and 21 d) groups after autologous ovarian transplantation and superovulatory effect of PMSG. [a,b]Different superscript letters show significant difference between different groups ($P < 0.05$).

to the surface of ovary [16]. On the other hand, oocyte metabolism was higher in primary follicles than at any subsequent stage [17]. Therefore, more reduction of primary follicles than secondary ones after one week (time between two samplings) may be the result of the effect of posttransplantation ischemia on reduction of early stages of follicles.

Complete removal of ovarian fat tissue before transplantation enhanced revascularization via facilitation of cell infiltration from the high blood supply muscular tissue. Formation of new blood vessels was initiated by elongation, sprouting, intussusception, or the incorporation of circulating endothelial cells of preexisting vasculature [18]. Most of these processes can be involved in angiogenesis of ovary [19]. Ischemic damage of ovarian tissue is unavoidable during postgrafting period and its effect is reduced after neo- and revascularization. Vascular connections between the murine ovary and transplanted site were observed 5 days after transplantation [20].

A cohort of primordial follicles within 10 to 12 d reaches the secondary follicle stage and by 6 to 12 d develop to the large antral stage in mice [21]. Considering the 5 d of posttransplantation angiogenesis, in the first sampling of 14 d, the evaluated tertiary follicles were the developed follicles from the primary and secondary follicles which suffered from posttransplantation ischemia, while in the second sampling of 21 d the sectioned tertiary follicles were related to the developed follicles from the primary and secondary follicles after angiogenesis. Therefore, the increase in mean of number or volume of tertiary follicles after 21 d in comparison with 14 d sampling in transplantation groups can be explained.

5. Conclusions

Primary and secondary follicles can survive after autologous transplantation but their reservoirs gradually get diminished by increasing the time of transplantation. However, number of tertiary follicles and their response to superovulation increased over time after transplantation. Therefore, it seems that early collection or superovulation of transplanted ovaries may result in more tertiary follicles.

Conflict of Interests

The authors declare that there is no conflict of interests regarding the publication of this paper.

References

[1] R. R. Santos, C. Amorim, S. Cecconi et al., "Cryopreservation of ovarian tissue: an emerging technology for female germline preservation of endangered species and breeds," *Animal Reproduction Science*, vol. 122, no. 3-4, pp. 151–163, 2010.

[2] P. Ghadjar, V. Budach, C. Köhler, A. Jantke, and S. Marnitz, "Modern radiation therapy and potential fertility preservation strategies in patients with cervical cancer undergoing chemoradiation," *Radiation Oncology*, vol. 10, no. 1, p. 50, 2015.

[3] S. Xie, X. Zhang, W. Chen et al., "Developmental status: impact of short-term ischemia on follicular survival of whole ovarian transplantation in a rabbit model," *PLoS ONE*, vol. 10, no. 8, Article ID e0135049, 2015.

[4] A. R. Rajabzadeh, H. Eimani, H. Mohseni Koochesfahani, A.-H. Shahvardi, and R. Fathi, "Morphological study of isolated ovarian preantral follicles using fibrin gel plus platelet lysate after subcutaneous transplantation," *Cell Journal*, vol. 17, no. 1, pp. 145–152, 2015.

[5] E. Torrents, I. Boiso, P. N. Barri, and A. Veiga, "Applications of ovarian tissue transplantation in experimental biology and medicine," *Human Reproduction Update*, vol. 9, no. 5, pp. 471–481, 2003.

[6] I. Demeestere, P. Simon, S. Emiliani, A. Delbaere, and Y. Englert, "Orthotopic and heterotopic ovarian tissue transplantation," *Human Reproduction Update*, vol. 15, no. 6, pp. 649–665, 2009.

[7] R. G. Gosden, "Ovary and uterus transplantation," *Reproduction*, vol. 136, no. 6, pp. 671–680, 2008.

[8] R. Garor, R. Abir, A. Erman, C. Felz, S. Nitke, and B. Fisch, "Effects of basic fibroblast growth factor on in vitro development of human ovarian primordial follicles," *Fertility and Sterility*, vol. 91, no. 5, pp. 1967–1975, 2009.

[9] C. S. Wright, O. Hovatta, R. Margara et al., "Effects of follicle-stimulating hormone and serum substitution on the in-vitro growth of human ovarian follicles," *Human Reproduction*, vol. 14, no. 6, pp. 1555–1562, 1999.

[10] I. Demeestere, A. K. Streiff, J. Suzuki et al., "Follicle-stimulating hormone accelerates mouse oocyte development in vivo," *Biology of Reproduction*, vol. 87, no. 1, p. 3, 2012.

[11] D. Bhartiya, K. Sriraman, P. Gunjal, and H. Modak, "Gonadotropin treatment augments postnatal oogenesis and primordial follicle assembly in adult mouse ovaries?" *Journal of Ovarian Research*, vol. 5, no. 1, article 32, 2012.

[12] M. S. Salehi, M. R. J. Shirazi, M. J. Zamiri et al., "Hypothalamic expression of KiSS1 and RFamide-related peptide-3 mRNAs during the estrous cycle of rats," *International Journal of Fertility and Sterility*, vol. 6, no. 4, pp. 304–309, 2013.

[13] M. Azarnia, H. Koochesfahani, M. Rajabi, Y. Tahamtani, and A. Tamadon, "Histological examination of endosulfan effects on follicular development of BALB/C mice," *Bulgarian Journal of Veterinary Medicine*, vol. 12, no. 1, pp. 33–41, 2008.

[14] M. Qiu, F. Quan, C. Han et al., "Effects of granulosa cells on steroidogenesis, proliferation and apoptosis of stromal cells and theca cells derived from the goat ovary," *The Journal of Steroid Biochemistry and Molecular Biology*, vol. 138, pp. 325–333, 2013.

[15] A. David, A. Van Langendonckt, S. Gilliaux, M.-M. Dolmans, J. Donnez, and C. A. Amorim, "Effect of cryopreservation and transplantation on the expression of kit ligand and anti-Müllerian hormone in human ovarian tissue," *Human Reproduction*, vol. 27, no. 4, pp. 1088–1095, 2012.

[16] J. B. Kerr, R. Duckett, M. Myers, K. L. Britt, T. Mladenovska, and J. K. Findlay, "Quantification of healthy follicles in the neonatal and adult mouse ovary: evidence for maintenance of primordial follicle supply," *Reproduction*, vol. 132, no. 1, pp. 95–109, 2006.

[17] S. E. Harris, H. J. Leese, R. G. Gosden, and H. M. Picton, "Pyruvate and oxygen consumption throughout the growth and development of murine oocytes," *Molecular Reproduction and Development*, vol. 76, no. 3, pp. 231–238, 2009.

[18] G. D. Yancopoulos, S. Davis, N. W. Gale, J. S. Rudge, S. J. Wiegand, and J. Holash, "Vascular-specific growth factors and blood vessel formation," *Nature*, vol. 407, no. 6801, pp. 242–248, 2000.

[19] G. Macchiarelli, J.-Y. Jiang, S. A. Nottola, and E. Sato, "Morphological patterns of angiogenesis in ovarian follicle capillary networks. A scanning electron microscopy study of corrosion cast," *Microscopy Research and Technique*, vol. 69, no. 6, pp. 459–468, 2006.

[20] A.-S. Van Eyck, B. F. Jordan, B. Gallez, J.-F. Heilier, A. Van Langendonckt, and J. Donnez, "Electron paramagnetic resonance as a tool to evaluate human ovarian tissue reoxygenation after xenografting," *Fertility and Sterility*, vol. 92, no. 1, pp. 374–381, 2009.

[21] J. J. Eppig, K. Wigglesworth, and F. L. Pendola, "The mammalian oocyte orchestrates the rate of ovarian follicular development," *Proceedings of the National Academy of Sciences of the United States of America*, vol. 99, no. 5, pp. 2890–2894, 2002.

A Retrospective Analysis of 5,195 Patient Treatment Sessions in an Integrative Veterinary Medicine Service: Patient Characteristics, Presenting Complaints, and Therapeutic Interventions

Justin Shmalberg[1] and Mushtaq A. Memon[2]

[1]Small Animal Clinical Sciences, College of Veterinary Medicine, University of Florida, Gainesville, FL 32608, USA
[2]Department of Veterinary Clinical Sciences, College of Veterinary Medicine, Washington State University, Pullman, WA 99164, USA

Correspondence should be addressed to Justin Shmalberg; shmalberg@ufl.edu

Academic Editor: Pedro J. Ginel

Integrative veterinary medicine, the combination of complementary and alternative therapies with conventional care, is increasingly prevalent in veterinary practice and a focus of clinical instruction in many academic teaching institutions. However, the presenting complaints, therapeutic modalities, and patient population in an integrative medicine service have not been described. A retrospective analysis of 5,195 integrative patient treatment sessions in a veterinary academic teaching hospital demonstrated that patients most commonly received a combination of therapeutic modalities (39% of all treatment sessions). The 274 patients receiving multiple modalities were most frequently treated for neurologic and orthopedic disease (50.7% versus 49.6% of all presenting complaints, resp.). Older neutered or spayed dogs (mean age = 9.0 years) and Dachshunds were treated more often than expected based on general population statistics. Acupuncture, laser therapy, electroacupuncture, and hydrotherapy were frequently administered (>50% patients). Neurologic patients were more likely to receive acupuncture, electroacupuncture, and therapeutic exercises but less likely than orthopedic patients to receive laser, hydrotherapy, or therapeutic ultrasound treatments ($P < 0.05$). The results suggest that the application of these specific modalities to orthopedic and neurologic diseases should be subjected to increased evidence-based investigations. A review of current knowledge in core areas is presented.

1. Introduction

Integrative medicine describes an increasingly popular form of medicine combining conventional medical practice with alternative or complementary therapies, which is based on the best available scientific evidence [1]. Alternative or complementary therapies are broadly defined in human medical practice but may include nutrition, acupuncture, laser therapy, hyperbaric oxygen, rehabilitation, and other interventions not typically considered mainstream medical practice. Integrative *veterinary* medicine is poorly described both in definition and in practice although the term occasionally appears in the scientific literature [2]. However, a similar definition as to that used in integrative human medical practice characterizes the concept in veterinary medicine. Alternate and historical terms used to describe unconventional therapies inadequately distort the purpose of such treatments. Alternative veterinary medicine suggests that certain therapies are a replacement or a mutually exclusive option to conventional care, which disregards the potential for synergistic effects. Complementary medicine implies that the therapies can and should only be used in tandem, when in some cases a modality may be the preferred or exclusive treatment available. Finally, holistic medicine suggests that conventional veterinary practice does not consider the impacts of treatment on the whole animal, an obviously flawed assumption.

The prevalence of integrative medical interventions in veterinary medicine has not been established. A survey of owners of veterinary oncology patients found a robust usage of therapies regarded as alternative or complementary [3]. A survey of one school's veterinary graduates identified that more than two-thirds of these veterinarians encountered clinical situations involving these therapies at least monthly and over 25% experienced them on a weekly or daily basis [4]. These findings served as a framework for that study's authors to suggest, with evidence from surveys of AVMA-accredited colleges of veterinary medicine, that a comprehensive curriculum should be available to veterinary students. The need for education and information in integrative medicine is highlighted by the fact that nearly one-third of the general population has used a complementary or alternative medical approach for their own health [5].

The purpose of this study was to retrospectively evaluate the caseload from within a busy academic integrative veterinary medicine service to determine the frequency with which specific modalities were used and the relationships of such modalities to presenting complaint, breed, age, and other factors. Study findings provide critical information to other integrative medicine services and for researchers investigating specific modalities within the scope of the service's practice. Future randomized controlled trials are needed to further evaluate a number of the modalities.

2. Material and Methods

The electronic medical records were collected from a mixed animal integrative medicine service at an academic teaching hospital over a 400-day period from July 2014 to August 2015. The total number of patient visits in each hospital service was tabulated. The presenting complaints for integrative medicine visits were recorded along with the species of patient, body condition score, outpatient or inpatient status, and the date of treatment.

The records of small animal patients receiving more than one therapeutic modality at a visit were further analyzed to determine whether each patient had seen another service in the 6 months before treatment and to calculate the number of integrative visits for each patient. If patients were seen more than once during the retrospective period, a visit was randomly selected to determine which therapeutic modalities the patient received.

The differences between groups were evaluated using one-way ANOVA and commercially available statistical software (Minitab 17.1). Results were considered statistically significant if the probability of error was less than 5% ($P <$ 0.05). Post hoc analysis was performed with Fisher's test for pairwise comparisons. Odds ratios were calculated, using commercial software (Microsoft Excel 2010), to assess if specific patient populations, grouped by condition or breed, had a different likelihood of receiving each modality or of presenting with a particular complaint. A result was considered statistically significant if the 95% confidence interval for the odds ratio excluded the value 1.0. The Pearson correlation coefficients (r) were calculated for the potential relationships between age, body weight, number of treatments, and the number of modalities used for each patient; results were considered significant if $P < 0.05$.

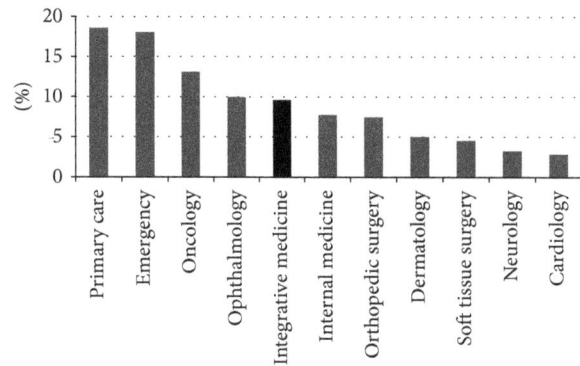

FIGURE 1: Comparative caseload of the study site's Academic Veterinary Hospital.

3. Results

The integrative medicine service attended to 5,195 patient treatment sessions during the study period. The distribution of species from greatest to least was as follows: dogs (95.6%), cats (3.0%), horses (0.8%), and exotic species or wildlife (0.6%). The majority of these cases were managed as outpatients (90.2%), with the remainder receiving inpatient treatment (9.8%) over an average inpatient rehabilitation period of 3.0 days. Recorded treatments included those performed during business hours (93.3%) and after hours (6.7%). The integrative medicine service received 9.6% of total hospital caseload (Figure 1).

A number of different therapies are included in the total treatment sessions. Outpatient integrative medicine sessions, which included multiple modalities, were the most prevalent ($n = 2,042$ or 39.3%), followed by rehabilitation-exclusive appointments (20.5%) and nutrition visits (11.1%). The complete distribution of service caseload is provided (Figure 2).

The patients who received multiple therapies were selected for additional analysis. The multiple modality treatment sessions were most commonly utilized for patients ($n = 274$) with neurological and orthopedic conditions (50.7% and 49.6%, resp.). 17.4% of patients presenting with primary neurologic disease had concurrent orthopedic abnormalities, and 15.6% of patients presenting with orthopedic disease had concurrent neurologic disorders. Patients also presented with issues related to internal medicine, oncology, soft tissue surgery, critical care, dermatology, and other conditions (Figure 3). Each patient receiving multiple modalities visited the service an average of 7.6 ± 10.5 times during the study period with a range of 1–106 visits. Orthopedic conditions were treated on average with more visits (10.1 ± 14.2) than were neurologic conditions (6.7 ± 8.9) ($P = 0.007$). The number of visits did not differ by breed ($P = 0.128$) or by age ($P = 0.68$).

The majority of small animal patients that presented for multiple modality visits were of ideal body condition (body condition score (BCS) = 4-5/9, 41.6%) but a significant number were classified as overweight (BCS = 6, 31.8%) or obese (BCS ≥ 7, 25%) (Figure 4). No statistical difference

Distribution of service caseload

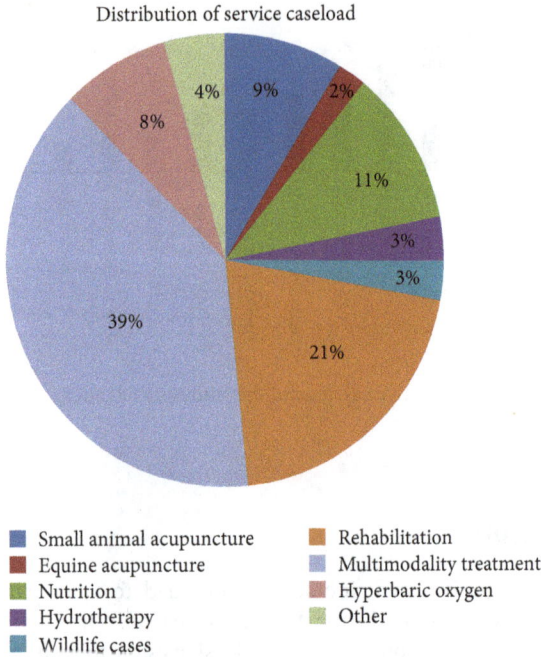

- Small animal acupuncture
- Equine acupuncture
- Nutrition
- Hydrotherapy
- Wildlife cases
- Rehabilitation
- Multimodality treatment
- Hyperbaric oxygen
- Other

FIGURE 2: Distribution of integrative medicine patient visits of the study site's Academic Veterinary Hospital.

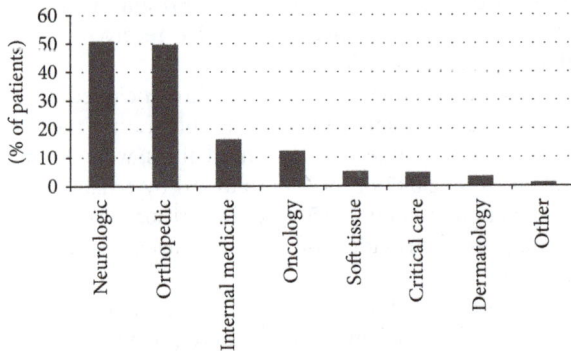

FIGURE 3: Presenting complaints of veterinary patients receiving multiple therapeutic modalities in the study site's integrative medicine service.

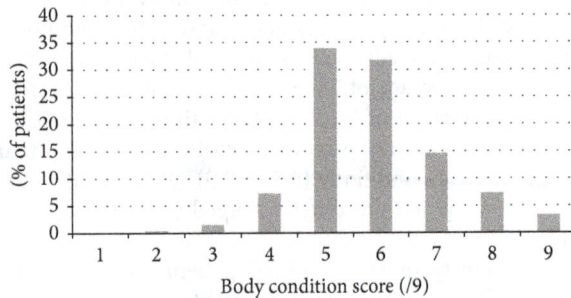

FIGURE 4: Body condition of veterinary patients receiving multiple integrative therapeutic modalities at the study site's Academic Veterinary Hospital.

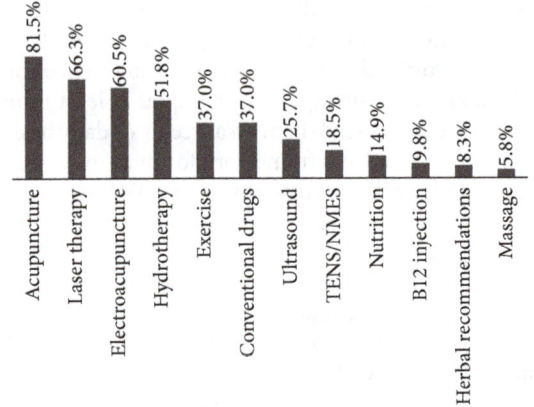

FIGURE 5: The percentage of patients receiving each integrative therapeutic modality at the study site's integrative medicine service.

was noted in the body condition scores of those patients presenting for neurologic, orthopedic, or other conditions ($P = 0.15$). A weak negative correlation was observed between the body condition score of the patient and the number of visits ($r = -0.12$, $P = 0.04$).

Patients receiving multiple modalities received 4.1 ± 1.6 different therapies at a visit, with a range of 1–11 modalities. No statistically significant differences were identified in the number of modalities used in patients with neurologic, orthopedic, or other conditions ($P = 0.19$). A weak positive correlation was identified between the number of modalities employed and the number of visits ($r = 0.21$, $P = 0.001$). No differences were detected in the number of modalities any breed category received ($P = 0.07$).

Four modalities were used in greater than half of the treatment sessions analyzed. These included acupuncture (81.5% of all treatment sessions), laser therapy (66.3%), electroacupuncture (60.5%), and hydrotherapy (51.8%). Eight other interventions were used for the mixed modality patients but less frequently (Figure 5).

Neurologic patients were significantly more likely to receive acupuncture, electroacupuncture, and rehabilitation exercises as compared to orthopedic patients ($P < 0.05$, Figure 6). These patients were less likely to receive laser therapy, hydrotherapy, and ultrasound. There was no difference in the odds of either group receiving transcutaneous electrical nerve stimulation (TENS) or neuromuscular electrical stimulation (NMES), nutritional or herbal recommendations, massage, conventional drugs, or cyanocobalamin injections.

Sixty-two breeds of dogs were treated. Mixed breed dogs were most commonly presented (27.0%). Both Dachshunds and Labrador retrievers were overrepresented in the patient population when compared to other breeds, amounting to 15.2% and 7.4% of the study population, respectively. German Shepherds comprised 3.3% of patients, and the remainder of breeds accounted for less than 2.2% of the dogs treated.

Analysis of the five major breed categories (Dachshunds, Labrador retrievers, mixed breeds, German Shepherds, and a group of all other breeds) did not show any statistically significant difference in age ($P = 0.12$). Labrador retrievers

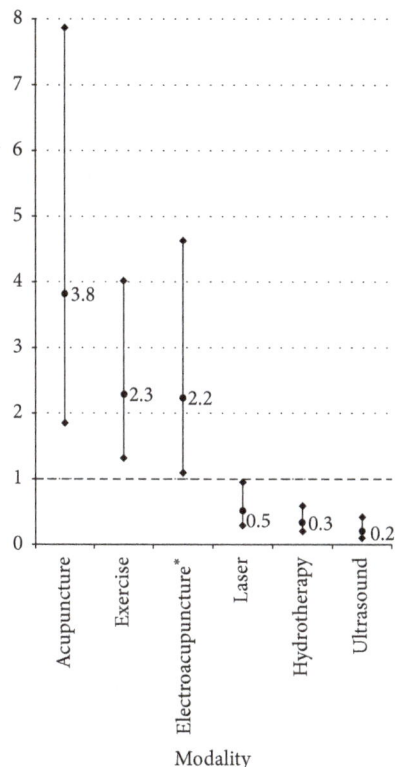

FIGURE 6: The odds of receiving six modalities were different in neurologic as compared to orthopedic patients (OR, 95% CI) of the veterinary patients at the study site's integrative medicine service. * The odds ratio was calculated by comparing the odds of neurologic patients with acupuncture receiving electroacupuncture as compared to orthopedic patients with acupuncture receiving electroacupuncture. Electroacupuncture was always performed with acupuncture, and therefore this comparison normalizes for the observed differences in the odds of receiving acupuncture alone.

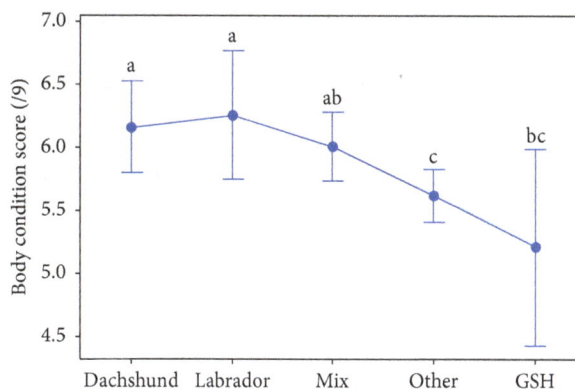

FIGURE 7: Breed differences in body condition score at the study site's integrative medicine service (breeds with different letters are statistically different).

and German Shepherds were heavier than mixed and other breeds in this study, and all four groups were more massive than Dachshunds. Statistically significant differences were noted between breeds and average body condition scores ($P = 0.008$, Figure 7).

Multiple modality treatments were employed primarily for dogs ($n = 270$) and also for cats ($n = 4$). The mean age of cats was 14.0 years (10–17) with a body weight of 4.6 kg (3.5–5.9). All cats were neutered males. The mean age for dogs ($n = 270$) was 9.0 ± 3.9 years (1–18) with a body weight of 19.2 kg ± 12.8 (1.2–63.2 kg). The genders of dogs were as follows: 23 intact males, 127 neutered males, 11 intact females, and 109 spayed females. The majority of the animals treated were seen either concurrently or within the previous six months by another service in the same academic teaching hospital (92.2%, $n = 249$).

Statistically significant differences were determined between dogs grouped by presenting condition. Dogs presenting for orthopedic conditions weighed less than those presenting for neurologic or for other conditions (14.9 ± 13.1 versus 23.3 ± 11.3 and 19.8 ± 12.5 kg, resp. $P < 0.001$). Dogs were younger if treated for orthopedic as opposed to other

conditions (8.3 ± 3.4 years versus 9.8 ± 3.6 years) ($P = 0.048$) but were not different in age from those treated for neurologic diseases. No difference was detected in the body condition scores of dogs when grouped by presenting complaint ($P = 0.12$). There was no difference in the number of modalities received for dogs presenting with orthopedic, neurologic, or other problems ($P = 0.57$).

Dachshunds were substantially more likely to present with a neurologic condition than with orthopedic or other conditions (OR 23.6; 7.47–74.5). Conversely, Labrador retrievers were more likely to be treated for a primary orthopedic complaint as opposed to a neurologic issue (OR 6.0; 1.46–24.7). Predictably, Dachshunds were more likely to present with neurologic conditions than were Labradors (OR 19.4; 4.96–76.1), mixed breed dogs (OR 14.8; 5.61–39.2), or other breeds (OR 7.48; 3.08–18.2). No Dachshunds presented with orthopedic complaints and they were therefore the least likely of the breeds to present with this condition.

The odds ratios for dogs receiving some modalities differed significantly among the breed categories (Dachshunds, Labradors, German Shepherds, mixed breed dogs, and the group of other dog breeds). Dachshunds were less likely to receive B12 injections than were German Shepherds (OR 0.10; 0.01–0.74) and were less likely to receive therapeutic ultrasound than mixed breed dogs (OR 0.21; 0.07–0.60). They were, however, more likely than other breeds to receive TENS/NMES (OR 2.51; 1.08–5.79) and also more likely than mixed breeds (OR 2.98; 1.33–6.68) and Labrador retrievers (OR 5.95; 1.51–23.5) to receive therapeutic exercises. Mixed breeds were more likely to receive therapeutic ultrasound than other breeds (OR 2.44; 1.30–4.60) and less likely to receive B12 injections than were German Shepherds (OR 0.15; 0.04–0.49). Other breeds were less likely than German Shepherds to receive conventional prescription drug recommendations (OR 0.21; 0.05–0.90).

4. Discussion

The integrative medicine service from which data was derived is unique in several respects. The academic mission of the veterinary college necessitates a model that incorporates student experiential learning, the training of house officers, and an emphasis on inter-specialty cooperation and on evidence-based medicine. The service was staffed during the study period by 1.25–2.25 full-time-equivalent faculty, 1-2 house officers, and two certified rehabilitation veterinary technicians. Four to five students were present in rotating two-week elective rotations for the entire year. The integrative nature of the service is supported by data in the present investigation; a large number of patients also presented to other hospital services (92%), and a recommendation of conventional therapies was made in 36.6% of multimodality treatment visits. Comparative data from integrative services at other institutions are unavailable, and no other service combines the same therapeutic options. Therefore, additional data and descriptions from other services are required before comparative conclusions can be made.

The service offers four of the five most commonly taught modalities in veterinary schools: nutrition, rehabilitation, acupuncture, and herbal therapy [4]. The notable exception is veterinary spinal manipulative therapy, also referred to as veterinary chiropractic. This practice, based on a principle that manually applied forces induce joint mobility and subsequent myofascial effects, has been objectively studied in horses but not in dogs [6]. Anecdotal concerns about mobilization and worsening of intervertebral discs exist, and practitioners of the modality do advise caution [7]. The absence of evidence-based testing and the lack of training by the service clinicians precluded the use of this technique. Other therapies discussed in the context of integrative medicine were also not a component of the service, including homeopathy, which is derived from foundational principles that "like treats like" and that serial dilutions of a compound increase the potency of a remedy. A recent meta-analysis of veterinary homeopathy found only scant data supporting its use in randomized controlled trials, and the two acceptable studies focused on bovine and porcine treatments [8]. Philosophical arguments surround the plausibility of the therapy, but nevertheless integration into a conventional veterinary hospital is both difficult and questionable given the competing tenets [9, 10].

The study data suggest that multimodality therapies were the most frequent treatment intervention elected by the attending clinicians. The patients receiving a multimodality therapy session were treated in the absence of the owners, from whom a brief history was obtained at the start of the visit and who were updated at the conclusion of the visit. The clients were charged a flat treatment fee irrespective of the number of modalities performed in order to eliminate the appearance of any financial incentive to expand a treatment protocol. Therefore, the patients in this study, which received a range of 1–11 modalities, were all charged equally, and patients on average received four of the available modalities based on clinician assessments. The students were permitted to assist with these patients, and the overall efficiency and case volume was managed by having the patients in the service for several hours.

4.1. Acupuncture, Electroacupuncture, and Vitamin B12 Injections.

Acupuncture and electroacupuncture were two of the four most frequently administered treatments. Acupuncture remains a source of significant controversy in veterinary medicine. Much of this controversy is derived from debates surrounding the antiquity of acupuncture, and available evidence suggests that modern veterinary acupuncture is a recent invention [11]. Veterinarians may place acupuncture needles based on traditional Chinese practices, on medical explanations and published studies of clinical effects or on a combination of the two approaches [12, 13]. A dated systematic review found there was insufficient evidence to recommend acupuncture in small animal patients like those of the study population [14]. Admittedly, two studies failed to document a significant benefit in dogs with both acute and chronic orthopedic injury [15, 16]. However, studies of varying methodological quality suggested an improvement in neurologic function of dogs affected by intervertebral disc disease when treated with electroacupuncture [17–19]. Interestingly, dogs treated in the retrospective period of this study were more likely to receive acupuncture and electroacupuncture when presenting with neurologic as opposed to orthopedic issues. Some studies of naturally occurring canine pain support an analgesic effect of acupuncture which could be beneficial for many conditions [20, 21]. A number of mechanisms have been postulated for the effects of acupuncture, including endogenous opioid release, substance P modulation, myofascial input, cannabinoid receptor modulation, and other cellular mediators. However, detailed evidence-based discussions should inform the location, effects, and utility of acupoints, several examples of which have been recently published [22, 23].

Cyanocobalamin injections (vitamin B12) were administered infrequently in patients (<10%). The technique has been recommended as an adjunctive method of acupoint stimulation [13], although it has not been scientifically validated. Cobalamin requires intrinsic factor, produced in the stomach and pancreas of dogs and in the pancreas of cats, for intestinal absorption and is a critical cofactor in enzymes for carbon rearrangement and methyl donation [24]. Cyanocobalamin injections have a wide margin of safety, and physiologic and cellular deficiencies have been reported in various conditions [24]. The finding that German Shepherds received B12 injections more commonly than some other breeds is likely unintentional. The fact that oncology patients accounted for the largest number of injections may suggest an intentional supplementation of this group due to perceived neoplasia-related true or relative deficiencies [25]. No animals were tested for their B12 status prior to supplementation so the effectiveness of such an approach remains unclear.

The application of electrical current to a patient's soft tissues is not unique to electroacupuncture. However, electroacupuncture has been shown in multiple species to augment therapeutic response by enhancing the release of endogenous opioids [26]. The best available data suggests that low frequency (2 Hz) acupuncture releases μ-acting opioids whereas high frequency stimulation (100 Hz) affects κ receptors. Veterinary studies frequently employ a mixed low and high frequency treatment of at least 20-minute duration [15,

17, 20]. Release of β-endorphins was documented three hours after treatment in dogs receiving an uncommon protocol of electroacupuncture (24 Hz and 43 Hz) [21]. Horses had a measurable rise of the same opioid in CSF for 2 hours following a 15–30 Hz treatment [27]. The most common protocol used in the present investigation was 2 Hz for 20 minutes in dogs, but additional studies are required to determine the optimal electroacupuncture frequency for the common neurologic and orthopedic conditions encountered during the study period.

4.2. TENS and NMES.

Transcutaneous electrical nerve stimulation (TENS) utilizes conductive pads to activate sensory nerve fibers and to modulate pain. This therapy was employed in only about 18% of the study patients and was often used in Dachshunds. A recent meta-analysis of human patients found some favorable evidence for TENS treatment of the pain associated with knee osteoarthritis, but subsequent small studies were unable to confirm the effect [28]. TENS treatments set to a frequency of 70 Hz improved ground reaction forces in osteoarthritic dogs [29]. TENS was also employed in a canine physiotherapy program but at unknown settings [30]. TENS units frequently contain a different program for neuromuscular electrical stimulation, which is employed in the treatment of atrophy by recruiting motor fibers. Increased muscle mass was documented in dogs receiving this type of stimulation following surgical repair of a cranial cruciate ligament repair [31]. TENS or NMES could be theorized to be more beneficial for the treatment of large areas given the greater current dispersal area over the pads whereas electroacupuncture might more effectively treat deep tissues; neither suggestion has been scientifically evaluated. Whether the clinical patients in the present retrospective would have benefited more from one therapy as opposed to the other remains unknown.

4.3. Laser Therapy (Photobiomodulation).

A therapeutic laser treatment was performed in a majority of the study population. The cellular effects of laser treatments, often referred to as photobiomodulation, are well established and include photonic changes to cytochrome c oxidase resulting in increased cellular energy (ATP) production, the release of nitric oxide, and the generation of free oxygen radicals which stimulates an endogenous antioxidant production [32]. The primary controversy of laser therapy is the dose needed to achieve such biologic effects given that water, melanin, and hemoglobin all absorb photons in a similar spectrum as the target cytochromes. Laser penetration has been poorly studied in dogs, although a study in horses showed consistent differences in penetration in shaved versus unshaved areas [33]. A single clinical trial of canine laser therapy found that dogs had a significantly reduced time to ambulation when treated with laser following a decompressive hemilaminectomy [34]. Therefore, the observation in this study that neurologic patients were less likely to receive laser therapy deserves attention because the strongest clinical evidence supports its use in these patients. Failure to provide this therapy may have been due to pragmatic considerations given

that a number of the postoperative patients treated by the service have an adhesive, absorbent, and poorly penetrable bandage over the surgical incision.

4.4. Hydrotherapy: Underwater Treadmill Walking and Swimming.

Hydrotherapy was more commonly used for orthopedic than neurologic patients, which may be because the service treats a large number of paralyzed dogs with no motor function at the outset of treatment. Neurosurgical patients in the academic teaching hospital typically have intravenous catheters for approximately 48 hours after surgery, and urinary catheters are frequently placed for lower motor neuron bladder dysfunction. The presence of either catheter complicates hydrotherapy, but the degree to which this influenced the odds ratio of hydrotherapy in orthopedic as compared to neurologic patients could not be quantified from the retrospective data available. Additionally, the available evidence for hydrotherapy is presently limited to orthopedic pathology although some authors advocate introduction of the technique 3 to 5 days after surgery for intervertebral disc disease and other neurologic conditions [35]. Underwater treadmill therapy reduces concussive forces on joints and promotes increased joint flexion and full active extension [36]. It has been used for both weight loss protocols and for postoperative rehabilitation of dogs following a tibial plateau leveling osteotomy [37, 38]. Hydrotherapy was defined as either swimming or underwater treadmill therapy in this study, and the exact distribution of each was not collected. Swimming, however, can be used to maximize active range of motion; hip, stifle, and hock flexion were all increased in a pool as compared to a ground treadmill after cranial cruciate ligament repair and in healthy dogs [39]. Conversely, hip and stifle extension angles were reduced by about 13 and 19 degrees, respectively, in swimming dogs after cruciate repair as compared to healthy controls. This was not observed in the same dogs when walking at two speeds on a land (nonaquatic) treadmill [39]. Severely osteoarthritic dogs often exercised more comfortably in a pool because they are completely nonweight bearing. Additional data is required to better inform the optimal time for starting hydrotherapy and the clinical benefits, if any, in neurologic patients.

4.5. Therapeutic Exercise.

Therapeutic exercises were performed less frequently than hydrotherapy, presumably because the service first exercises patients in water before advancing them to weight-bearing activities with the aid of ground treadmills or other interventions, such as cavaletti poles, weaves, balance ball, and related rehabilitation techniques. Several authors have advocated early limb use after injury in animals, and the kinematics of many techniques are described for dogs [40–43]. However, no study has yet independently associated any one particular exercise with any improvement in clinical outcome. Dachshunds and neurologic patients in the present study were interestingly more likely to receive therapeutic exercises than Labrador retrievers, mixed breeds, and those with orthopedic conditions. This may be due to the fact that many neurologic dogs were paretic and therefore more difficult for owners to exercise when compared to those with orthopedic pathology.

4.6. Therapeutic Ultrasound. Therapeutic ultrasound provides energy in the form of sound, which is absorbed by tissues of high protein content such as skeletal muscle, thereby providing deep heating to target tissues. Short-term (<10 minutes) heating of 1.6–4.6 degrees Celsius was reported in the caudal thigh muscles of dogs following ultrasound, with results dependent on the selected power (1–1.5 W/cm^2). Calcaneal tendon extensibility and tarsal flexion also increased for 5 minutes following a similar protocol in dogs [44]. The short-term effects of ultrasound are likely most beneficial when followed by range of motion exercises. Repeated and frequent administration may produce faster rates of healing in tendons and in other tissues, but this approach is often constrained by logistical and financial considerations in clinical practice [45]. The facilitation of tissue stretching and thermal heating was used more often in orthopedic as opposed to neurologic patients, likely due to the more severe range of motion restrictions noted in many orthopedic conditions, such as cranial cruciate ligament rupture [15].

4.7. Massage Therapy. Massage therapy may have similar effects as to the aforementioned modalities. The techniques and goals of such manipulations are similar to those described in humans, although there is minimal scientific literature regarding the efficacy of massage in dogs and cats [46]. The principles by which massage might benefit an integrative medicine patient, based on available human studies, include increased lymphatic flow, modulation of local pain mediators such as substance P and prostaglandins, positive cortical responses, increased local circulation, reductions in muscle spasms and pain, and reduction of tissue adhesions [46]. Massage was the least frequently applied therapeutic modality, which may be related to the time required for the treatment or to the perception that manual therapies are less effective than other interventions. The latter cannot be determined until further veterinary studies are performed.

4.8. Herbal Interventions. Herbal recommendations were made to a small number of clients for a number of different conditions. A discussion of the merits of herbal supplements is outside the scope of this investigation, but there are a number of herbs and herbal formulas suggested to impart a clinical effect in veterinary species [47, 48]. Unfortunately, herbal veterinary products have minimal regulatory oversight, as neither the Association of American Feed Control Officials (AAFCO) nor the United States Food and Drug Administration (FDA) controls these products. A previous study of Chinese herbal formulas identified variable amounts of minerals and potential contaminants, and some contain small amounts of potentially toxic compounds [49, 50]. The herbal recommendations in this study were made by the supervising clinician based on a review of the conventional therapies and with a risk-benefit discussion with the owner, recognizing that interactions with drugs or unpredictable reactions are of real concern [51].

4.9. Nutritional Recommendations and Obesity Prevalence. Nutritional recommendations were provided to the owners in approximately 15% of cases. This is in contrast to current recommendations that every patient receives a nutritional assessment and recommendation [52]. All audited patient records except for one contained a weight and body condition score, and the multiple modality visits were nearly all recheck examinations. Therefore, it is likely that the collected data underestimates the percentage of patients receiving nutritional recommendations in the service. The importance of communication is stressed in current consensus guidelines and as such a revision of the patient discharge form to reinforce nutritional plans and monitoring appears warranted.

More than half of the dogs treated were overweight or obese. This prevalence is consistent with a recent study in the United Kingdom but higher than a dated study performed in the United States [53, 54]. Nevertheless, the animals in this study do not appear to be more overweight than the general population. A limitation of the collected retrospective data is that the same clinician did not perform all body condition scoring, but a validated nine-point system was available to all service clinicians. Dachshunds and Labrador retrievers were both more likely to be overweight than were other breeds in this study. A previous study identified that both breeds had increased risk of being overweight (OR = 1.6) and that Dachshunds also displayed increased risk for obesity (OR = 1.7) [53]. An association between body condition score and the number of visits or the presenting complaint was not detected, suggesting either that body condition did not contribute to the observed pathologies or, more likely, that excess adiposity contributed equally to the patients' conditions.

4.10. Breed, Age, and Gender Distribution of the Study Population. The breed distributions observed in this study are remarkably similar to a previous survey of general breed prevalence [55]. Mixed breeds accounted for 27% of this patient population and the same amount was reported in a national survey. Labrador retrievers comprised 7.4% and German Shepherds 3.3% which is again similar to the 7.9% and 3%, respectively, reported in the previous population study. Therefore, only the Dachshund appears overrepresented when compared to available data; they were 15.2% of the treated dogs, which dramatically contrasts with published statistics that they are less than 1.5% of the general population.

The predisposition of Labradors to orthopedic disease in this study is consistent with previous reports [56, 57], as is the predisposition of Dachshunds to intervertebral disc disease [57, 58]. The Dachshund accounted for 31.8% of all cases with a primary neurologic complaint, and a previous report found that Dachshunds comprised 48.0% of all canine intervertebral disc disease cases [58]. In the present study, intervertebral disc disease was included in a broader category of all neurologic disease and therefore a definitive comparison between the reported prevalence data cannot be made. The average age of the treated Dachshunds (7.9 years) is older than the age of highest risk for IVDD in chondrodystrophic breeds of 4–6 years [58], which could represent an anomaly. The finding could also suggest that older Dachshunds are more likely to require rehabilitation or those owners are more likely to elect therapy for this population.

Treated dogs were older (median = 9) and more likely to be neutered when compared to general population statistics (median age = 4.8) [55]. Intact males comprised 8.5% of caseload, neutered males 47%, intact females 4%, and spayed females 40.5% as compared to 21.2%, 24.4%, 16.7%, and 37.1%, respectively. It is unclear if neutering is causally related to the orthopedic and neurologic diseases treated in this study although an association between early neutering and joint disorders has been suggested [59].

4.11. Treatment Differences between Orthopedic and Neurologic Patients. The present data demonstrates that more than 15% of patients presenting with orthopedic or neurologic disease will have concurrent pathology of the other type. Therefore, a thorough physical examination and inventory of all conditions should be performed in all integrative medicine patients. Given that neurologic and orthopedic patients received the same number of modalities, it is logical to suggest that the same amount of time can be dedicated to orthopedic and neurologic cases. However, orthopedic patients were treated with more sessions during the study period than were those with neurologic disease. It could be hypothesized that this is because some neurologic patients, particularly those with intervertebral disc disease, make a full and complete recovery whereas many orthopedic diseases are chronic. Identification of overweight and obese patients is equally important in both groups as neither was more predisposed to obesity than the other.

4.12. Study Limitations. The study is subject to several limitations. The medical record system did not allow for clear examination of efficacy across the range of conditions that were treated. Prospective studies of each modality are needed. As is true of most individualized patient rehabilitation protocols, the effectiveness of a combination protocol, as opposed to a single modality treatment, was not assessed. The combination of modalities selected by a clinician could act synergistically or could negate the benefits of other therapies. The reason for selection of modalities was not explored, and the bias of the different service clinicians may confound the presented results. Additionally, detailed data is not presented on other types of appointments although information on hyperbaric oxygen treatments performed by the service is available elsewhere [60].

The data are heavily skewed toward dogs, but this is not surprising given that more of the small animal publications in integrative medicine, especially rehabilitation, focus on dogs. Additional investigation is warranted in practices that support a higher feline caseload. Similarly, equine cases were insufficient to be compared to dogs and are likely different in the modalities elected and the patient demographics. A limitation of this study is that detailed data was only collected from one treatment sheet from each patient's record, and

therefore the audited data may not accurately reflect the characteristics of the patients despite randomization. However, the large volume of cases prohibited a more comprehensive analysis.

4.13. Controversies in Integrative Veterinary Medicine. General controversies regarding the efficacy and suitability of integrative medical practice exist, and this study may incite criticisms of the use of these modalities in integrative practice. The amount of evidence for each technique employed in this study is admittedly unknown. One prominent integrative medicine scholar in the human medical field has proposed that only 7.4% of complementary and alternative techniques have compelling evidence justifying their use [61]. No similar attempt has been made to characterize the evidence for integrative or conventional veterinary therapies. The veterinary profession has very few interventions which reach the highest evidence grade, and significant challenges of the application of evidence-based medicine to veterinary practice have been described [62]. These include the expense of randomized controlled trials, the reliance on retrospective studies, the smaller population of researchers and research funding, the inherent difficulties in searching available databases, and the veterinarian's reliance on clinical experience. Clearly, however, integrative veterinary medicine should adopt the recommendations of McKenzie that all interventions, whether integrative, complementary, alternative, or holistic, be subjected to the same investigative standards and that practitioners accept both the primacy of empirical evidence and willingness to modify their practice based on such evidence [63]. This conversely requires skeptics of integrative medicine to support evidence-based integrative medicine based on the available data and evidence rather than on a perceived scale of acceptability. The authors of this paper hope that the information contained herein can provide a starting point for continued research on the applicability of these and other modalities.

5. Conclusions

The collected data provide a foundation for future prospective evaluations of integrative veterinary medicine. The prevalence of acupuncture, laser, and hydrotherapy in this patient population suggests that these should be initial areas of research. Older dogs with neurologic or orthopedic diseases were the primary patient populations treated, and Dachshunds were overrepresented compared to national statistics. Therefore, these patients should likely serve as the target populations for additional study. The data further support that integrative medicine can be successfully incorporated into conventional multispecialty referral practices with a high degree of cooperation. Additional evidence-based outcome measures should be used to evaluate the efficacy of integrative therapies, and both veterinarians and veterinary students should be prepared to counsel owners in these areas.

Conflict of Interests

The authors declare that there is no conflict of interests regarding the publication of this paper.

Acknowledgments

The authors acknowledge participation of the University of Florida Integrative Medicine clinicians, interns, technicians, and veterinary students. The study was conducted during Dr. Memon's sabbatical leave from Washington State University to the University of Florida during July–December, 2015.

References

[1] B. Kligler, V. Maizes, S. Schachter et al., "Core competencies in integrative medicine for medical school curricula: a proposal," *Academic Medicine*, vol. 79, no. 6, pp. 521–531, 2004.

[2] D. M. Raditic and J. W. Bartges, "Evidence-based integrative medicine in clinical veterinary oncology," *Veterinary Clinics of North America: Small Animal Practice*, vol. 44, no. 5, pp. 831–853, 2014.

[3] S. E. Lana, L. R. Kogan, K. A. Crump, J. T. Graham, and N. G. Robinson, "The use of complementary and alternative therapies in dogs and cats with cancer," *Journal of the American Animal Hospital Association*, vol. 42, no. 5, pp. 361–365, 2006.

[4] M. A. Memon and L. K. Sprunger, "Survey of colleges and schools of veterinary medicine regarding education in complementary and alternative veterinary medicine," *Journal of the American Veterinary Medical Association*, vol. 239, no. 5, pp. 619–623, 2011.

[5] M. Frass, R. P. Strassl, H. Friehs, M. Müllner, M. Kundi, and A. D. Kaye, "Use and acceptance of complementary and alternative medicine among the general population and medical personnel: a systematic review," *The Ochsner Journal*, vol. 12, no. 1, pp. 45–56, 2012.

[6] K. K. Haussler, A. E. Hill, C. M. Puttlitz, and C. W. McIlwraith, "Effects of vertebral mobilization and manipulation on kinematics of the thoracolumbar region," *American Journal of Veterinary Research*, vol. 68, no. 5, pp. 508–516, 2007.

[7] L. L. Taylor and L. Romano, "Veterinary chiropractic," *The Canadian Veterinary Journal*, vol. 40, no. 10, pp. 732–735, 1999.

[8] R. T. Mathie and J. Clausen, "Veterinary homeopathy: meta-analysis of randomised placebo-controlled trials," *Homeopathy*, vol. 104, no. 1, pp. 3–8, 2015.

[9] D. Mastrangelo, "Hormesis, epitaxy, the structure of liquid water, and the science of homeopathy," *Medical Science Monitor*, vol. 13, no. 1, pp. SR1–SR8, 2007.

[10] C. Bayley, "Homeopathy," *Journal of Medicine and Philosophy*, vol. 18, no. 2, pp. 129–145, 1993.

[11] J. Shmalberg, *Acupuncture: History and Application*, Clinician's Brief, 2014.

[12] C. Chrisman and H. Xie, "Canine transpositional points," in *Xie's Veterinary Acupuncture*, V. Preast and H. Xie, Eds., pp. 129–216, Blackwell, Ames, Iowa, USA, 2007.

[13] S. L. Cantwell, "Traditional Chinese veterinary medicine: the mechanism and management of acupuncture for chronic pain," *Topics in Companion Animal Medicine*, vol. 25, no. 1, pp. 53–58, 2010.

[14] G. Habacher, M. H. Pittler, and E. Ernst, "Effectiveness of acupuncture in veterinary medicine: systematic review," *Journal of Veterinary Internal Medicine*, vol. 20, no. 3, pp. 480–488, 2006.

[15] J. Shmalberg and J. Burgess, "A randomized controlled blinded clinical trial of electro-acupuncture administered one month after cranial cruciate ligament repair in dogs," *American Journal of Traditional Chinese Veterinary Medicine*, vol. 9, no. 2, pp. 43–51, 2014.

[16] A. S. Kapatkin, M. Tomasic, J. Beech et al., "Effects of electrostimulated acupuncture on ground reaction forces and pain scores in dogs with chronic elbow joint arthritis," *Journal of the American Veterinary Medical Association*, vol. 228, no. 9, pp. 1350–1354, 2006.

[17] A. M. Hayashi, J. M. Matera, and A. C. B. de Campos Fonseca Pinto, "Evaluation of electroacupuncture treatment for thoracolumbar intervertebral disk disease in dogs," *Journal of the American Veterinary Medical Association*, vol. 231, no. 6, pp. 913–918, 2007.

[18] H.-J. Han, H.-Y. Yoon, J.-Y. Kim et al., "Clinical effect of additional electroacupuncture on thoracolumbar intervertebral disc herniation in 80 paraplegic dogs," *The American Journal of Chinese Medicine*, vol. 38, no. 6, pp. 1015–1025, 2010.

[19] J. G. F. Joaquim, S. P. L. Luna, J. T. Brondani, S. R. Torelli, S. C. Rahal, and F. P. De Freitas, "Comparison of decompressive surgery, electroacupuncture, and decompressive surgery followed by electroacupuncture for the treatment of dogs with intervertebral disk disease with long-standing severe neurologic deficits," *Journal of the American Veterinary Medical Association*, vol. 236, no. 11, pp. 1225–1229, 2010.

[20] A. Laim, A. Jaggy, F. Forterre, M. G. Doherr, G. Aeschbacher, and O. Glardon, "Effects of adjunct electroacupuncture on severity of postoperative pain in dogs undergoing hemilaminectomy because of acute thoracolumbar intervertebral disk disease," *Journal of the American Veterinary Medical Association*, vol. 234, no. 9, pp. 1141–1146, 2009.

[21] D. Groppetti, A. M. Pecile, P. Sacerdote, V. Bronzo, and G. Ravasio, "Effectiveness of electroacupuncture analgesia compared with opioid administration in a dog model: a pilot study," *British Journal of Anaesthesia*, vol. 107, no. 4, pp. 612–618, 2011.

[22] R. B. Koh, N. Isaza, H. Xie, K. Cooke, and S. A. Robertson, "Effects of maropitant, acepromazine, and electroacupuncture on vomiting associated with administration of morphine in dogs," *Journal of the American Veterinary Medical Association*, vol. 244, no. 7, pp. 820–829, 2014.

[23] N. Robinson, "The need for consistency and comparability of transitional acupuncture points across species," *American Journal of Traditional Chinese Veterinary Medicine*, vol. 1, no. 1, pp. 14–21, 2006.

[24] C. G. Ruaux, "Cobalamin in companion animals: diagnostic marker, deficiency states and therapeutic implications," *The Veterinary Journal*, vol. 196, no. 2, pp. 145–152, 2013.

[25] A. K. Cook, Z. M. Wright, J. S. Suchodolski, M. R. Brown, and J. M. Steiner, "Prevalence and prognostic impact of hypocobalaminemia in dogs with lymphoma," *Journal of the American Veterinary Medical Association*, vol. 235, no. 12, pp. 1437–1441, 2009.

[26] G. A. Ulett, S. Han, and J.-S. Han, "Electroacupuncture: mechanisms and clinical application," *Biological Psychiatry*, vol. 44, no. 2, pp. 129–138, 1998.

[27] R. T. Skarda, G. A. Tejwani, and W. W. Muir III, "Cutaneous analgesia, hemodynamic and respiratory effects, and β-endorphin concentration in spinal fluid and plasma of horses

after acupuncture and electroacupuncture," *American Journal of Veterinary Research*, vol. 63, no. 10, pp. 1435–1442, 2002.

[28] A. W. Rutjes, E. Nüesch, R. Sterchi et al., "Transcutaneous electrostimulation for osteoarthritis of the knee," *Cochrane Database of Systematic Reviews*, no. 4, Article ID CD002823, 2009.

[29] D. Levine, K. Johnson, M. Price et al., "The effect of TENS on osteoarthritic pain in the stifle of dogs," in *Proceedings of the 2nd International Symposium on Rehabilitation and Physical Therapy in Veterinary Medicine*, Knoxville, Tenn, USA, 2002.

[30] E. Mlacnik, B. A. Bockstahler, M. Müller, M. A. Tetrick, R. C. Nap, and J. Zentek, "Effects of caloric restriction and a moderate or intense physiotherapy program for treatment of lameness in overweight dogs with osteoarthritis," *Journal of the American Veterinary Medical Association*, vol. 229, no. 11, pp. 1756–1760, 2006.

[31] J. M. Johnson, A. L. Johnson, G. J. Pijanowski et al., "Rehabilitation of dogs with surgically treated cranial cruciate ligament-deficient stifles by use of electrical stimulation of muscles," *American Journal of Veterinary Research*, vol. 58, no. 12, pp. 1473–1478, 1997.

[32] H. Chung, T. Dai, S. K. Sharma, Y.-Y. Huang, J. D. Carroll, and M. R. Hamblin, "The nuts and bolts of low-level laser (Light) therapy," *Annals of Biomedical Engineering*, vol. 40, no. 2, pp. 516–533, 2012.

[33] T. Ryan and R. Smith, "An investigation into the depth of penetration of low level laser therapy through the equine tendon in vivo," *Irish Veterinary Journal*, vol. 60, no. 5, pp. 295–299, 2007.

[34] W. E. Draper, T. A. Schubert, R. M. Clemmons, and S. A. Miles, "Low-level laser therapy reduces time to ambulation in dogs after hemilaminectomy: a preliminary study," *Journal of Small Animal Practice*, vol. 53, no. 8, pp. 465–469, 2012.

[35] M. G. Drum, "Physical rehabilitation of the canine neurologic patient," *Veterinary Clinics of North America: Small Animal Practice*, vol. 40, no. 1, pp. 181–193, 2010.

[36] A. Jackson, D. Millis, M. Stevens et al., "Joint kinematics during underwater treadmill activity," in *Proceedings of the 2nd International Symposium on Rehabilitation and Physical Therapy in Veterinary Medicine*, Knoxville, Tenn, USA, 2002.

[37] M. L. Monk, C. A. Preston, and C. M. McGowan, "Effects of early intensive postoperative physiotherapy on limb function after tibial plateau leveling osteotomy in dogs with deficiency of the cranial cruciate ligament," *American Journal of Veterinary Research*, vol. 67, no. 3, pp. 529–536, 2006.

[38] A. Chauvet, J. Laclair, D. A. Elliott, and A. J. German, "Incorporation of exercise, using an underwater treadmill, and active client education into a weight management program for obese dogs," *Canadian Veterinary Journal*, vol. 52, no. 5, pp. 491–496, 2011.

[39] G. S. Marsolais, S. McLean, T. Derrick, and M. G. Conzemius, "Kinematic analysis of the hind limb during swimming and walking in healthy dogs and dogs with surgically corrected cranial cruciate ligament rupture," *Journal of the American Veterinary Medical Association*, vol. 222, no. 6, pp. 739–743, 2003.

[40] D. Millis and D. Levine, *Canine Rehabilitation and Physical Therapy*, Elsevier Health Sciences, 2013.

[41] R. P. Millard, J. F. Headrick, and D. L. Millis, "Kinematic analysis of the pelvic limbs of healthy dogs during stair and decline slope walking," *Journal of Small Animal Practice*, vol. 51, no. 8, pp. 419–422, 2010.

[42] M. G. Drum, D. J. Marcellin-Little, and M. S. Davis, "Principles and applications of therapeutic exercises for small animals," *Veterinary Clinics of North America: Small Animal Practice*, vol. 45, no. 1, pp. 73–90, 2015.

[43] P. J. Holler, V. Brazda, B. Dal-Bianco et al., "Kinematic motion analysis of the joints of the forelimbs and hind limbs of dogs during walking exercise regimens," *American Journal of Veterinary Research*, vol. 71, no. 7, pp. 734–740, 2010.

[44] J. Loonam, D. Millis, and M. Stevens, "The effect of therapeutic ultrasound on tendon heating and extensibility," in *Proceedings of the 30th Veterinary Orthopedic Society Conference*, Steamboat Springs, Colo, USA, February-March 2003.

[45] N. S. Saini, K. S. Roy, P. S. Bansal, B. Singh, and P. S. Simran, "A preliminary study on the effect of ultrasound therapy on the healing of surgically severed Achilles tendons in five dogs," *Journal of Veterinary Medicine Series A*, vol. 49, no. 6, pp. 321–328, 2002.

[46] A. Sutton and D. Whitlock, "Massage," in *Canine Rehabilitation and Physical Therapy*, D. Millis and D. Levine, Eds., pp. 464–483, Elsevier, Philadelphia, Pa, USA, 2014.

[47] D. C. Brown and J. Reetz, "Single agent polysaccharopeptide delays metastases and improves survival in naturally occurring hemangiosarcoma," *Evidence-Based Complementary and Alternative Medicine*, vol. 2012, Article ID 384301, 8 pages, 2012.

[48] K. A. Wirth, K. Kow, M. E. Salute, N. J. Bacon, and R. J. Milner, "In vitro effects of *Yunnan Baiyao* on canine hemangiosarcoma cell lines," *Veterinary and Comparative Oncology*, 2014.

[49] J. Shmalberg, R. C. Hill, and K. C. Scott, "Nutrient and metal analyses of Chinese herbal products marketed for veterinary use," *Journal of Animal Physiology and Animal Nutrition*, vol. 97, no. 2, pp. 305–314, 2013.

[50] J. Shmalberg, "Detection and quantification of neuroexcitatory alkaloids in modified Da Huo Luo Dan prescribed for paresis or paralysis in dogs," *American Journal of Traditional Chinese Veterinary Medicine*, vol. 10, no. 2, pp. 27–31, 2015.

[51] R. H. Poppenga, "Herbal medicine: potential for intoxication and interactions with conventional drugs," *Clinical Techniques in Small Animal Practice*, vol. 17, no. 1, pp. 6–18, 2002.

[52] K. Baldwin, J. Bartges, T. Buffington et al., "AAHA nutritional assessment guidelines for dogs and cats," *Journal of the American Animal Hospital Association*, vol. 46, no. 4, pp. 285–296, 2010.

[53] E. M. Lund, P. J. Armstrong, C. A. Kirk et al., "Prevalence and risk factors for obesity in adult dogs from private US veterinary practices," *International Journal of Applied Research in Veterinary Medicine*, vol. 4, no. 2, pp. 177–186, 2006.

[54] E. A. Courcier, R. M. Thomson, D. J. Mellor, and P. S. Yam, "An epidemiological study of environmental factors associated with canine obesity," *Journal of Small Animal Practice*, vol. 51, no. 7, pp. 362–367, 2010.

[55] E. M. Lund, P. J. Armstrong, C. A. Kirk, L. M. Kolar, and J. S. Klausner, "Health status and population characteristics of dogs and cats examined at private veterinary practices in the United States," *Journal of the American Veterinary Medical Association*, vol. 214, no. 9, pp. 1336–1341, 1999.

[56] J. M. Duval, S. C. Budsberg, G. L. Flo, and J. L. Sammarco, "Breed, sex, and body weight as risk factors for rupture of the cranial cruciate ligament in young dogs," *Journal of the American Veterinary Medical Association*, vol. 215, no. 6, pp. 811–814, 1999.

[57] E. LaFond, G. J. Breur, and C. C. Austin, "Breed susceptibility for developmental orthopedic diseases in dogs," *Journal of the*

American Animal Hospital Association, vol. 38, no. 5, pp. 467–477, 2002.

[58] W. A. Priester, "Canine intervertebral disc disease—occurrence by age, breed, and sex among 8,117 cases," *Theriogenology*, vol. 6, no. 2-3, pp. 293–303, 1976.

[59] B. L. Hart, L. A. Hart, A. P. Thigpen, and N. H. Willits, "Long-term health effects of neutering dogs: comparison of labrador retrievers with golden retrievers," *PLoS ONE*, vol. 9, no. 7, Article ID e102241, 2014.

[60] J. Shmalberg, W. Davies, S. Lopez, D. Shmalberg, and J. Zil-berschtein, "Rectal temperature changes and oxygen toxicity in dogs treated in a monoplace chamber," *Undersea & Hyperbaric Medicine*, vol. 42, no. 1, pp. 95–102, 2015.

[61] E. Ernst, "How much of CAM is based on research evidence?" *Evidence-Based Complementary and Alternative Medicine*, vol. 2011, Article ID 676490, 3 pages, 2011.

[62] J.-M. Vandeweerd, N. Kirschvink, P. Clegg, S. Vandenput, P. Gustin, and C. Saegerman, "Is evidence-based medicine so evident in veterinary research and practice? History, obstacles and perspectives," *Veterinary Journal*, vol. 191, no. 1, pp. 28–34, 2012.

[63] B. A. McKenzie, "Is complementary and alternative medicine compatible with evidence-based medicine?" *Journal of the American Veterinary Medical Association*, vol. 241, no. 4, pp. 421–426, 2012.

3

Prevalence of Neoplastic Diseases in Pet Birds Referred for Surgical Procedures

Patrícia F. Castro, Denise T. Fantoni, Bruna C. Miranda, and Julia M. Matera

Department of Surgery, School of Veterinary Medicine and Animal Science, University of São Paulo,
Avenida Prof. Orlando Marques de Paiva 87, Cidade Universitária, 05508-270 São Paulo, SP, Brazil

Correspondence should be addressed to Patrícia F. Castro; pfcastro@usp.br

Academic Editor: Giuliano Bettini

Neoplastic disease is common in pet birds, particularly in psittacines, and treatment should be primarily aimed at tumor eradication. Nineteen cases of pet birds submitted to diagnostic and/or therapeutic surgical procedures due to neoplastic disease characterized by the presence of visible masses were retrospectively analyzed; affected species, types of neoplasms and respective locations, and outcomes of surgical procedures were determined. All birds undergoing surgery belonged to the order Psittaciformes; the Blue-fronted parrot (*Amazona aestiva*) was the prevalent species. Lipoma was the most frequent neoplasm in the sample studied. Most neoplasms affected the integumentary system, particularly the pericloacal area. Tumor resection was the most common surgical procedure performed, with high resolution and low recurrence rates.

1. Introduction

Pet birds suffer from a wide variety of neoplastic diseases [1]. Growing understanding of avian medicine is increasingly turning neoplastic diseases into more than just a *postmortem* diagnosis; however, related scientific literature, particularly therapeutic data, remains scarce [2, 3] or is limited to case reports [4, 5].

Neoplastic diseases are common among pet birds, particularly psittacines [6]; lipomas, lymphomas, and fibrosarcomas are among the most common neoplasms seen in birds in the genus *Amazona* [7]. Therapeutic strategies should be aimed at tumor eradication and may involve several modalities, employed as either combined or staged treatments [8]. Whenever feasible, surgical resection of neoplastic masses is the treatment of choice [1, 9]; however, radiotherapy, photodynamic therapy, cryotherapy, and chemotherapy may also be used [8].

This study set out to determine which bird species, among those presented to our referral veterinary center, are most frequently affected with neoplastic diseases characterized by the presence of visible masses, as well as neoplasm types and locations. Outcomes of different surgical procedures performed in affected pet birds were also analyzed.

2. Materials and Methods

Data regarding bird species, type of neoplasm (according to histological diagnosis; Figure 1) and respective location, type of surgical procedure, and short- (one week) and long-term progression were collected from pet birds submitted to diagnostic and/or therapeutic surgical procedures at the Small Animal Surgery Department of the Veterinary Hospital of the School of Veterinary Medicine and Animal Science, University of São Paulo (FMVZ/USP), over an eight-year period.

The anesthetic protocol included preanesthetic medication with intramuscular diazepam (Compaz 10 mg injectable; Cristália, Itapira, SP) and ketamine (Dopalen injectable; Agribrands do Brasil, Paulínia, SP) (pectoral muscle; 1 mg/kg and 10 mg/kg, resp.) and induction with sevoflurane (Sevocris, Cristália; Itapira, SP) in 100% oxygen delivered via facial mask in a closed nonrebreathing circuit; an appropriate sized endotracheal tube was then passed for anesthetic maintenance. Birds received fluid therapy (lactated ringer solution; 10 mL/kg/h) via a catheter inserted into the brachial vein (Figure 2). Intramuscular flunixin-meglumine (Banamine injectable 10 mg; Schering-Plough, Rio de Janeiro, RJ)

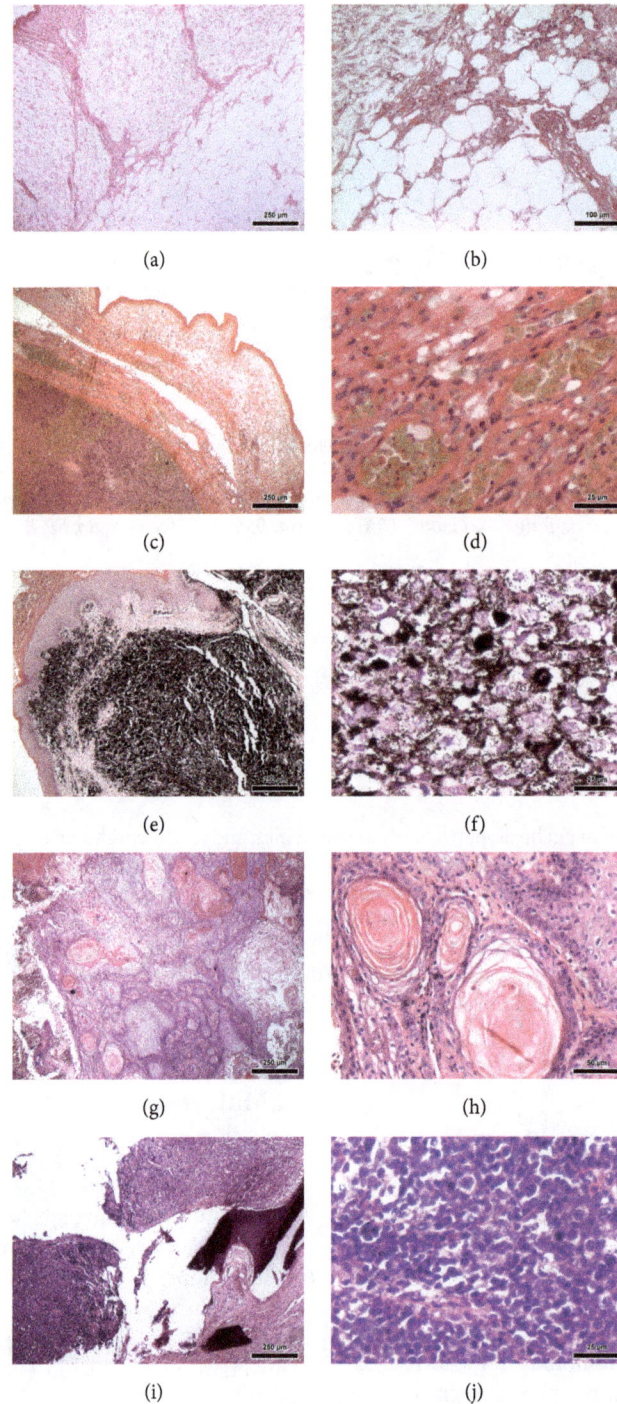

FIGURE 1: Histological photomicrographs of avian neoplasms—Hematoxylin and Eosin stain (H&E). (a) and (b) Case number 1: pericloacal lipoma (*A. aestiva*). (c) and (d) Case number 2: well-differentiated hemangiosarcoma in pelvic limb (*A. aestiva*). (e) and (f) Case number 3: mandibular melanoma (*Ara ararauna*). (g) and (h) Case number 11: oral squamous cell carcinoma (*Diopsittaca nobilis*). (i) and (j) Case number 15: distal tibiotarsal lymphoma (*Amazona* sp.).

(5 mg/kg) was given for immediate postoperative pain management.

Anesthetized birds were further prepared for surgery. Following feather plucking and removal from the surgical field, birds were placed in the required position for the procedure at hand and skin antisepsis performed with 70%

alcohol and povidone iodine, taking care to avoid excessive wetting and potential body temperature loss. Intramuscular enrofloxacin (Baytril 5% injectable; Bayer, São Paulo, SP) (pectoral muscle; 15 mg/kg) was also given. Surgical procedures were performed according to recommendations given in literature regarding minimal surgical trauma and bleeding

TABLE 1: Numerical (N) and percentage (%) distribution of soft tissue neoplasms in different species of Psittaciformes submitted to surgical interventions at the FMVZ/USP Veterinary Hospital between 2000 and 2008, São Paulo, Brazil.

Common name *Scientific name*	Lipoma		Lymphoma		Liposarcoma		Hemangiosarcoma		Squamous cell carcinoma		Melanoma		Total	
	N	%	N	%	N	%	N	%	N	%	N	%	N	%
Blue-fronted parrot *Amazona aestiva*	4	21.05	1	5.26	1	5.26	1	5.26	0	0.00	0	0.00	7	36.84
Orange-winged parrot *Amazona amazonica*	6	31.57	0	0.00	0	0.00	0	0.00	0	0.00	0	0.00	6	31.57
Parrot *Amazona* sp.	2	10.52	1	5.26	0	0.00	0	0.00	0	0.00	0	0.00	3	15.78
Blue-and-yellow macaw *Ara ararauna*	0	0.00	0	0.00	0	0.00	0	0.00	0	0.00	1	5.26	1	5.26
Red-shouldered macaw *Diopsittaca nobilis*	0	0.00	0	0.00	0	0.00	0	0.00	1	5.26	0	0.00	1	5.26
Eastern rosella *Platycercus eximius*	1	5.26	0	0.00	0	0.00	0	0.00	0	0.00	0	0.00	1	5.26
Total	13	68.42	2	10.52	1	5.26	1	5.26	1	5.26	1	5.26	19	100.00

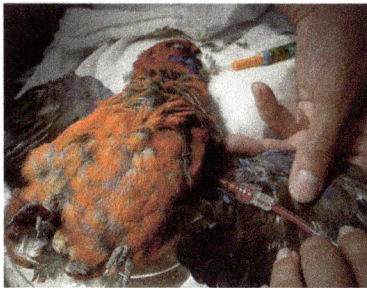

FIGURE 2: Case number 16: eastern rosella (*Platycercus eximius*) undergoing preoperative procedures. Note the endotracheal tube (adapted urinary catheter) in place and the catheterization of the brachial vein for intraoperative fluid therapy.

[9–11]. Skin closure was achieved with 4-0/5-0 nylon, 4-0 poliglecaprone, or 4-0 polyglactin 910, in a simple interrupted pattern.

Short-term progression was graded *excellent* (complete resolution), *satisfactory* (resolution not achieved but diagnosis confirmed), *unsatisfactory* (deterioration of patient's clinical condition), or *death* (death within 24 hours of surgery). Long-term progression was characterized as *no* (no recurrence along the experimental period), *yes* (recurrence along the experimental period), *death, lost to follow-up,* or *euthanasia.*

3. Results

Nineteen diagnostic and/or therapeutic surgical procedures were performed in pet birds during the eight-year experimental period, which then led to patient identification; one bird was operated on three times, each accounting for one procedure in the sample. All birds belonged to the order Psittaciformes, with birds in the genus *Amazona*

accounting for 84.21% (16/19) of cases. The Blue-fronted parrot (*Amazona aestiva*) was the most prevalent species (36.84%, 7/19). Malignant and benign tumors accounted for 31.57% (6/19) and 68.42% (16/19) of lesions, respectively. All benign tumors in this sample were lipomas and were more commonly diagnosed in birds in the genus *Amazona* (92.30%, 12/13) (Table 1).

Most neoplasms affected the integumentary system. Neoplastic lesions were limited to the pericloacal area in 42.10% of cases (8/19; Figure 3(a)) and extended to the abdominal area or the pelvic limb in three (15.78%, 3/19) and one case (5.26%, 1/19), respectively. With the exception of one case (liposarcoma), integumentary pericloacal lesions were diagnosed as lipomas. Other sites affected by neoplasms in this study were the abdominal area (lipoma; 5.26%, 1/19), the dorsal area near the tail (lipoma; 5.26%, 1/19; Figure 3(b)), the chest (lymphoma; 5.26%, 1/19; Figure 3(c)), the distal tibiotarsal area (lymphoma; 5.26%, 1/19), the oral cavity (well-differentiated squamous cell carcinoma; 5.26%, 1/19), the pelvic limb (well-differentiated cutaneous hemangiosarcoma; 5.26%, 1/19; Figure 3(d)), and the mandible (melanoma; 5.26%, 1/19).

Short-term postoperative data were lacking in two cases; therefore, those were excluded from the analysis. Analysis of the remaining cases revealed the following surgical interventions: resection, resection and cryotherapy, incisional biopsy, and collection of samples for histopathological and/or culture and sensitivity testing. No birds showed deterioration of clinical condition (*unsatisfactory*) or died within 24 hours of surgery (*death*). Resection (Figure 4) was the most common surgical procedure performed (82.35%, 14/17), with excellent short-term outcomes in 100% of cases (14/14; complete resolution). These included all lipomas (12/14), one well-differentiated hemangiosarcoma (1/14), and one liposarcoma (1/14), with a 14.28% recurrence rate over the long-term (2 lipomas out of 14 tumors resected; Table 2).

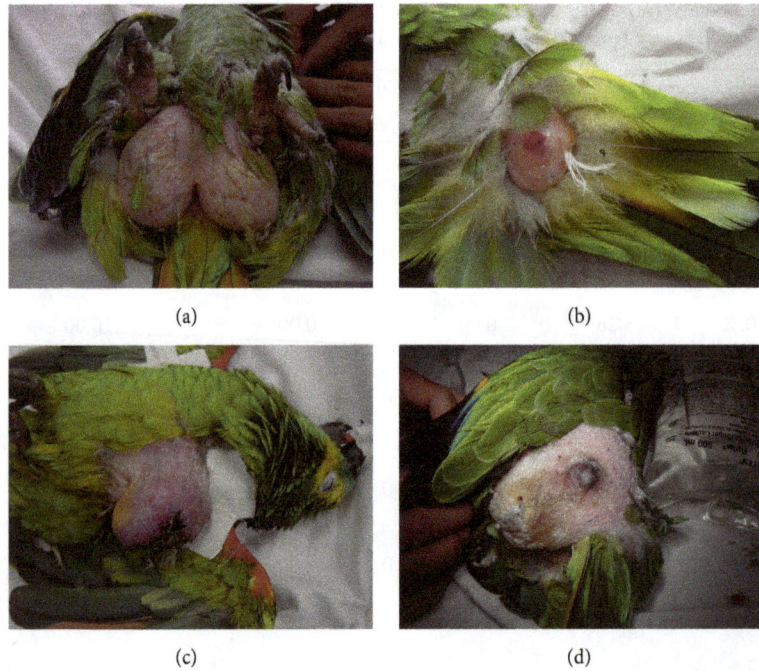

FIGURE 3: Neoplasms affecting the integumentary system of birds in the genus *Amazona*. (a) Pericloacal lipoma (*A. aestiva*). (b) Lipoma affecting the dorsal area near the tail (*Amazona* sp.). (c) Cutaneous lymphoma (*A. aestiva*). (d) Well-differentiated hemangiosarcoma affecting the pelvic limb (*A. aestiva*).

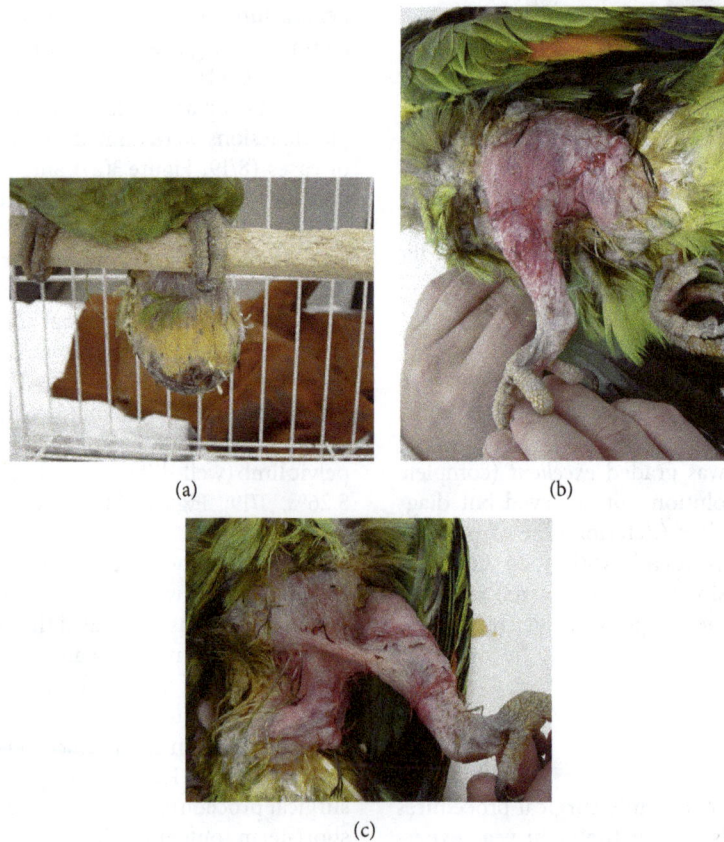

FIGURE 4: Case number 13: lipoma affecting the pelvic limb and pericloacal area (*Amazona* sp.). (a) Caudal, ulcerated, pendulum-like neoplasm. ((b) and (c)) Immediate postoperative appearance: skin closure on the lateral (b) and medial (c) aspects of the pelvic limb, extending to the pericloacal area (simple interrupted sutures, 4-0 polyglactin 910).

TABLE 2: Distribution of 17 cases of neoplastic disease operated on between 2000 and 2008 at FMVZ/USP, São Paulo, Brazil, according to surgical outcomes.

Case number	Common name (Scientific name)	Soft tissue neoplasm	Surgical procedure	Short-term progression		Long-term progression				
				E	S	No	Yes	D	NI	Eut
1	Blue-fronted parrot (Amazona aestiva)	Pericloacal lipoma	Resection	x		x				
2	Blue-fronted parrot (Amazona aestiva)	Well-differentiated hemangiosarcoma in pelvic limb	Resection	x		x				
3	Blue-and-yellow macaw (Ara ararauna)	Mandibular melanoma	Incisional biopsy		x			x		
4	Orange-winged parrot (Amazona amazonica)	Pericloacal lipoma	Resection	x			x			
5	Orange-winged parrot (Amazona amazonica)	Pericloacal lipoma	Resection	x			x			
6	Orange-winged parrot (Amazona amazonica)	Pericloacal lipoma	Resection	x		x				
7	Blue-fronted parrot (Amazona aestiva)	Pericloacal liposarcoma	Resection	x		x				
8	Orange-winged parrot (Amazona amazonica)	Abdominal and pericloacal lipoma	Resection	x		x				
9	Orange-winged parrot (Amazona amazonica)	Pericloacal lipoma	Resection	x		x				
10	Blue-fronted parrot (Amazona aestiva)	Abdominal ventral lipoma	Resection	x		x				
11	Red-shouldered macaw (Diopsittaca nobilis)	Oral squamous cell carcinoma	SC (HP, CST)		x					x
12	Blue-fronted parrot (Amazona aestiva)	Abdominal and pericloacal lipoma	Resection	x		x				
13	Parrot (Amazona sp.)	Pelvic limb and pericloacal lipoma	Resection	x		x				
14	Blue-fronted parrot (Amazona aestiva)	Pericloacal lipoma	Resection	x		x				
15	Parrot (Amazona sp.)	Distal tibiotarsal lymphoma	Incisional biopsy		x			x		
16	Eastern rosella (Platycercus eximius)	Pericloacal lipoma	Resection	x					x	
17	Parrot (Amazona sp.)	Lipoma on dorsum near the tail	Resection and cryotherapy	x		x				
			Total	14	3	11	2	2	1	1

Surgical procedure: SC: sample collection (HP: histopathology; CST: culture and sensitivity testing); *short-term progression*: E: excellent (complete resolution); S: satisfactory (resolution not achieved but diagnosis confirmed); *long-term progression*: no: no recurrence along the experimental period; yes: recurrence along the experimental period; D: death; NI: information not available; Eut: euthanasia.

4. Discussion

In this study, all birds affected with neoplastic disease belonged to the order Psittaciformes; the Blue-fronted parrot (*Amazona aestiva*) was the prevalent species. A study conducted at Northwest ZooPath specialty diagnostic service (Monroe, WA) reported higher prevalence of tumors in Anseriformes; Psittaciformes was the fifth most prevalent order, with cockatiels (*Nymphicus hollandicus*) and parrots (*Amazona* sp.) accounting for the first and second most frequently affected species [12]. Prevalence and popularity of different birds around the world [13] may explain these discrepancies; birds in the genus *Amazona* are likely the best known among New World psittacines and 27 members of this genus can be found throughout the Caribbean and Central and South America [7]. Results of this study are further supported by scientific data suggesting higher prevalences of neoplasia in Psittaciformes [8, 9, 14, 15], which possibly reflects the global popularity of psittacines as pets birds [16].

As reported elsewhere [17, 18], lipomas were the most common neoplasms in this study and tended to affect primarily birds in the genus *Amazona* [7]. The fact that most of these birds were obese suggests that high energy diets may play a role in the etiology of lipomas, along with genetic predisposition [1–3]. Lipomas have often been reported in budgerigars [3] and cockatoos [6, 19, 20]. Population composition clearly influenced the outcomes of this study. Native parrots are ubiquitous pet birds in Brazil [21]; therefore birds in the genus *Amazona* accounted for most cases of neoplasia in this sample. Also, higher surgical morbidity and mortality in small sized birds [22] translates into lower numbers of such patients (e.g., budgerigars) being submitted to surgical procedures given the high risk of death and related owner concerns.

Most neoplasms in this sample affected the integumentary system. A literature survey of neoplasia in pet birds, including cases diagnosed at a Veterinary Medical Teaching Hospital (University of California, Davis) over a 10-year period, revealed that tumors arising in the integument (31.7%) were more common than from other organ systems [6]. Lipomas were more frequently reported in the sternum, abdomen, and inner face of the thigh [8]; in contrast, in our study the pericloacal area was the most commonly affected site.

Resection was the most common surgical procedure [1, 9] performed (14/17), with excellent short-term outcomes (i.e., complete resolution) in 100% of cases. The long-term recurrence rate following surgical resection was 14.28% (2/14) and reflected disease progression in the same patient (cases numbers 4, 5, and 6; Table 2), operated on three times over the course of the eight-year experimental period for resection of pericloacal lipomas. Lipomas tend not to have well-defined margins, with tumor blood vessels often infiltrating the surrounding adipose tissue; resection is therefore more difficult and recurrence more common in such cases [2, 17]. In case 17, the neoplasm (lipoma) was treated with a combination of surgical resection and cryotherapy and did not recur. Aspiration cytology findings in this case suggested liposarcoma, but tumor location close to the cloaca precluded resection with sufficiently wide surgical margins. Hence a combined procedure was performed. Cryotherapy is indicated for treatment of tumors located around the oral cavity and nares, or as an ancillary technique in cases involving resection of wide-based or malignant tumors such as fibrosarcoma [8].

Short-term outcomes of incisional biopsies (2/17) and collection of samples for histopathology or culture/sensitivity testing (1/17) were satisfactory (i.e., resolution not achieved but diagnosis confirmed) in 100% of cases in this study. In the long-term, all (100%) of these cases progressed to death and/or were euthanized; this was not surprising given the diagnoses of melanoma, lymphoma (cases numbers 3 and 15, resp.; Table 2), and advanced oral squamous cell carcinoma (case number 11; Table 2), all malignant tumors, with limited possibilities of quality of life improvement via palliative and/or specific antineoplastic treatment. Different from birds suffering from benign conditions (e.g., lipomas), in the aforementioned cases, surgical procedures were intended for diagnosis rather than disease eradication. Still surgical interventions provided support for therapeutic decisions aimed at quality of life improvement and are therefore indicated in cases of neoplastic disease with a poor prognosis in birds.

Deeper understanding of neoplastic diseases amenable to surgical treatment in pet birds, as well as data on affected species, tumor prevalence, preferential location of neoplasms, and potential outcomes of related surgical interventions, constitutes relevant information for clinicians specializing in avian medicine. Also important is the fact that such knowledge may serve as a basis for future studies in avian oncology.

5. Conclusion

All birds operated on due to neoplastic disease in this study belonged to the order Psittaciformes, with a higher prevalence of birds in the genus *Amazona*. Lipoma was the most prevalent neoplasm and the pericloacal area the most commonly affected site. Lipomas responded well to surgical resection, with high complete resolution and low recurrence rates. Diagnostic procedures such as incisional biopsy provided support for therapeutic planning in cases with a poor prognosis.

Conflict of Interests

The authors declare that there is no conflict of interests regarding the publication of this paper.

Acknowledgments

The authors thank Dr. Marta Brito Guimarães (DVM, Ph.D., Veterinary Hospital, FMVZ/USP) for the referral of surgical cases compiled in the Master's Thesis entitled "Afecções Cirúrgicas em Aves: Estudo Retrospectivo," which gave rise to the present paper, and Dr. Danilo Marin Rodrigues (DVM, Veterinary Hospital, FMVZ/USP) for histological photomicrographs.

References

[1] R. E. Schmidt and K. Quesenberry, "Neoplasia. Neoplastic diseases," in *Avian Medicine and Surgery*, R. B. Altman, S. L. Clubb, G. M. Dorrestein, and K. Quesenberry, Eds., pp. 590–603, WB Saunders, Philadelphia, Pa, USA, 1997.

[2] D. R. Reavill, "Tumors of pet birds," *Veterinary Clinics of North America. Exotic Animal Practice*, vol. 7, no. 3, pp. 537–560, 2004.

[3] T. L. Lightfoot, "Clinical avian neoplasia and oncology," in *Clinical Avian Medicine*, G. L. Harrison and T. L. Lightfoot, Eds., vol. 2, pp. 560–565, Spix, Palm Beach, Fla, USA, 2006.

[4] S. J. Mehler, J. A. Briscoe, M. J. Hendrick, and K. L. Rosenthal, "Infiltrative lipoma in a blue-crowned conure (*Aratinga acuticaudata*)," *Journal of Avian Medicine and Surgery*, vol. 21, no. 2, pp. 146–149, 2007.

[5] C. Bradford, A. Wack, S. Trembley, T. Southard, and E. Bronson, "Two cases of neoplasia of basal cell origin affecting the axillary region in anseriform species," *Journal of Avian Medicine and Surgery*, vol. 23, no. 3, pp. 214–221, 2009.

[6] M. W. Leach, "A survey of neoplasia in pet birds," *Seminars in Avian and Exotic Pet Medicine*, vol. 1, no. 2, pp. 52–64, 1992.

[7] B. S. Levine and Companion Animal Practice, "Common disorders of Amazons, Australian parakeets, and African grey parrots," *Seminars in Avian and Exotic Pet Medicine*, vol. 12, no. 3, pp. 125–130, 2003.

[8] L. J. Filippich, "Tumor control in birds," *Seminars in Avian and Exotic Pet Medicine*, vol. 13, no. 1, pp. 25–43, 2004.

[9] B. H. Coles, "Surgery," in *Essentials of Avian Medicine and Surgery*, B. H. Coles, Ed., pp. 142–182, Blackwell Publishing, Oxford, UK, 3rd edition, 2007.

[10] R. B. Altman, "General surgical considerations," in *Avian Medicine and Surgery*, R. B. Altman, S. L. Clubb, G. M. Dorrestein, and K. Quesenberry, Eds., pp. 691–703, WB Saunders, Philadelphia, Pa, USA, 1997.

[11] H. L. Bowles, E. Odberg, G. J. Harrison, and J. J. Kottwitz, "Surgical resolution of soft tissue disorders," in *Clinical Avian Medicine*, G. J. Harrison and T. L. Lightfoot, Eds., pp. 775–829, Spix, Palm Beach, Fla, USA, 2006.

[12] M. M. Garner, "A retrospective study of case submissions to a specialty diagnostic service," in *Clinical Avian Medicine*, G. L. Harrison and T. L. Lightfoot, Eds., vol. 2, pp. 566–571, Spix, Palm Beach, Fla, USA, 2006.

[13] F. B. Gill, *Ornithology*, W. H. Freeman and Company, New York, NY, USA, 2nd edition, 1995.

[14] R. L. Reece, "Observations on naturally occurring neoplasms in birds in the state of Victoria, Australia," *Avian Pathology*, vol. 21, no. 1, pp. 3–32, 1992.

[15] D. K. Blackmore, "The clinical approach to tumours in cage birds. I. The pathology and incidence of neoplasia in cage birds," *Journal of Small Animal Practice*, vol. 7, no. 3, pp. 217–223, 1966.

[16] N. A. Forbes and M. P. C. Lawton, "Introduction," in *Manual of Psittacine Birds*, P. H. Beynon, N. A. Forbes, and M. P. C. Lawton, Eds., pp. 7–10, Bsava, Cheltenham, UK, 1996.

[17] R. B. Altman, "Soft tissue surgical procedures," in *Avian Medicine and Surgery*, R. B. Altman, S. L. Clubb, G. M. Dorrestein, and K. Quesenberry, Eds., pp. 704–732, W.B. Saunders Company, Philadelphia, Pa, USA, 1997.

[18] K. S. Latimer, "Oncology," in *Avian Medicine: Principles and Application*, B. W. Ritchie, G. J. Harrison, and L. R. Harrison, Eds., pp. 640–669, Wingers Publishing, Lake Worth, Fla, USA, 1994.

[19] R. A. Perry, J. Gill, and G. M. Cross, "Disorders of the avian integument," *Veterinary Clinics of North America: Small Animal Practice*, vol. 21, no. 6, pp. 1307–1327, 1991.

[20] M. A. Koski, "Dermatologic diseases in psittacine birds: an investigational approach," *Seminars in Avian and Exotic Pet Medicine*, vol. 11, no. 3, pp. 105–124, 2002.

[21] H. Sick, *Ornitologia Brasileira*, Nova Fronteira, Rio de Janeiro, Brazil, 1997.

[22] P. Helmer and P. T. Redig, "Surgical resolution of orthopedic disorders," in *Clinical Avian Medicine*, G. L. Harrison and T. L. Lightfoot, Eds., vol. 2, pp. 761–773, Spix, Palm Beach, Fla, USA, 2006.

4

Bayesian Estimation of Sensitivity and Specificity of Rose Bengal, Complement Fixation, and Indirect ELISA Tests for the Diagnosis of Bovine Brucellosis in Ethiopia

T. Getachew, G. Getachew, G. Sintayehu, M. Getenet, and A. Fasil

National Animal Health Diagnostic and Investigation Center (NAHDIC), Ethiopian Ministry of Livestock and Fisheries Development, P.O. Box 04, Sebeta, Ethiopia

Correspondence should be addressed to G. Sintayehu; sintayehuguta_guta@yahoo.com

Academic Editor: Timm C. Harder

Test evaluation in the absence of a gold standard test was conducted for the diagnosis and screening of bovine brucellosis using three commercially available tests including RBPT, CFT, and I-ELISA in National Animal Health Diagnostic and Investigation Center (NAHDIC) Ethiopia. A total of 278 sera samples from five dairy herds were collected and tested. Each serum sample was subjected to the three tests and the results obtained were recorded and the test outcomes were cross-classified to estimate the sensitivity and specificity of the tests using Bayesian model. Prior information generated on the sensitivity and specificity of bovine brucellosis from published data was used in the model. The three test-one population Bayesian model was modified and applied using WinBug software with the assumption that the dairy herds have similar management system and unknown disease status. The Bayesian posterior estimate for sensitivity was 89.6 (95% PI: 79.9–95.8), 96.8 (95% PI: 92.3–99.1), and 94 (95% PI: 87.8–97.5) and for specificity was 84.5 (95% PI: 68–94.98), 96.3 (95% PI: 91.7–98.8), and 88.5 (95% PI: 81–93.8) for RBT, I-ELISA, and CFT, respectively. In this study I-ELISA was found with the best sensitivity and specificity estimates 96.8 (95% PI: 92.3–99.1) and 96.3 (95% PI: 91.7–98.8), compared to both CFT and RBPT.

1. Introduction

Brucellae are Gram-negative, facultative intracellular bacteria that can infect many species of animals and man. Ten species are recognized within the genus *Brucella*. There are 6 "classical" species: *B. abortus*, *B. melitensis*, *B. suis*, *B. ovis*, *B. canis*, and *B. neotomae* [1, 2] and, more recently, other four species have been recognized [3]. The principal manifestations of brucellosis are reproductive failure such as abortion or birth of unthrifty newborn and infertility [4, 5]. Brucellosis in animals and humans is still common in the Middle East, Asia, Africa, South and Central America, the Mediterranean Basin, and the Caribbean. *Brucella melitensis* is particularly common in the Mediterranean basin and it has also been reported in Africa, India, and Mexico [6].

Previous studies carried out in Ethiopia on bovine brucellosis using Rose Bengal and complement fixation tests described higher prevalence in intensive and semi-intensive dairy farms than extensive farms [1, 7, 8]. In 1987, the World Organization for Animal Health reported 20% prevalence of brucellosis, being higher around large towns than in rural areas [9]. In central highlands of Ethiopia, 4.2% prevalence of brucellosis was reported in zebu cattle [7]. Eshetu et al. [10] reported a prevalence of 10% in smallholder farms of central Ethiopia (Wuchale-Jida district) near Addis Ababa in 2005. Kebede et al. [11] reported a prevalence of 11% in cattle under extensive management systems. Studies conducted in different regions in 2003 and 2005 have reported animal level prevalence of 0.8% and 3.2% and herd prevalence of 2.9% and 42.3% [8, 12]. Another study in Ethiopia from 2003 to 2004 has reported a prevalence of 1.6% and a herd level prevalence of 13.7% [1]. A more recent study from 2011 to 2012 on exotic and crossbred dairy cattle and breeding farms has reported animal level prevalence of 1.9% and herd level prevalence of 10.6% in Ethiopia [13].

Serological tests are widely used to conduct several epidemiological studies and diagnostic purposes, but there is no perfect serological test [14, 15]. However, the diagnostic performance and discriminative ability of a test could be evaluated by comparing the sensitivity and specificity of several tests analytically [14, 16]. The diagnostic performance of a test could be evaluated by comparison with standard reference test and analyzed using latent models [17–19]. The objective of this study was to evaluate diagnostic performance and discriminative ability of Rose Bengal Plate Test (RBPT), complement fixation test (CFT), and indirect enzyme linked immunosorbent assay (I-ELISA) tests used for screening and confirmatory diagnosis of bovine brucellosis in Ethiopia using Bayesian method. This study is one of a kind in the context of field diagnostic test evaluation for bovine brucellosis in Ethiopia which has significant importance for disease surveillance and future control endeavors.

2. Materials and Methods

2.1. Study Area and Population. The study was conducted in five dairy farms, namely, Sululta, Awash, Wonji, Adami Tulu, and Alage located at 35, 100, 90, 170, and 200 km from Addis Ababa, respectively. The management system and breed of the farms were similar and the disease status was unknown. Thus, the farms were assumed as one population. All animals aged above six months in the farm were included in the sampling and the total number of the study animals was 278 pure and crossbreed Holstein Frisian dairy cows.

The farm history during sampling showed that there was no vaccination against brucellosis in all farms. Blood samples of 5–7 mL were collected in plain vacutainer tube from the jugular vein. The samples were allowed to clot for 2-3 h at room temperature. Then the serum was extracted by spinning at 2500 rpm for five minutes and kept in refrigerator at −20°C until the test is conducted. All farms except Sululta are located in the Great Rift Valley area of Ethiopia.

2.2. Diagnostic Tests. All serological tests conducted for test evaluation were performed at NAHDIC, Sebeta, Ethiopia (Bacterial Serology Laboratory).

2.2.1. Rose Bengal Test. Rose Bengal Test was conducted following the procedure described by OIE 2009. Antigen for the Rose Bengal Test was prepared from *B. abortus* strain 99 stained with Rose Bengal dye and suspended in acid buffer pH 3.65. Equal volume (30 μL) of antigen and test serum is brought together using a micropipette channel; then after thorough mixing it was rocked for four minutes; finally the result was read using magnifying glass and recorded as positive or negative based on the absence or presence of agglutination due to antigen-antibody reaction in the serum. Rose Bengal antigen was purchased from Lillidale Diagnostics, UK.

2.2.2. Complement Fixation Test. Complement fixation test was conducted using Alton et al. [20] Method. As a principle, if a specific antibody against bovine *Brucella* is present in

the serum, then antigen-antibody complex is formed and the complement will bind. The positive result of the test was when no hemolysis of the sheep RBC occurs. If there is no specific antibody against *Brucella*, the free complement exists which will cause sensitization of sheep RBC and lead to hemolysis. The validation of the result was done using positive and negative controls. Result interpretation based on the titration scale considered strong reaction when more than 75% fixation of the complement (3+) occurred at a dilution of 1 : 5 and the reaction was classified as weak positive with 50% fixation of complement (2+) that occurred at a dilution of 1 : 10 and above. *Brucella* antigen for the complement fixation test was prepared from *B. abortus* S99 and standardized against the OIEISS to give 50% fixation at a dilution of 1/200. *Brucella* antigen and positive control for complement fixation test were obtained from AH-VLA (Animal Health Veterinary Laboratory Agency), UK. Hemolytic serum and guinea pig complement was obtained from ID VET (Innovative Veterinary Diagnostic) Company.

2.2.3. Indirect ELISA Test. Test was performed according to the manufacturer's instructions and procedures. Indirect ELISA kit obtained from VLA Lillidale Animal Health Limited, Badbury View, Bothenwood, Wimborne, Dorset BH214HU, UK (https://www.gov.uk/government/organisations/animal-health-and-veterinary-laboratories-agency).

Reagent Preparation. The dilution buffer was prepared by adding 5 tablets PBS 0.5 mL phenol red indicator and 250 μL of Tween 20 to 500 mL distilled water; the pH was adjusted to 7.2. Then solution was prepared by adding the contents of the ampoule of Na_2HPO_4 and 1 mL of Tween 20 to 10 liters of distilled water. The substrate buffer prepared was by dissolving 1 tablet in 120 mL distilled water. The chromogen was prepared by dissolving 2 tablets in 1 mL of sterile distilled water. The stopping solution was prepared by diluting the ampoule of sodium azide with 500 mL of distilled water. Antigen was prepared from approved smooth lipopolysaccharides *B. abortus* strain 99 1 μg/m/L coated in 0.05 M carbonate/bicarbonate buffer, pH 9.6 onto flat bottom microplate wells. Positive and negative controls were reconstituted with 1 mL sterile distilled water and allowed until an even suspension is obtained before use. The test procedure, first a 1/40 predilution of all tests and control sera was made; then the plate was prepared by adding 80 μL of diluting buffer to wells followed by transferring of 20 μL of prediluted samples into a 96-well microplate coated with *Brucella* lipopolysaccharides (LPS). The optical density (OD0) was set at 405 nanometers blanked on well H12 and the presence or absence of antibodies against LPS of *Brucella* was determined by comparing the mean OD of positive controls. Color development within a well indicates that the sample has antibodies to *Brucella*. The validation criteria are as follows the cut-off value for positive/negative was calculated as 10% of the mean OD of positive control wells. Any test sample giving an OD equal to or above this value should be considered positive.

2.2.4. Test Evaluation Using Bayesian Model. Estimation of diagnostic test sensitivity and specificity through Bayesian

TABLE 1: Prior information used for sensitivity and specificity of RBT, I-ELISA, and CFT.

	RBT	I-ELISA	CFT	
Se	81.2 (66.4–96)	96 (90.2–99.8)	89 (81.3–96.7)	Gall and Nielsen (2004) [15]
Sp	86.3 (71.64–99)	93.8 (88–99.6)	83.5 (75.8–91.2)	
Se	100 (96.7–100)	98.9 (96.2–99.8)	100 (96.7–100)	Mainar-Jaime et al. (2005) [23]
Sp	86.4 (79.1–91.9)	100 (97.1–100)	94.4 (88.8–97.7)	
Âse	90.6 (81.6–98)	97.4 (93.2–99.9)	94.5 (89–98.3)	Mean Se and Sp
ÂSp	86.4 (71–99)	96.9 (92.5–99.8)	89 (82.3–94.4)	

modeling has an advantage to provide more stable point and interval estimates without the necessity of large sample sizes [21, 22]. One of the reasons why Bayesian approach was employed was that it can give good estimates of sensitivity and specificity in the absence of gold standard method like culture and isolation. The Bayesian approach is a well-established methodology for robust diagnostic test evaluation. We could not culture samples for bacterial isolation of *Brucella* in our laboratory because of biorisk and biosecurity concern. Finally, we consider that this does not affect the results of our study.

The sensitivity and specificity of the three tests were evaluated using a total of 278 sera samples collected from five dairy farms. Each serum sample was subjected to the three tests and the results were entered into the computer. The observed data of the three tests' results was summarized in cross tabulation. Bayesian model without gold standard was applied to estimate the sensitivity and specificity estimates. Prior information for the unknown data in the model was used from published data on bovine brucellosis [15, 23].

Gall and Nielsen [15] reviewed over 50 publications in which sensitivity and specificity values of assays used for the detection of exposure to *Brucella abortus* where the sum of sensitivity and specificity values for each test was averaged to give a performance index. Similarly, comparison was made of sensitivity and specificity of I-ELISA RBT that thus we used as prior information for our data analysis.

The uncertainty of an average sensitivity and specificity obtained from the published data was transformed to the beta distribution using Betabuster free software (http://www.epi .ucdavis.edu/diagnostictests [22]). The prior information for sensitivity of RBP, I-ELISA, and CFT was of modes 0.91, 0.97, and 0.94, respectively, and the transformed beta (a, b) was beta (49.4, 6.0); (103.2, 3.73); and (89.27, 6.14), respectively. Prior mode for specificity of RBP, I-ELISA, and CFT was 0.86, 0.97, and 0.89, respectively, and the transformed beta distribution (a, b) was (22.76, 4.43); (102.1, 4.23); and (83.05, 11.14), respectively (Table 1).

The Bayesian model for one population-three tests was modified and applied for the data using WinBUGS free software. The median value of the posterior distributions was built after 50,000 iterations and the burnout of the initial 5,000 iterations. The model sensitivity was checked using kernel density and autocorrelation graphs that showed the posterior distribution fit fairly to the data. Conditional dependence of the tests was also checked because the tests are based on

TABLE 2: Cross tabulation of the three tests' results.

	CFT pos.		CFT neg. I-ELISA		Total
	I-ELISA pos.	I-ELISA neg.	Pos.	neg.	
RBT pos.	2	0	2	1	5
RBT neg.	0	0	4	269	273
Total	2	0	6	270	278

similar biological basis which might lead to correlated errors leading to incorrect estimation of sensitivity and specificity [22]. Then, conditional independent Bayesian model was applied which allowed us to estimate the conditional correlations (rhoD and rhoDc) for Se and Sp, respectively, for the three tests.

3. Results

All sera samples were tested blindly by all the three tests (RBT, I-ELISA, and CF) independently. The tests result showed 5/278; 8/278 and 2/278 positive for RBT, I-ELISA, and CF, respectively; this indicated that I-ELISA is superior in sensitivity and specificity, followed by CF. Kappa test of the three tests showed moderate agreement (kappa = 0.70); the rhoD and rhoDc values were small and clustered around zero which indicates that the tests are conditionally independent (Table 2).

The posterior inference for the true sensitivity of RBT, I-ELISA, and CFT was 89.6 (95% PI: 79.9–95.8), 96.8 (95% PI: 92.3–99.1), and 94 (95% PI: 87.8–97.5) and true specificity was 84.5 (95% PI: 68–94.98), 96.3 (95% PI: 91.7–98.8), and 88.5 (81–93.8), respectively. In this study, the true sensitivity and specificity of I-ELISA (96.8 95% PI (92.3–99.1) and 96.3 95% PI (91.7–98.8), resp.) were found higher than RBPT and CFT. The seroprevalence of brucellosis in these farms was estimated to be 4 (95% PI: 0.8–11.45).

The conditional correlation to evaluate conditional dependence of the three tests showed that the value estimate for both rhoD (for sensitivity) and rhoDc (for specificity) was small with the probability interval clustering around zero which showed the tests were conditionally independent. The sensitivity analysis based on the posterior distribution kernel density and autocorrelation graphs showed that the observed data fairly fit the model and prior information has not significantly influenced the median estimate (Table 3).

TABLE 3: Observed estimate of sensitivities and specificities.

Test	Parameter	Posterior estimation
RBT	Se	89.6 (95% PI: 79.9–95.8)
	Sp	84.5 (95% PI: 68–94.8)
I-ELISA	Se	96.8 (95% PI: 92.3–99.1)
	Sp	96.3 (95% PI: 91.7–98.8)
CFT	Se	94 (95% PI: 87.8–97.5)
	Sp	88.5 (95% PI: 81–93.8)
Prevalence		4 (95% PI: 0.8–11.45)
rhoD		0.22 (95% PI: −0.05–0.71)
rhoDc		0.176 (95% PI: −0.082–0.64)

95% PI = 95% probability interval.

4. Discussion

Screening and confirmatory diagnostic tests are the primary tools for successful epidemiological study. In Ethiopia, although many papers were published to determine the prevalence of bovine brucellosis in different farm settings, we could not find any published data on sensitivity and specificity of the serological tests. The knowledge on the diagnostic sensitivity and specificity of a test would help to limit diagnostic errors in classifying infected and noninfected animals correctly and to prevent excessive economical losses when the animals are wrongly classified by the tests [24].

No single serological test is appropriate in all epidemiological situations and all animal species; all tests have limitations especially when screening individual animals. Consideration should be given to all factors that impact on the relevance of the test method and test results to a specific diagnostic interpretation or application. Antigen for the Rose Bengal Test was prepared by depositing killed *B. abortus* strain 99 (Weybridge) cells stained with Rose Bengal dye and suspended in acid buffer pH 3.65. Antigen for complement fixation test was prepared from *B. abortus* strain 99 (Weybridge) and standardized against the OIEISS to give 50% fixation at a dilution of 1/200. The same *B. abortus* strain 99 (Weybridge) was also used as a source of soluble antigen extracts (smooth lipopolysaccharide (S-LPS) for the indirect ELISA). Therefore, antigen for indirect ELISA was prepared from approved smooth lipopolysaccharides *B. abortus* strain 99 $1 \mu g/m/L$ coated in 0.05 M carbonate/bicarbonate buffer, pH 9.6, onto flat bottom microplate wells. All the three antigens are used to detect infections due to smooth *Brucella* species as per information obtained from the manufacturer. All diagnostic kit components (i.e., antigen, reference sera, and complements) used for the test evaluation purpose were of highest quality obtained from VLA, UK, internationally recognized diagnostic kit supplier with good manufacturing practice.

Estimation of diagnostic sensitivity and specificity of a test requires knowledge of the true disease status of the animals on which the test is to be applied using the gold standard test; however, in the absence of such a gold standard test a Bayesian approach is a useful tool to evaluate the characteristics of the tests [18, 19, 25].

Bayesian method has an advantage as it provides a stable point and interval estimates without the necessity of large sample size [21, 26]. It is widely accepted that screening tests should have a higher sensitivity but could have a lower specificity. The sensitivity of RBT in the current study was fairly high (89.6 (95% PI: 79.9–95.8)) which was higher than the previous finding by Sanogo et al. (2013) [27] (54.9% (cr 23.5–95.1)).

Previous studies suggested that CFT is an appropriate confirmatory test with high specificity [16] but this was not consistent with the current finding that the specificity of CFT was moderate (88.5 (95% PI: 81–93.8)) which might be due to small population size in our study. However, Gall and Nielsen (2004) [15] reported the sensitivity and specificity of CFT as Se 81.2 and Sp 83.5, respectively, which is in agreement with our current finding. The I-ELISA was found to be the best sensitive and specific test (95% PI: 92.3–99.1 and 95% PI: 91.7–98.8, resp.) for bovine brucellosis compared to both CFT and RBPT. The possible reason for this high accuracy might be due to the fact that I-ELISA detects all isotopes of immunoglobulin IgG while CFT cannot detect them [14]. The mean sensitivity and specificity for indirect ELISA were reported as Se 96.0 and Sp 93.8 by Gall and Nielsen (2004) which was in agreement with our estimates.

The conditional dependence of the tests is that the conditional correlation rhoD and rhoDc values for sensitivity and specificity, respectively, were small and clustered around zero which indicates that the tests are conditionally independent and could be an advantage while using in test combinations [28]. The sensitivity analysis using different prior information showed that the posterior distribution kernel density and autocorrelation graphs showed that the observed data fairly fit the model and prior information has not significantly influenced the median estimates.

5. Conclusion and Recommendation

Based on this observation I-ELISA had the best performance followed by CFT and RBPT in descending order of accuracy. However, the decision for the choice of diagnostic test for different purposes not only does rely on the accuracy, but also should take into consideration the capacity for the test throughput, technical complexity, and cost effectiveness. Regardless of its lower sensitivity, RBT remains the most widely used screening test because of its rapid result and cost effectiveness. Therefore, conducting test verification is very essential to know the test characteristics and to determine the type of test we require to use for the study purpose, epidemiological surveillance, or international trade. We recommend further studies should be conducted on the performance of these tests in the field setting for the diagnosis of sheep and goat brucellosis to generate sufficient information.

Competing Interests

The authors of the submitted paper have no conflict of interests.

Acknowledgments

The research team acknowledges the National Animal Health Diagnostic and Investigation Center for facilitating field programs and Mr. Belachew Dura, Mr. Mengistu Nemera, and Mr. Tafesse Koran for collecting serum samples from different dairy farms for the study.

References

[1] K. Asmare, Y. Asfaw, E. Gelaye, and G. Ayelet, "Brucellosis in extensive management system of Zebu cattle in Sidama Zone, Southern Ethiopia," *African Journal of Agricultural Research*, vol. 5, no. 3, pp. 257–263, 2010.

[2] M. J. Corbel, M. Banai, and I. Genus, "Brucella Meyer and Shaw 1920, 173AL," in *Bergey's Manual of Systematic Bacteriology*, D. J. Brenner, N. R. Krieg, and J. T. Staley, Eds., pp. 370–386, Springer, New York, NY, USA, 2005.

[3] V. L. Atluri, M. N. Xavier, M. F. de Jong, A. B. den Hartigh, and R. M. Tsolis, "Interactions of the human pathogenic *Brucella* species with their hosts," *Annual Review of Microbiology*, vol. 65, pp. 523–541, 2011.

[4] O. M. Radostits, C. C. Gay, D. C. Blood, and K. W. Hinchcliff, *Veterinary Medicine: A Textbook of the Diseases of Cattle, Sheep, Pigs, Goats and Horses*, WB Saunders, London, UK, 9th edition, 2000.

[5] World Organization for Animal Health (OIE), "Ovine and Caprine Brucellosis," 2009, http://web.oie.int/eng/normes/MMANUAL/2008/pdf/2.07.02_CAPRINE_OVINE_BRUC.pdf.

[6] Center for Food Security and Public Health (CFSPH), 2009, http://www.cfsph.iastate.edu/Factsheets/pdfs/brucellosis.pdf.

[7] B. Tekleye, O. B. Kassali, M. Mugurewa, R. G. Sholtens, and Y. Tamirat, "The prevalence of brucellosis in indigenous cattle in central Ethiopia," *Bulletin of Animal Health and Production in Africa*, vol. 37, pp. 97–98, 1989.

[8] T. Tolosa, F. Regassa, K. Belihu, and Inter-African Bureau for Animal Resources, "Sero-prevalence study of bovine brucellosis in extensive management system in selected sites of Jimma zone, Western Ethiopia," *Bulletin of Animal Health and Production in Africa*, vol. 56, pp. 25–37, 2008.

[9] World Organization for Animal Health (OIE), "Bovine brucellosis and brucellosis of small ruminants," *Technical Series Office International des Epizooties*, vol. 6, pp. 48–49, 1987.

[10] Y. Eshetu, J. Kassahun, P. Abebe, M. Beyene, B. Zewdie, and A. Bekele, "Seroprevalence study of Brucellosis on dairy cattle in Addis Ababa, Ethiopia," *Bulletin of Animal Health and Production in Africa*, vol. 53, pp. 211–214, 2005.

[11] T. Kebede, G. Ejeta, G. Ameni, and École Nationale Vétérinaire de Toulouse, "Seroprevalence of bovine brucellosis in smallholder farms in central Ethiopia (Wuchale-Jida district)," *Revue de Médecine Vétérinaire*, vol. 159, pp. 3–9, 2008.

[12] G. Berhe, K. Belihu, and Y. Asfaw, "Seroepidemiological investigation of bovine brucellosis in the extensive cattle production system of Tigray region of Ethiopia," *International Journal of Applied Research in Veterinary Medicine*, vol. 5, pp. 65–71, 2007.

[13] K. Asmare, B. Sibhat, W. Molla et al., "The status of bovine brucellosis in Ethiopia with special emphasis on exotic and cross bred cattle in dairy and breeding farms," *Acta Tropica*, vol. 126, no. 3, pp. 186–192, 2013.

[14] F. P. Poester, K. Nielsen, L. E. Samartino, and W. L. Yu, "Diagnosis of Brucellosis," *The Open Veterinary Science Journal*, vol. 4, pp. 46–60, 2010.

[15] D. Gall and K. Nielsen, "Serological diagnosis of Bovine brucellosis: a review of test performance and cost comparison," *Revue Scientifique et Technique*, vol. 23, no. 3, pp. 989–1002, 2004.

[16] I. R. Dohoo, P. F. Wright, G. M. Ruckerbauer, B. S. Samagh, F. J. Robertson, and L. B. Forbes, "A comparison of five serological tests for bovine brucellosis," *Canadian Journal of Veterinary Research*, vol. 50, no. 4, pp. 485–493, 1986.

[17] R. Poulloit and R. Gerbier, "A Bayesian method for the evaluation of the sensitivity and specificity of correlated diagnostic tests in the absence of gold standard," in *Proceeding of the 9th International Symposium on Veterinary Epidemiology and Economics*, 2000, http://www.sciquest.org.nz/.

[18] R. Pouillot, G. Gerbier, and I. A. Gardner, "'TAGS', a program for the evaluation of test accuracy in the absence of a gold standard," *Preventive Veterinary Medicine*, vol. 53, pp. 67–81, 2002.

[19] C. Enøe, S. Andersen, V. Sørensen, and P. Willeberg, "Estimation of sensitivity, specificity and predictive values of two serologic tests for the detection of antibodies against *Actinobacillus pleuropneumoniae* serotype 2 in the absence of a reference test (gold standard)," *Preventive Veterinary Medicine*, vol. 51, no. 3-4, pp. 227–243, 2001.

[20] G. G. Alton, L. M. Jones, R. D. Angus, and J. M. Verger, *Techniques for the Brucellosis Laboratory*, Institut National de la Recherche Agronomique, Paris, France, 1988.

[21] C. Enøe, M. P. Georgiadis, and W. O. Johnson, "Estimation of sensitivity and specificity of diagnostic tests and disease prevalence when the true disease state is unknown," *Preventive Veterinary Medicine*, vol. 45, no. 1-2, pp. 61–81, 2000.

[22] A. J. Branscum, I. A. Gardner, and W. O. Johnson, "Estimation of diagnostic-test sensitivity and specificity through Bayesian modeling," *Preventive Veterinary Medicine*, vol. 68, no. 2–4, pp. 145–163, 2005.

[23] R. C. Mainar-Jaime, P. M. Muñoz, M. J. de Miguel et al., "Specificity dependence between serological tests for diagnosing bovine brucellosis in Brucella-free farms showing false positive serological reactions due to *Yersinia enterocolitica O:9*," *Canadian Veterinary Journal*, vol. 46, no. 10, pp. 913–916, 2005.

[24] B. W. Stemshorn, L. B. Forbes, M. D. Eaglesome, K. H. Nielsen, F. J. Robertson, and B. S. Samagh, "A comparison of standard serological tests for the diagnosis of bovine brucellosis in Canada," *Canadian Journal of Comparative Medicine*, vol. 49, no. 4, pp. 391–394, 1985.

[25] N. Toft, E. Jørgensen, and S. Højsgaard, "Diagnosing diagnostic tests: evaluating the assumptions underlying the estimation of sensitivity and specificity in the absence of a gold standard," *Preventive Veterinary Medicine*, vol. 68, no. 1, pp. 19–33, 2005.

[26] G. Gari, F. Biteau-Croller, C. Le Goff, P. Caufour, and F. Roger, "Evaluation of the indirect fluorescent antibody test for the diagnosis and screening of lumpy skin disease," *Veterinary Microbiology*, vol. 129, no. 3-4, pp. 269–280, 2008.

[27] M. Sanogo, E. Thys, Y. L. Achi et al., "Bayesian estimation of the true prevalence, sensitivity and specificity of the Rose Bengal and indirect ELISA tests in the diagnosis of bovine brucellosis," *Veterinary Journal*, vol. 195, no. 1, pp. 114–120, 2013.

[28] N. Dendukuri and L. Joseph, "Bayesian approaches to modeling the conditional dependence between multiple diagnostic tests," *Biometrics*, vol. 57, no. 1, pp. 158–167, 2001.

5

Assessment of *Pasteurella multocida* A Lipopolysaccharide, as an Adhesin in an In Vitro Model of Rabbit Respiratory Epithelium

Carolina Gallego, [1,2] **Stefany Romero,** [3] **Paula Esquinas,** [4] **Pilar Patiño,** [5] **Nhora Martínez,** [5] **and Carlos Iregui** [5]

[1]*Laboratory of Veterinary Pathology, Universidad de Ciencias Aplicadas y Ambientales, Calle 222 No. 55-37, Bogotá, Colombia*
[2]*Faculty of Science, Pontificia Universidad Javeriana, Carrera 7 No. 43-82, Bogotá, Colombia*
[3]*Academic Assistant, Veterinary Medicine Program, Universidad de La Salle, Cra. 7 No. 179-03, Bogotá, Colombia*
[4]*Laboratory of Cytogenetics and Genotyping of Domestic Animal UGA, Faculty of Veterinary Medicine,*
 National University of Colombia, Bogotá, Colombia
[5]*Laboratory of Veterinary Pathology, Faculty of Veterinary Medicine, National University of Colombia, Bogotá, Colombia*

Correspondence should be addressed to Carlos Iregui; caireguic@unal.edu.co

Academic Editor: Douglas Morck

The role of the *P. multocida* lipopolysaccharide (LPS) as a putative adhesin during the early stages of infection with this bacterium in the respiratory epithelium of rabbits was investigated. By light microscopy and double enzyme labeling of nasal septa tissues, the amount of bacteria attached to the respiratory epithelium and the amount of LPS present in goblet cells at different experimental times were estimated. Transmission electron microscopy (TEM) and LPS labeling with colloidal gold particles were also used to determine the exact location of LPS in the cells. Septa that were challenged with LPS of *P. multocida* and 30 minutes later with *P. multocida* showed more adherent bacteria and more severe lesions than the other treatments. Free LPS was observed in the lumen of the nasal septum, forming bilamellar structures and adhering to the cilia, microvilli, cytoplasmic membrane, and cytoplasm of epithelial ciliated and goblet cells. The above findings suggest that *P. multocida* LPS plays an important role in the process of bacterial adhesion and that it has the ability of being internalized into host cells.

1. Introduction

Pasteurella multocida is considered the most important causal agent of respiratory diseases in rabbits and in other species; this group of microorganisms is responsible for the largest economic losses in production farm animals [1]. Under production conditions, rabbits are frequently subjected to overcrowding, drastic changes in temperature and humidity, or stress, all of which contribute to the appearance of respiratory pathologies caused by *P. multocida* [2–5].

Bacterial adhesion to the mucosal surfaces of a host results from physicochemical interactions between the pathogens and the host epithelial cells, and the ultimate colonization of deeper layers of the mucosa and the successful establishment of an infection depends on this interaction. Therefore, adhesion is considered the first essential step that a pathogen must overcome to cause disease [6–9]. Such interactions occur between molecules located on the surface of host epithelial cells as well as molecules on the bacteria. Lipopolysaccharide (LPS) is the most abundant superficial constituent of Gram-negative bacteria. This glycolipid molecule is fundamental for the survival of these microorganisms and is responsible for causing severe systemic effects in the hosts, such as endotoxemia; therefore, LPS is considered an important virulence factor of these pathogens [10–13]. However, studies on the involvement of LPS during the first steps of infection, namely, during adhesion and colonization of the surface epithelia before the bacteria causes systemic effects, are rare and most are devoted to other bacterial adhesive structures, such as the fimbria [14–17].

Bélanger et al. [18] proposed that the LPS of *Actinobacillus pleuropneumoniae* would be responsible for the adhesion of the bacterium to the respiratory epithelial cells of swine; later, studies of *E. coli, Salmonella enterica* subsp. *enterica* serovar Typhimurium, *Helicobacter pylori, Klebsiella pneumonia,* and *Pseudomonas aeruginosa* showed that it was possible to block the adhesion of the corresponding microorganisms to different cell surfaces by suppressing or modifying the structure of their respective LPS molecules and by employing monoclonal antibodies against the O antigen of the molecule [16, 17, 19–23].

Recently, Bravo et al. [16] showed that the core of *S. typhimurium* LPS plays an important role in the interaction of the bacteria with HeLa epithelial cells, as well as BHK and IB3 cells lines. The inner core of the molecule has Glc I and Gal I residues, which are essential for adhesion and entry of the microorganism into epithelial cells in vitro. The authors speculate that a lectin type receptor could be involved in the interaction of the host cells with the outer core structure, which is composed of (Gal I α 1-3 Glu) [16].

In addition, a role for *Helicobacter pylori* LPS O antigen in adhesion and colonization of the gastric mucosa of mice has also been proposed. Moreover, it has been shown that the core of *H. pylori* LPS is involved in pathogen binding to laminin, an extracellular matrix and basement membrane glycoprotein of the epithelium that is essential for the process of bacterial adhesion [17].

On the other hand, few reports document the mechanism by which LPS is internalized into the cytoplasm of the host cells; caspases 4, 5, and 11 are considered intracytoplasmic receptors for *E. coli* and *S. typhimurium* LPS in macrophage cell cultures and somatic cells such as mouse enterocytes in which they induce pyroptosis and apoptosis [23]. In addition, LPS can be internalized by the lipopolysaccharide binding protein (LBP) into the cytoplasm of monocytes and macrophages, as well as by nonimmune human cells such as the HEK293 cell line. These findings have led to the hypothesis that LPS plays an important role in the regulation of intracellular pro- and anti-inflammatory signals [24].

In *P. multocida,* different studies reported the significance of several surface structures such as adhesins, including highly hydrated polyanionic polysaccharides on the capsule that are covalently bound to the surface of bacteria through phospholipids or lipid A. Other structures also include outer membrane proteins (OMPs), which may serve as adhesins or invasins or participate in the formation of biofilms such as type IV fimbriae, the fibronectin binding protein, and filamentous hemagglutinin [25]; however, no study has been devoted to exploring the role of *P. multocida* LPS as an adhesion molecule. For the first time, we show that the LPS of *P. multocida* significantly increases the adhesion of the microorganism to the apical surface of the respiratory epithelium of the rabbit nasal septum and that the increased number of adhered microorganisms causes more severe damage to the host cells. We also show that LPS is internalized into the cytoplasm of respiratory cells and that goblet cells play an important role during these first steps of infection.

2. Materials and Methods

2.1. Pasteurella multocida Strain. Pasteurella multocida A strain 001 was obtained from turbinates, trachea, and lungs of rabbits with signs of rhinitis and pneumonia from farms in the Sabana de Bogotá (Colombia). The organism was grown in brain heart infusion (BHI) agar; gray nonhemolytic colonies with a round morphology were selected. The colonies were identified as bipolar-staining, Gram-negative coccobacilli and were shown to be catalase-, oxidase-, indole-, ornithine decarboxylase-, glucose-, sucrose-, and mannitol-positive using biochemical tests. The colonies did not grow on MacConkey agar and were urease-negative [1]. Molecular identification of *P. multocida* of capsular serogroup A was performed by expanding the sequence of the hyaD cap gene locus with the following primers: F: 5′ TGC CAA AAT CGC AGT CAG 3′; R: 5′ TTG CCA TCA TTG TCA GTG 3′ [26].

2.2. Extraction, Purification, Quantification, and Biological Activity of P. multocida LPS. LPS was extracted using the phenol/hot water method [30]. *Pasteurella multocida* (5.8 g) were resuspended in 29 mL of ultrapure water. The aqueous phase was dialyzed against sterile water and then lyophilized. The sample was reconstituted in 10 mL of 0.1 M Tris buffer containing 0.15 M NaCl and 1 N HCl, pH 7, and treated with RNase (0.5 mg/mL), DNase (0.05 mg/mL), and 100 μL of 4 mM $MgCl_2$ for 2 hours at 60°C. The sample was then treated with proteinase K (0.05 mg/mL) and 100 μL of 1 mM $CaCl_2$ for 18 hours at 37°C. The extract was frozen at −80°C and lyophilized for 48 h. A mass of 70.4 mg was obtained and was then subjected to gel permeation chromatography; briefly, the extract was resuspended in 5 mL of 0.05 M Tris buffer containing 1.5% sodium deoxycholate and 1 mM EDTA, pH 9.5, and passed through a GE Healthcare HiPrep™ 16/60 Sephacryl™ S-200 HR column (Sigma Aldrich, St. Louis, MO, USA). Fractions of 2.5 mL were collected at a flow rate of 0.8 mL/min and measured at 220 nm, 260 nm, and 280 nm using spectrophotometry. At each stage of purification and characterization, aliquots were sampled and were analyzed with a spectrophotometer by scanning between 200 nm and 600 nm (NanoDrop 2000 Spectrophotometer Thermo Scientific, Wilmington, DE, USA).

The resolving gel for electrophoresis was prepared at 12%, the stacking gel was prepared at 4%, and the electrophoresis conditions were 0.03 A/45 min and 0.02 A/1 h, respectively. The lyophilized fractions were reconstituted in pyrogen-free water to a final concentration of 1 mg/mL, prepared in 1x Laemmli buffer, and heated at 95°C for 5 minutes before they were added to the gel. Staining was performed with silver nitrate and Coomassie blue [31].

The amount of polysaccharide in the extract was quantified using the Purpald test; a reference curve was constructed with a standard of 3-deoxy-α-D-mannooctulosonic acid (Kdo) (Sigma Co., St. Louis, MO, USA) in concentrations ranging from 0.8 mM to 0.025 mM. Commercial *Escherichia coli 0111:B4, S. typhimurium* and *Rhodobacter sphaeroides* DSM 158 LPSs were diluted to two concentrations: 0.4 mg/mL and 0.2 mg/mL. Different concentrations of the *P. multocida* LPS fractions were used, ranging from 1 mg/mL to

0.125 mg/mL. Duplicates of each sample were placed in a 96-well microplate containing 32 mM sodium periodate; the plates were incubated at room temperature for 25 min. Subsequently, 136 mM Purpald reagent was added to each well and incubated for 20 min at room temperature. Immediately, 64 mM of sodium periodate was added and incubated at room temperature for 20 min. Then, 20 μL of 2-isopropanol was added. Spectrophotometry was performed at 550 nm.

The sterility of the LPS was confirmed with cultures in agar BHI in the presence and absence of 5% ovine blood, which was incubated at 37°C and observed daily for six days.

The biological activity of LPS was determined in mice by evaluating its pathogenic effects. Twenty-five μg of LPS diluted in 100 μL of PSS was intraperitoneally inoculated in five mice; 125 μL of PSS was also IP injected in 5 additional mice as a negative control. After eight hours, the animals were euthanized and the lungs and liver were evaluated by histopathology.

2.3. Simultaneous and Sequential Exposure of Rabbit Nasal Septa Explants to P. multocida and to LPS (H&E). The nasal septa of rabbit fetuses were cultured ex vivo using the methods reported by [32, 33]. Briefly, fetuses were obtained by cesarean on gestational day 26 under anesthesia and were immediately euthanatized by medullar sectioning; two sequential approximately 2 mm thick cross sections of the nasal cavity were maintained in Dulbecco's minimal essential medium (MEM) during the experiment. All procedures were approved and authorized by the Bioethics Committee of the Faculty of Veterinary Medicine and Animal Science, National University of Colombia (Act 006/2010).

Experimental Design. The tissues were treated as described in Table 1.

The tissues were immersed in 10 mL of MEM in 5 cm wide × 2 cm high Petri dishes; the tissues were incubated in a humid chamber at 37°C with a 5% CO_2 atmosphere for 2 h. At the appropriate times, the tissues were immersed in McDowell and Trump fixative (commercial 4% formaldehyde and 1% glutaraldehyde) diluted in Sorenson's sodium phosphate buffer.

The lesions on the respiratory epithelium were evaluated with a 100x objective and were semiquantitatively assessed. The severity and extent of the lesions were graded using the scale reported by Bernet et al. [29] (Table 2).

The following changes or lesions were evaluated: desquamated cells (DC), activity of goblet cells (AGC), cilia loss (CL), the presence of intracytoplasmic vacuoles (IV), and dead cells (DC).

2.4. Evaluating the Amount of P. multocida LPS on the Apical Surface of Respiratory Epithelial Cells and within the Cytoplasm of Goblet Cells, as well as the Number of P. multocida That Adhered to the Respiratory Epithelium (LH-IIP). P. multocida and P. multocida LPS were simultaneously detected on the respiratory epithelium of nasal septa by a double labeling technique using indirect immunoperoxidase (IIP) for the bacterium and lectin histochemistry (LH) for LPS. Briefly, polyclonal ovine antibodies labeled with

horseradish peroxidase (HRP) were employed to detect *P. multocida*; a specific commercial *Limulus polyphemus* lectin (LPA) conjugated with alkaline phosphatase was added to the nasal explants (alkaline phosphatase-conjugated *Limulus polyphemus* lectin, horseshoe crab, EY Laboratories Inc., San Mateo, CA, USA). This lectin specifically binds the 2-keto-3-deoxyoctanate (KDO) sugar of the core of LPS [34]. The peroxidase technique was performed first, and then the tissues were incubated with the LPA lectin.

2.5. Analysis of the Images of LPS Lectin Histochemistry and Indirect Immunoperoxidase Staining of Pasteurella multocida. The program ImageJ version 1.41 GPL (General Public License), which is available for all systems and platforms and is widely used for analyzing biomedical images, was implemented to evaluate the quantity of LPS on the apical surface of epithelial cells and the number of *P. multocida* that had adhered to the ciliated border of the respiratory epithelium and within the cytoplasm of goblet cells [35].

2.6. Transmission Electron Microscopy. The tissues were dehydrated in an ascending ethanol series from 50% to 90% and were then embedded in LR White resin. Ultrathin sections (90 to 100 nm) were cut and mounted on nickel grids or nickel-covered 200 mesh Formvar grids; the samples were rehydrated in distilled water. Nonspecific sites were blocked with 10% bovine serum albumin in PBS for 15 minutes, incubated on a drop of lectin *Limulus polyphemus* diluted 1 : 3 in a buffer solution, and conjugated to 5 nm wide colloidal gold particles for 30 minutes at 37°C. The grids were washed and contrasted with 1% uranyl acetate for 3–5 minutes and observed with a Jeol 1400 Plus transmission electron microscope at 80 kV [36]. No IIP was necessary because bacteria are more easily visible with this technique than with light microscopy.

2.7. Statistical Analysis. For the model assumptions, the Shapiro-Wilk test was used to determine the normality of the errors and Levene's test was used to determine the homogeneity of the variance. Analysis of variance (ANOVA) with a confidence interval of 95% and Tukey's multiple comparison test were used to determine the differences between treatments [37].

3. Results

3.1. Pasteurella multocida Strain. According to the taxonomic tools of SeqMatch classification from the RDP, the comparison of the BlastN of Greengens, and the basic alignment in NCBI, the strain of *P. multocida* used in this study shares 99% identity with the genus and species *Pasteurella multocida* subsp. *multocida*.

3.2. Extraction, Purification, Quantification, and Biological Activity of P. multocida LPS. A purified smooth chemotype of *P. multocida* LPS with the presence of KDO and heptoses in its core was obtained. It was also protein-free (Figure 1).

3.3. Simultaneous and Sequential Exposure of Rabbit Nasal Septa Explants to P. multocida LPS (H&E). Nasal septa that

TABLE 1: Experimental protocol for exposing fetal rabbit nasal septa to *P. multocida* and LPS: IIP (indirect immunoperoxidase), LH (lectin histochemistry), TEM (transmission electron microscopy), and C (−) (negative control)* [27, 28].

| Treatment | Negative control | | *P. multocida* | | LPS + *P. multocida* simultaneously | LPS + *P. multocida* 30 min later | | *P. multocida* + LPS 30 min later | LPS |
	Treatment 1		Treatment 2		Treatment 3	Treatment 4		Treatment 5	Treatment 6
Technique	IIP-LH	TEM	IIP-LH	TEM	IIP-LH	IIP-LH	TEM	IIP-LH	TEM
Number of explants	7	3	7	3	7	7	3	7	3
Dose*	MEM	MEM	1×10^8 cfu/mL	1×10^8 cfu/mL	$10\,\mu g/mL + 1 \times 10^8$ cfu/mL	$10\,\mu g/mL + 1 \times 10^8$ cfu/mL	$10\,\mu g/mL + 10^8$ cfu/mL	1×10^8 cfu/mL + $10\,\mu g/mL$	$10\,\mu g/mL$
Exposure time	2 h	2 h	2 h	2 h	2 h	2 h	2 h	2 h	2 h

TABLE 2: Grading the severity of the lesions using H&E, adapted from Bernet et al. [29].

(a)

Grade	Severity	Description
−	Absent	(i) Cells with normal activity (ii) Normal architecture is readily visible
+	Light	(i) Cells with scant activity (ii) Lesions are observed with some difficulty
++	Moderate	(i) Cells with moderate activity (ii) Lesions are easily observed, with normal architecture still visible
+++	Severe	(i) Cells are very active (ii) Lesions are easily observed; the normal architecture is not identified

(b)

Extension	Description
Focal	F: lesion in an area comprising less than 10% of the section
Multifocal	M: lesions in more than two areas, each comprising less than 10% of the section
Diffuse	G: multiple areas or an area greater than 50% of the section

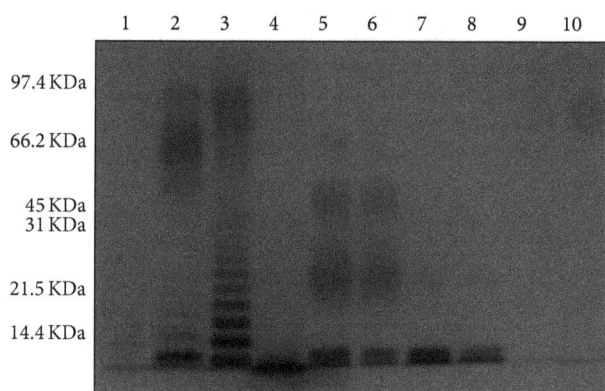

FIGURE 1: Electrophoretic profile of LPS of *P. multocida* A UN001: 1, low molecular weight marker; 2, commercial LPS of *Escherichia coli* O111:B4 (InvivoGen, San Diego, CA, USA) (0.06 mg/well); 3, commercial lipopolysaccharide of *S. typhimurium* ATCC 7823 (Sigma Co., St. Louis, MO, USA) (0.1 mg/well); 4, commercial LPS of *Rhodobacter sphaeroides* DSM 158 (InvivoGen, San Diego, CA, USA); 5, LPS of *P. multocida* A UN001 (0.06 mg/well); 6, LPS of *P. multocida* A UN001 (0.03 mg/well); 7, LPS of *P. multocida* A UN001 (0.06 mg/well); 8, LPS of *P. multocida* A UN001 (0.06 mg/well); 9, LPS of *P. multocida* A UN001 (0.06 mg/well); 10, LPS of *P. multocida* A UN001 (0.03 mg/well).

were only challenged with *P. multocida* showed moderate cell desquamation and increased goblet cells activity, consisting of dilatation of the cytoplasm. Most of these cells exhibited this change. Slight cilia loss was present in ciliated cells; in some, the cytoplasm was vacuolated, and others were dead.

TABLE 3: Grading of the lesions after each treatment (H&E): desquamated cells (DQ); increased goblet cells activity (AGC); cilia loss (CL); presence of intracytoplasmic vacuoles (IV); and dead cells (DC).

Treatment	DQ	AGC	CL	IV	DC
(1) Negative control	−	−	−	−	−
(2) Exposure to *P. multocida*	++	++	+	+	+
(3) Simultaneous exposure to *P. multocida* LPS and *P. multocida*	+++	+++	++	++	++
(4) Exposure to *P. multocida* LPS followed by *P. multocida* 30 min later	+++	+++	++	++	++
(5) Exposure to *P. multocida* followed by *P. multocida* LPS 30 min later	++	++	++	++	++
(6) Exposure to LPS of *P. multocida*	+++	+++	+	+	+

The changes and lesions in the respiratory epithelium of treatments 3 and 4, that is, simultaneous exposure to *P. multocida* LPS and *P. multocida* and exposure to *P. multocida* LPS followed by *P. multocida* 30 min later, were more severe. These changes consisted of desquamated cells and the presence of detritus in the septal lumen. In addition, increased dilatation of the cytoplasm of goblet cells and a notorious extrusion of their secretion were common findings in many others; moderate loss of cilia, cytoplasmic vacuolization, and death of the ciliated cells were more abundant. No such changes or lesions were observed in the nasal septa of the control group (treatment 1) that was only incubated with MEM without bacteria or LPS (Table 3).

3.4. Evaluating the Amount of P. multocida LPS on the Apical Surface of Respiratory Epithelial Cells and within the Cytoplasm of Goblet Cells, as well as the Number of P. multocida That Adhered to the Respiratory Epithelium (LH-IIP). The quantity of *P. multocida* LPS on the apical surface of goblet cells and ciliated cells and within their cytoplasm and the number of bacteria that adhered to the respiratory epithelium are recorded in Table 4. The results correspond to the mean of pixels of seven repetitions for each treatment; the colorimetric information is transformed to numeric information under the color model RGB (Red-Green-Blue). Based on the previous analysis, the intensity and extent of the labeling for LPS and for *P. multocida* were increased in the treatment group in which *P. multocida* LPS and *P. multocida* were administered simultaneously, followed by the challenge with *P. multocida* LPS and 30 min later with *P. multocida*, the challenge with *P. multocida* and 30 min later with its LPS, and finally the tissues that were only exposed to *P. multocida*.

Positive *P. multocida* staining was brown and had a granular appearance, whereas the LPS staining was reddish and of diffuse character; in experiments 2 and 3 (Table 1), both colors were adjacent at the interface (Figure 2). On the other hand, in tissues that were only exposed to *P. multocida* (Figure 2(b)), the brown color was mainly observed on the ciliated border of the corresponding cells and free in the lumen of the

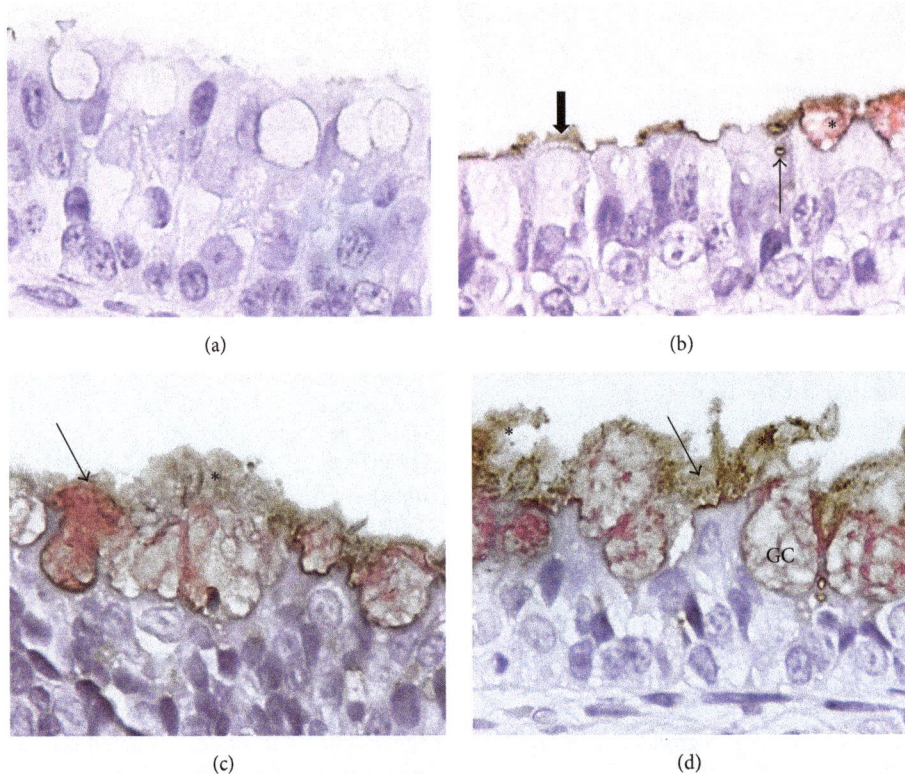

FIGURE 2: Simultaneous and sequential exposure to *P. multocida* and to its LPS and to *P. multocida* alone in nasal septa explants: LH and IIP. (a) Tissue cultures that were not exposed to LPS or *P. multocida*; ciliated cells and goblet cells were not labeled. (b) Tissues that were only exposed to *P. multocida* (thick arrow). LPS is visible within the cytoplasm of goblet cells (∗); faint LPS labeling lines the apical border of apparently ciliated cells that have lost their cilia; an apparent brown color is located intracytoplasmically in a nonidentifiable cell (thin arrow). (c) Simultaneous exposure to *P. multocida* LPS and *P. multocida* (∗). Most of the LPS labeling is located within the cytoplasm of goblet cells; several goblet cells are extruding their content along with LPS (arrow). (d) Tissues that were exposed to *P. multocida* LPS followed by *P. multocida* (∗) 30 min later show a similar appearance and signs as in (c); note the clearer interface between LPS and the bacteria (thin arrows); GC: goblet cell. H&E: 100x.

TABLE 4: Mean estimated quantity of LPS on the apical surface of epithelial cells and within the goblet cells and the number of bacteria that adhered to the ciliated border (mean of 7 repetitions for each experiment).

Treatment	Estimated number of bacteria (pixels) (mean ± SD)	Estimated LPS quantity (pixels) (mean ± SD)
(1) Negative control	0	0
(2) *P. multocida*	59897.6 ± 12.81	1247 ± 4.65
(3) LPS and *P. multocida* simultaneously	1024041.1 ± 32.41	2080027 ± 89.50
(4) LPS and 30 min later *P. multocida*	1020481.7 ± 1188.70	2079876 ± 333.80
(5) *P. multocida* and 30 min later its LPS	634092.6 ± 6.94	31586 ± 4.80
(6) LPS *P. multocida*	0	1998847 ± 550.56

tissue. Interestingly, the characteristic reddish LPS staining was also visible within the goblet cells and apparently lining the apical border of nonidentifiable epithelial cells.

Moreover, both colors, the brown *P. multocida* and the reddish LPS, were also observed in close proximity to each other in the treatment groups where both the bacterium and its LPS were administered, albeit to a lesser extent (Figures 2(c) and 2(d)).

No positive labeling was observed for either antigen, *P. multocida* or its LPS, in tissue that was not exposed to the antigens (Figure 2(a)).

A confidence interval of 95% ($\alpha = 0.05$) was used for all statistical analyses.

3.5. *Transmission Electron Microscopy (TEM)*. Tissues from the negative control (treatment 1) that were only cultured with MEM, explants that were only exposed to *P. multocida* (treatment 2), explants that were exposed to LPS and then to *P. multocida* 30 minutes later (treatment 4), and explants that were only treated with LPS (treatment 6) were processed for TEM and LH (Table 1).

A *Pasteurella multocida gatF* mutant (AL2116) was also used that was unable to assemble the external core of LPS beyond Glc IV; GatF is the galactosyltransferase which adds Gal I to the 4th position of the Glc IV [38]; in these experiments no bacteria were seen to adhere to the respiratory nasal

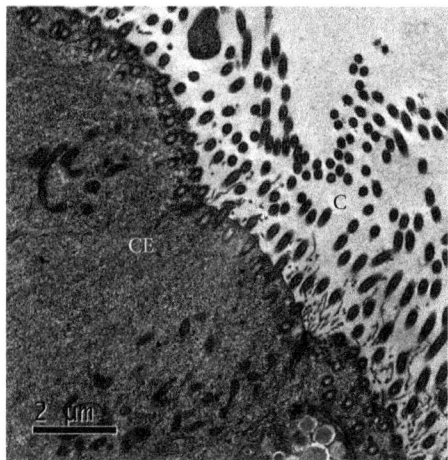

FIGURE 3: Respiratory epithelium of the nasal septum (treatment 1). Negative control (treatment 1). Ciliated epithelial cell (CE) and cilia (C). MET and gold-labeling of LPS using a lectin of *Limulus polyphemus*.

epithelium; moreover, LPS staining with *Limulus polyphemus* colloidal gold-labeled lectin was very poor or was completely absent, and no ultrastructural changes in the respiratory epithelium were observed after challenge with the mutant strain (kindly donated by Dr. Ben Adler, Bacterial Pathogenesis Research Group, Department of Microbiology, Monash University).

No ultrastructural changes or positive labeling with colloidal gold was observed in tissues that were not treated with *P. multocida* or its LPS (Figure 3).

3.6. Location of the Ultrastructural Changes in the Nasal Septa Caused by P. multocida at Two Hours after Incubation (Treatment 2). In nasal septa that were only exposed to *P. multocida* for two hours, the bacteria adhered to the microvilli and cilia of the corresponding cells. In bacterial culture, the external bacterial membrane and, even more so, the capsule were LPS-positive as they reacted with colloidal gold-labeled lectin (Figure 4(a)). In tissue culture, LPS is localized at the interface of the bacterium and the cell membrane of microvilli of ciliated cells, which are also LPS-positive (Figures 4(b) and 4(c)). Moreover, in the lumen of the organ, thread-like structures resembling a cellular bilayer membrane were also evident and were associated with the microvilli and cilia and even within the cytoplasm of epithelial cells (Figures 4(d), 4(e), and 4(f)); many of these threads spanned the distance between cilia, microvilli, and the apical membrane, building an apparent scaffold. No or only a few ultrastructural changes were observed in the epithelial cells of these septa.

3.7. Location of the Ultrastructural Changes in Epithelial Cells Caused by Exposure to P. multocida LPS and Then to P. multocida 30 Minutes Later (Treatment 3). Nasal septa that were sequentially exposed to *P. multocida* LPS and to *P. multocida* 30 min later showed increased numbers of bacteria attached to the cilia of epithelial cells; positive labeling for

LPS (colloidal gold nanoparticles of 5 nm in diameter) was also visible on the outer membrane of the bacteria, as well as in the cilia and cytoplasm of ciliated cells. The bacteria lost their capsule. Moderate ultrastructural changes such as epithelial cell cytoplasmic vacuolization were more evident in this experiment (Figure 5).

3.8. Location of the Ultrastructural Changes in Nasal Septa Induced by P. multocida LPS at Two Hours after Incubation (Treatment 6). Intense labeling in the cilia and within the cytoplasm of goblet cells and ciliated cells was observed in nasal septa that were exposed to *P. multocida* LPS for two hours. Severe cytoplasmic vacuolization was observed in epithelial cells that were only exposed to LPS (Figure 6).

4. Discussion

The LPS of Gram-negative bacteria is considered one of the main virulence factors of these pathogens, causing severe systemic damage in the interaction with their hosts [39–41]; a similar role has been recognized for the LPS of *P. multocida* [39–42]. Accordingly, most studies with these molecules have been devoted to understanding the systemic effects caused by LPS once it reaches the circulatory stream [11, 41, 43, 44]. In contrast, much less effort has been dedicated to investigating the role of LPS in its respective bacteria during the first phases of an infection and attachment to the mucosal surfaces of the corresponding hosts [45]. In an in vitro model, we provide morphological evidence that *P. multocida* A LPS mediates the adherence of the bacterium to the apical surface of the nasal respiratory epithelium in rabbits; to our knowledge, this finding has not been reported for this pathogen.

It is considered that a Gram-negative bacterium possesses approximately 3.5×10^6 LPS molecules that occupy an area of $4.9 \, \mu m^2$ on its outer membrane. Given that the approximate surface of one of these microorganisms ranges from 6 to $9 \, \mu m^2$, the LPS would cover approximately 75% of its surface, constituting the main component of the outer membrane of these agents [11, 46, 47]. Taking into account the amount of LPS on the surface of a Gram-negative bacterium, its privileged localization on the surface of the microorganism, and its rich content of carbohydrates, some of which have adhesive properties, and so forth, it is surprising that the role of this molecule during the first steps of infection with these microorganisms has not been more thoroughly investigated. Recently, the role of the core oligosaccharide of *Helicobacter pylori* LPS in mediating the adhesion of the bacterium to laminin, an extracellular matrix glycoprotein in host basement membrane that is believed to be essential in the cellular adhesion process, was suggested [17]. In the same vein, Bravo et al. [16] showed that the outer core of *S. typhi* LPS, which is composed of Glc I, Gal I, and Glc II, was required for effective adhesion and bacterial entry into HEp-2 cells.

Based on these findings and on our own previous results [48] we proposed that the LPS of *P. multocida* could be a good adhesive candidate for mediating pathogen attachment to the respiratory epithelium of rabbits during the first phases of infection. Accordingly, by simultaneously and sequentially exposing the nasal septa of fetal rabbits to *P. multocida* LPS

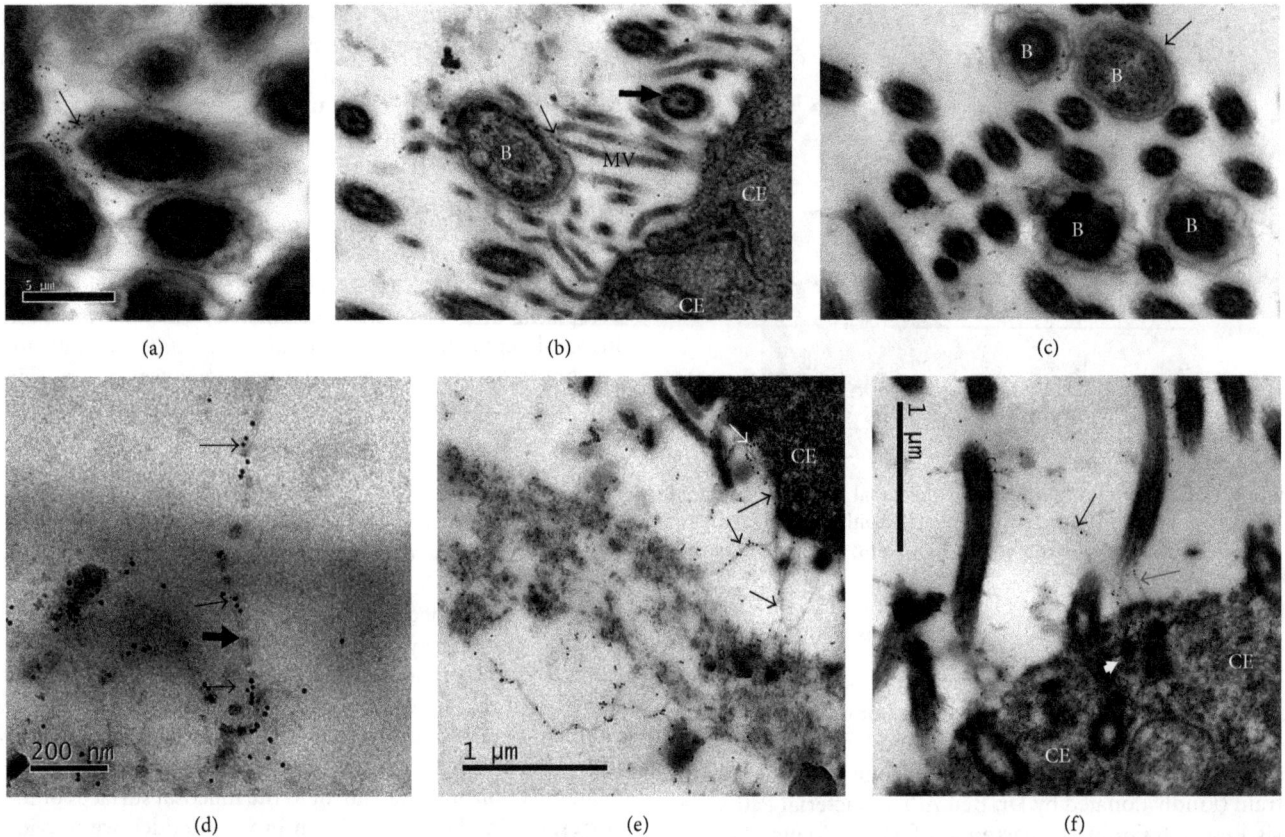

FIGURE 4: Respiratory epithelium of the nasal septum that was exposed to *P. multocida* A UN001 (treatment 2). MET and gold-labeling of LPS using a lectin of *Limulus polyphemus*. (a) Bacterial structure with positive labeling on the outer membrane (thin arrow). Note the abundant capsule that surrounds each bacteria. Bacterial culture. (b) Note the interface of the LPS between the bacterium (B) and microvilli (thin arrow). Some LPS is free in the lumen admixed with amorphous material but is also visible at the surface of some microvilli. Microvilli (MV) of a ciliated epithelial cell (CE) and cilia (thick arrows). (c) This particular bacterium has lost its capsule (arrow) compared with three other bacteria (B). (d) Thread-like bilaminar structure (thick arrow) located in the lumen of the nasal septum that is positively labeled with LPS (thin arrows). (e) Multiple thread-like LPS-positive bilaminar structures are associated with the cytoplasmic membrane and microvilli of an ciliated epithelial cell (CE) (black arrows); some gold particles seem to ingress into the cell (white arrow). (f) A bilaminar structure bridges two cilia (black arrow), and similar thread-like bilaminar structures bridge the cilia and the cytoplasm of the same cell where the base of a cilia was not included (red arrow); large numbers of gold particles are already present within the cytoplasm of the same cell (arrowheads).

and to the bacterium, it was possible to show that the LPS of *P. multocida* significantly increases the amount of *P. multocida* that attaches to the respiratory epithelial cells of the nasal septa compared with the septa that were only exposed to the pathogen. This result was confirmed by TEM experiments, which showed that higher numbers of bacteria adhered to the cilia of epithelial cells when the septa were previously exposed to LPS (Figure 5).

Using lectin histochemistry (LH), *P. multocida* LPS was more visible within the cytoplasm of goblet and ciliated cells, on their apical border, surrounding the cilia and in the extracellular medium. This result was confirmed by TEM. On the other hand, as shown in Figure 2, larger numbers of bacteria adhered to goblet cells ($P < 0.05$); moreover, in the two treatments where nasal septa cultures were simultaneously and sequentially exposed to the LPS and the bacterium, the severity of the lesions in the respiratory epithelial cells was significantly increased ($P < 0.001$), compared with the septa

that were only treated with *P. multocida* or were treated with the microorganism and then its LPS 30 min later (Table 3).

However, and perhaps more importantly, an unexpected finding in this study was that the explants that were only exposed to *P. multocida* were also positively labeled for its LPS by LH, understandably, in a lower amount compared with the explants that were exposed to the molecule and the bacterium. This staining included the same structures as when the LPS and the bacterium were added simultaneously or sequentially, that is, within the cytoplasm of goblet cells and ciliated cells, as well as a thin film over their respective apical membrane. Previous findings were corroborated by TEM, where, in addition to the surface of the bacterium, the molecule seems to join the microorganism to the microvilli and cilia of ciliated cells (Figures 4 and 5). More detailed location and relationship of the molecule with the apical membrane of goblet cells and ciliated cells were shown by this technique, where it was observed to adhere to the cilia, the

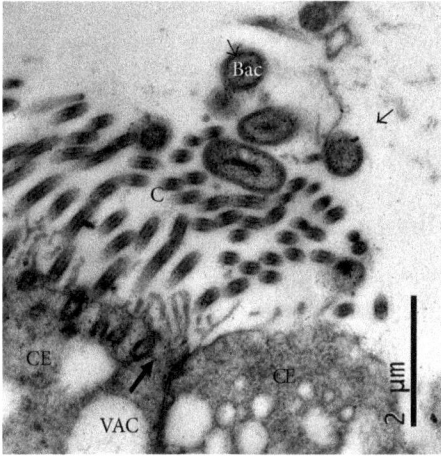

FIGURE 5: Respiratory epithelium of the nasal septum that was exposed to *P. multocida* LPS and then to *P. multocida* 30 min later (Treatment 4). MET and gold-labeling of LPS using a lectin of *Limulus polyphemus*. Bacterial structures (Bac) were positively labeled on their outer membrane (arrows) and were associated with the cilia (C) of a ciliated epithelial cell (CE); all microorganisms have lost their capsule. Large numbers of colloidal gold particles are visible at the apical cytoplasm of the cell. Cytoplasmic vacuolization (VAC).

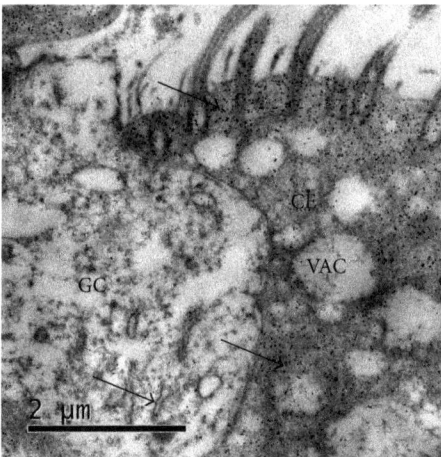

FIGURE 6: Respiratory epithelium of the nasal septum that was exposed to *P. multocida* AUN001 LPS (treatment 6). MET and gold-labeling of LPS using a lectin of *Limulus polyphemus*. Intense *P. multocida* LPS-positive labeling is associated with the cilia, cytoplasmic membrane, and cytoplasm (arrows) of a ciliated epithelial cell (CE) and with a goblet cell; severe intracytoplasmic vacuolization (VAC) is observed.

microvilli, the apical membrane, or even spanning two neighboring cilia (Figure 4), building a mesh-like structure that may favor bacterial adherence; finally, the molecule reached the cytoplasm of the epithelial cells. One possible explanation for this finding would be that *P. multocida* spontaneously releases its LPS from its outer membrane from the very first incubation time [49, 50] or from the very first moment of its interaction with the respiratory epithelium, as shown in this work. Interestingly, the experiment in which the most

significant number of bacteria adhered was the experiment in which nasal septa cultures were simultaneously exposed to the LPS and to *P. multocida*. This finding suggests that, under natural conditions, the adherence of the bacterium to the respiratory epithelium would occur in a matter of minutes. This result fits well with the experimental results of infection in rabbits, which develop clinical signs after two hours. In any case, the unexpected release of LPS under the experimental conditions indirectly favors the suggested adhesive role of the *P. multocida* LPS under natural conditions.

Notably, in this work, the microorganisms display an abundant capsule immediately before they are added to the nasal septa cultures compared to the bacteria adhering to microvilli or cilia, which have completely lost their capsule, or when only a small amount of the capsule remains (Figures 4 and 5). The presence of a capsule on Gram-negative and Gram-positive bacteria has repeatedly been reported as an impediment for their ability to adhere to mucosal surfaces. One mechanism proposed for this interference is that the capsule masks adhesin(s) that might be located deeper on the bacterial surface [10, 51, 52]; this mechanism works well in the case of *P. multocida* in this study.

Lipopolysaccharide-positive labeling of the same *P. multocida* A within the cytoplasm of goblet cells in the same experimental model used in this research has been already reported [32]; the only difference was that the previous study labeled the LPS with polyclonal antibodies instead of with *Limulus polyphemus* lectin, as in this work. Using TEM, Esquinas et al. [53] showed that myelin-like structures were contained within the vacuoles in the cytoplasm of ciliated cells and suggested that these structures might correspond to *P. multocida* LPS; this study confirms that the LPS of *P. multocida* effectively reaches the cytoplasm of these cells and that cytoplasmic vacuoles are formed in these cells, which may be caused by this molecule. There are some possibilities to explain how the molecule reaches the cytoplasm of goblet cells and ciliated cells. One is that the LPS of *P. multocida*, similar to the LPS of other Gram-negative pathogens, would be recognized by free, mucus- and glycocalyx-located CD14 receptors that would be internalized by activation of the TLR4/MD2 complex [24, 54–56]. Another soluble receptor is LPS binding protein (LBP); this receptor binds LPS in the blood plasma and transfers it to cellular receptors, thus increasing the activation of cells that lack mCD14 [57, 58]. The mechanisms for the internalization and intracellular transport of the endotoxin are not clear, but some authors propose that it travels after interacting with CD14 [59], whereas others suggest that the internalization involves a clathrin-dependent pathway through which it is transported via lipid rafts to the Golgi apparatus to bind intracellular TLR4 [15, 60–62].

Recent studies report that LBP catalyzes the intercalation of LPS into the reconstituted phospholipid bilayers, providing an additional mechanism of LBP-mediated transport of LPS into host cell membranes and the cytoplasm of human monocytes and macrophages [24]. In this regard, it is quite interesting that the LPS of *P. multocida* adopted a thread-like bilaminar appearance and was observed in direct interaction with the cell membrane of the ciliated cells and their cilia in this work (Figures 4(d), 4(e), and 4(f)), which could be evidence of the intercalation described by [24]. It should be noted that these bilamellar structures were only observed in the LPS that was spontaneously released by the bacteria (treatment 2, Table 1) and were not observed in experiments that used purified LPS (treatments 3 and 4, Table 1), which is more similar to the natural conditions of the infection.

In experiments with purified LPS (treatments 3 and 4, Table 1), it was found that LPS induced ultrastructural changes of the respiratory epithelium, such as cytoplasmic vacuolization and dilated interepithelial spaces of the nasal septa; the changes induced by *P. multocida* LPS alone were more severe than the changes caused by the bacterium alone (Figures 5 and 6). This finding could be explained by the LPS dose to which the explants were exposed; surely, the amount of LPS that is spontaneously released by the bacteria is much lower than the amount of purified LPS used in the experiments. Studies exist that show that the effect of LPS is dose-dependent. It is possible that, in the first instance, the pathogen does not try to activate mechanisms that lead to tissue damage but induces intracellular signals that stimulate the immune system. Some authors argue that this upregulation may occur in the body in response to high doses of LPS or by a state of hyperreactivity to LPS. On the other hand, when there is contact with low levels of LPS, beneficial effects on the host such as the development of resistance to infections may be triggered [24, 63–66].

Yan et al. [67] proposed a mechanism by which LPS upregulates mucin genes such as MUC5AC and MUC2 expression in human epithelial cells; they demonstrated that bacterial LPS utilizes reactive oxygen species (ROS) for transmitting signals to provoke the host defense response and upregulate MUC5AC mucin expression. Gram-negative bacteria would use some substrates present in glycoproteins produced by goblet cells as the first binding site to initiate adhesion. It is proposed that the mechanism would start from metaplasia of mucus-producing cells induced by proinflammatory cytokines such as TNF alpha released from leukocytes by the action of LPS [32, 67–71].

More recently, the PLUNC (palate, lung, and nasal epithelium clone) protein, which is related to the LPS binding protein (LBP) family, has been demonstrated in epithelial cells, goblet cells, and glandular airway cells [72, 73], and it has been suggested that it is stored and released from the granules of neutrophils [74]. PLUNC recognizes and binds to LPS, and it is proposed that PLUNC may play a role in the innate immune response of the upper airways [73, 75]. Consistent with these findings, our results might suggest that the positive labeling for *P. multocida* LPS mixed with mucus, in the cytoplasm of inflammatory cells that accompany this mucus, and inside the glandular and epithelial cells could be explained in part by the binding of the endotoxin to this substance [45].

It can be concluded that the LPS of *P. multocida* A UN001 plays an important role in the adhesion of bacteria to the rabbit respiratory epithelium by increasing the number of adherent bacteria in the presence of LPS. Lipopolysaccharide is spontaneously released by the bacteria and interacts with structures such as the cilia, microvilli, and cytoplasmic membrane to achieve internalization into the cytoplasm of

epithelial ciliated and goblet cells. These results should be the foundation of new research focused on determining exactly which components of *P. multocida* LPS interact with the host cell not only to advance the understanding of the pathogenesis of this disease but also to propose mechanisms to inhibit this interaction.

Competing Interests

The authors declare that there is no conflict of interests regarding the publication of this paper.

Authors' Contributions

Carolina Gallego and Stefany Romero are lead authors because they made contributions of equal importance in this research.

Acknowledgments

This study was financed by Colciencias, the National University of Colombia, and the University of Applied and Environmental Sciences.

References

[1] F. Dziva, A. P. Muhairwa, M. Bisgaard, and H. Christensen, "Diagnostic and typing options for investigating diseases associated with *Pasteurella multocida*," *Veterinary Microbiology*, vol. 128, no. 1-2, pp. 1–22, 2008.

[2] E. Kawamoto, T. Sawada, and T. Maruyama, "Evaluation of transport media for *Pasteurella multocida* isolates from rabbit nasal specimens," *Journal of Clinical Microbiology*, vol. 35, no. 8, pp. 1948–1951, 1997.

[3] H. Takashima, H. Sakai, T. Yanai, and T. Masegi, "Detection of antibodies against *Pasteurella multocida* using immunohistochemical staining in an outbreak of rabbit pasteurellosis," *The Journal of Veterinary Medical Science*, vol. 63, no. 2, pp. 171–174, 2001.

[4] Z. Jaglic, E. Jeklova, L. Leva et al., "Experimental study of pathogenicity of *Pasteurella multocida* serogroup F in rabbits," *Veterinary Microbiology*, vol. 126, no. 1–3, pp. 168–177, 2008.

[5] A. B. J. Stahel, R. K. Hoop, P. Kuhnert, and B. M. Korczak, "Phenotypic and genetic characterization of *Pasteurella multocida* and related isolates from rabbits in Switzerland," *Journal of Veterinary Diagnostic Investigation*, vol. 21, no. 6, pp. 793–802, 2009.

[6] M. Jacques, "Role of lipo-oligosaccharides and lipopolysaccharides in bacterial adherence," *Trends in Microbiology*, vol. 4, no. 10, pp. 408–410, 1996.

[7] S. N. Abraham, B. L. Bishop, N. Sharon, and I. Ofek, "Adhesion of bacteria to mucosal surfaces," *Mucosal Immunology, Two-Volume Set*, pp. 35–48, 2005.

[8] E. Fadda and R. J. Woods, "Molecular simulations of carbohydrates and protein-carbohydrate interactions: motivation, issues and prospects," *Drug Discovery Today*, vol. 15, no. 15-16, pp. 596–609, 2010.

[9] S. Sattin and A. Bernardi, "Glycoconjugates and glycomimetics as microbial anti-adhesives," *Trends in Biotechnology*, vol. 34, no. 6, pp. 483–495, 2016.

[10] M. Jacques, M. Kobisch, M. Belanger, and F. Dugal, "Virulence of capsulated and noncapsulated isolates of *Pasteurella multocida* and their adherence to porcine respiratory tract cells and mucus," *Infection and Immunity*, vol. 61, no. 11, pp. 4785–4792, 1993.

[11] E. T. Reitschel, T. Kirikae, F. U. Shade et al., "Bacterial endotoxin: molecular relationships of structure to activity and function," *The FASEB Journal*, vol. 8, no. 2, pp. 217–225, 1994.

[12] C. Erridge, E. Bennett-Guerrero, and I. R. Poxton, "Structure and function of lipopolysaccharides," *Microbes and Infection*, vol. 4, no. 8, pp. 837–851, 2002.

[13] L. N. López-Bojórquez, A. Z. Dehesa, and G. Reyes-Terán, "Molecular mechanisms involved in the pathogenesis of septic shock," *Archives of Medical Research*, vol. 35, no. 6, pp. 465–479, 2004.

[14] C. Risco, J. L. Carrascosa, and M. A. Bosch, "Uptake and subcellular distribution of Escherichia coli lipopolysaccharide by isolated rat Type II pneumocytes," *Journal of Histochemistry and Cytochemistry*, vol. 39, no. 5, pp. 607–615, 1991.

[15] M. W. Hornef, B. H. Normark, A. Vandewalle, and S. Normark, "Intracellular recognition of lipopolysaccharide by toll-like receptor 4 in intestinal epithelial cells," *The Journal of Experimental Medicine*, vol. 198, no. 8, pp. 1225–1235, 2003.

[16] D. Bravo, A. Hoare, A. Silipo et al., "Different sugar residues of the lipopolysaccharide outer core are required for early interactions of *Salmonella enterica* serovars Typhi and Typhimurium with epithelial cells," *Microbial Pathogenesis*, vol. 50, no. 2, pp. 70–80, 2011.

[17] P.-C. Chang, C.-J. Wang, C.-K. You, and M.-C. Kao, "Effects of a HP0859 (rfaD) knockout mutation on lipopolysaccharide structure of Helicobacter pylori 26695 and the bacterial adhesion on AGS cells," *Biochemical and Biophysical Research Communications*, vol. 405, no. 3, pp. 497–502, 2011.

[18] M. Bélanger, S. Rioux, B. Foiry, and M. Jacques, "Affinity for porcine respiratory tract mucus is found in some isolates of Actinobacillus pleuropneumoniae," *FEMS Microbiology Letters*, vol. 97, no. 1-2, pp. 119–125, 1992.

[19] E. L. Fletcher, S. M. J. Fleisig, and N. A. Brennan, "Lipopolysaccharide in adherence of *Pseudomonas aeruginosa* to the cornea and contact lenses," *Investigative Ophthalmology & Visual Science*, vol. 34, no. 6, pp. 1930–1936, 1993.

[20] S. K. Gupta, R. S. Berk, S. Masinick, and L. D. Hazlett, "Pili and lipopolysaccharide of Pseudomonas aeruginosa bind to the glycolipid asialo GM1," *Infection and Immunity*, vol. 62, no. 10, pp. 4572–4579, 1994.

[21] G. B. Pier, N. L. Koles, G. Meluleni, K. Hatano, and M. Pollack, "Specificity and function of murine monoclonal antibodies and immunization- induced human polyclonal antibodies to lipopolysaccharide subtypes of Pseudomonas aeruginosa serogroup 06," *Infection and Immunity*, vol. 62, no. 4, pp. 1137–1143, 1994.

[22] A. Venable, M. Mitalipova, I. Lyons et al., "Lectin binding profiles of SSEA-4 enriched, pluripotent human embryonic stem cell surfaces," *BMC Developmental Biology*, vol. 5, article no. 15, 2005.

[23] J. Yang, Y. Zhao, and F. Shao, "Non-canonical activation of inflammatory caspases by cytosolic LPS in innate immunity," *Current Opinion in Immunology*, vol. 32, pp. 78–83, 2015.

[24] F. Kopp, S. Kupsch, and A. B. Schromm, "Lipopolysaccharide-binding protein is bound and internalized by host cells and colocalizes with LPS in the cytoplasm: implications for a role of LBP in intracellular LPS-signaling," *Biochimica et Biophysica Acta&Molecular Cell Research*, vol. 1863, no. 4, pp. 660–672, 2016.

[25] T. Hatfaludi, K. Al-Hasani, J. D. Boyce, and B. Adler, "Outer membrane proteins of *Pasteurella multocida*," *Veterinary Microbiology*, vol. 144, no. 1-2, pp. 1–17, 2010.

[26] K. M. Townsend, J. D. Boyce, J. Y. Chung, A. J. Frost, and B. Adler, "Genetic organization of *Pasteurella multocida* cap loci and development of a multiplex capsular PCR typing system," *Journal of Clinical Microbiology*, vol. 39, no. 3, pp. 924–929, 2001.

[27] S. L. Brockmeier and K. B. Register, "Expression of the dermonecrotic toxin by Bordetella bronchiseptica is not necessary for predisposing to infection with toxigenic *Pasteurella multocida*," *Veterinary Microbiology*, vol. 125, no. 3-4, pp. 284–289, 2007.

[28] D. J. Halloy, N. A. Kirschvink, J. Mainil, and P. G. Gustin, "Synergistic action of E. coli endotoxin and *Pasteurella multocida* type A for the induction of bronchopneumonia in pigs," *Veterinary Journal*, vol. 169, no. 3, pp. 417–426, 2005.

[29] D. Bernet, H. Schmidt, W. Meier, P. Burkhardt-Holm, and T. Wahli, "Histopathology in fish: proposal for a protocol to assess aquatic pollution," *Journal of Fish Diseases*, vol. 22, no. 1, pp. 25–34, 1999.

[30] O. Westphal and K. Jann, "Bacterial lipopolysaccharides: extraction with phenol-water further applications of this procedure," *Methods in Carbohydrate Chemistry*, vol. 5, p. 9, 1965.

[31] D. Gualtero, J. E. Castellanos, and G. I. Lafaurie, "*Porphyromonas gingivalis* libre de polisacáridos utilizando cromatografía de alta resolución sephacryl S-200," *Acta Biológica Colombiana*, vol. 13, no. 3, pp. 147–160, 2008.

[32] P. Esquinas, "Comparación ultraestructural de fosa nasal y nasofaringe de Conejos sanos y enfermos con el síndrome de neumonía enzoótica," in *Abstracts IV Reunión Anual de Patología*, 2004.

[33] C. Gallego, A. M. Middleton, N. Martínez, S. Romero, and C. Iregui, "Interaction of *Bordetella bronchiseptica* and its lipopolysaccharide with in vitro culture of respiratory nasal epithelium," *Veterinary Medicine International*, vol. 2013, Article ID 347086, 9 pages, 2013.

[34] T. G. Pistole, "Interaction of bacteria and fungi with lectins and lectin-like substances," *Annual Review of Microbiology*, vol. 35, pp. 85–112, 1981.

[35] M. D. Abràmofff, P. J. Magalhães, and S. J. Ram, "Image processing with ImageJ Part II," *Biophotonics International*, vol. 11, no. 7, pp. 36–43, 2005.

[36] S. E. Wong, C. E. Winbanks, C. S. Samuel, and T. D. Hewitson, "Lectin histochemistry for light and electron microscopy," *Methods in Molecular Biology*, vol. 611, pp. 103–114, 2010.

[37] R. Martínez, N. Martinez, and M. V. Martinez, *Diseño de Experimentos en Ciencias Agropecuarias y Biológicas con SAS, SPSS, R Y STATISTIX*, Fondo Nacional Universitario—Institución Auxiliar del Cooperativismo, 2011.

[38] M. Harper, F. St Michael, M. John et al., "Pasteurella multocida heddleston serovar 3 and 4 strains share a common lipopolysaccharide biosynthesis locus but display both inter- and intrastrain lipopolysaccharide heterogeneity," *Journal of Bacteriology*, vol. 195, no. 21, pp. 4854–4864, 2013.

[39] K. Le Blay, P. Gueirard, N. Guiso, and R. Chaby, "Antigenic polymorphism of the lipopolysaccharides from human and animal isolates of *Bordetella bronchiseptica*," *Microbiology*, vol. 143, no. 4, pp. 1433–1441, 1997.

[40] E. T. Harvill, A. Preston, P. A. Cotter, A. G. Allen, D. J. Maskell, and J. F. Miller, "Multiple roles for Bordetella lipopolysaccharide molecules during respiratory tract infection," *Infection and Immunity*, vol. 68, no. 12, pp. 6720–6728, 2000.

[41] M. Harper, F. St Michael, M. John et al., "*Pasteurella multocida* Heddleston serovars 1 and 14 express different lipopolysaccharide structures but share the same lipopolysaccharide biosynthesis outer core locus," *Veterinary Microbiology*, vol. 150, no. 3-4, pp. 289–296, 2011.

[42] M. Harper, J. D. Boyce, and B. Adler, "Pasteurella multocida pathogenesis: 125 years after Pasteur," *FEMS Microbiology Letters*, vol. 265, no. 1, pp. 1–10, 2006.

[43] J. C. Hodgson, "Endotoxin and mammalian host responses during experimental disease," *Journal of Comparative Pathology*, vol. 135, no. 4, pp. 157–175, 2006.

[44] K. Singh, J. W. Ritchey, and A. W. Confer, "*Mannheimia haemolytica*: bacterial-host interactions in bovine Pneumonia," *Veterinary Pathology*, vol. 48, no. 2, pp. 338–348, 2011.

[45] P. Patiño, *Efectos morfológicos y distribución del lipopolisacárido de Pasteurella multocida en el tracto respiratorio de conejos expuestos intranasalmente [M.S. thesis]*, Universidad Nacional de Colombia, 2016.

[46] R. Y. Hampton and C. R. H. Raetz, "Macrophage catabolism of lipid A is regulated by endotoxin stimulation," *Journal of Biological Chemistry*, vol. 266, no. 29, pp. 19499–19509, 1991.

[47] P. G. Adams, L. Lamoureux, K. L. Swingle, H. Mukundan, and G. A. Montaño, "Lipopolysaccharide-induced dynamic lipid membrane reorganization: tubules, perforations, and stacks," *Biophysical Journal*, vol. 106, no. 11, pp. 2395–2407, 2014.

[48] M. P. Carrillo, N. M. Martinez, M. D. P. Patiño, and C. A. Iregui, "Inhibition of pasteurella multocida adhesion to rabbit respiratory epithelium using lectins," *Veterinary Medicine International*, vol. 2015, Article ID 365428, 10 pages, 2015.

[49] E. T. Rietschel and H. Brade, "Bacterial endotoxins," *Scientific American*, vol. 267, no. 2, pp. 54–61, 1992.

[50] I. W. Devoe and J. E. Gilchrist, "Release of endotoxin in the form of cell wall blebs during in vitro growth of *Neisseria meningitidis*," *Journal of Experimental Medicine*, vol. 138, no. 5, pp. 1156–1167, 1973.

[51] H. Al-Haj Ali, T. Sawada, H. Hatakeyama, Y. Katayama, N. Ohtsuki, and O. Itoh, "Invasion of chicken embryo fibroblast cells by avian *Pasteurella multocida*," *Veterinary Microbiology*, vol. 104, no. 1-2, pp. 55–62, 2004.

[52] T. O. Schaffner, J. Hinds, K. A. Gould et al., "A point mutation in cpsE renders *Streptococcus pneumoniae* nonencapsulated and enhances its growth, adherence and competence," *BMC Microbiology*, vol. 14, no. 1, article no. 210, 2014.

[53] P. Esquinas, L. Botero, M. D. P. Patiño, C. Gallego, and C. Iregui, "Ultrastructural comparison of the nasal epithelia of healthy and naturally affected rabbits with pasteurella multocida A," *Veterinary Medicine International*, vol. 2013, Article ID 321390, 8 pages, 2013.

[54] N. Mukaida, Y. Ishikawa, N. Ikeda et al., "Novel insight into molecular mechanism of endotoxin shock: biochemical analysis of LPS receptor signaling in a cell-free system targeting NF-κB and regulation of cytokine production/action through β2 integrin in vivo," *Journal of Leukocyte Biology*, vol. 59, no. 2, pp. 145–151, 1996.

[55] M. Yarim, S. Karahan, and N. Kabakci, "Immunohistochemical investigation of CD14 in experimental rabbit pneumonic pasteurellosis," *Revue de Medecine Veterinaire*, vol. 156, no. 1, pp. 13–19, 2005.

[56] M. Lu, A. W. Varley, S. Ohta, J. Hardwick, and R. S. Munford, "Host inactivation of bacterial lipopolysaccharide prevents prolonged tolerance following gram-negative bacterial infection," *Cell Host and Microbe*, vol. 4, no. 3, pp. 293–302, 2008.

[57] J. Pugin, C.-C. Schürer-Maly, D. Leturcq, A. Moriarty, R. J. Ulevitch, and P. S. Tobias, "Lipopolysaccharide activation of human endothelial and epithelial cells is mediated by lipopolysaccharide-binding protein and soluble CD14," *Proceedings of the National Academy of Sciences of the United States of America*, vol. 90, no. 7, pp. 2744–2748, 1993.

[58] A. Haziot, E. Ferrero, F. Köntgen et al., "Resistance to endotoxin shock and reduced dissemination of gram-negative bacteria in CD14-deficient mice," *Immunity*, vol. 4, no. 4, pp. 407–414, 1996.

[59] T. Vasselon, E. Mailman, R. Thieringer, and P. A. Detmers, "Internalization of monomeric lipopolysaccharide occurs after transfer out of cell surface CD14," *Journal of Experimental Medicine*, vol. 190, no. 4, pp. 509–521, 1999.

[60] L. Guillott, S. Medjane, K. Le-Barillec et al., "Response of human pulmonary epithelial cells to lipopolysaccharide involves toll-like receptor 4 (TLR4)-dependent signaling pathways: evidence for an intracellular compartmentalization of TLR4," *Journal of Biological Chemistry*, vol. 279, no. 4, pp. 2712–2718, 2004.

[61] C. M. Greene and N. G. McElvaney, "Toll-like receptor expression and function in airway epithelial cells," *Archivum Immunologiae et Therapiae Experimentalis*, vol. 53, no. 5, pp. 418–427, 2005.

[62] S. W. Wong, M.-J. Kwon, A. M. K. Choi, H.-P. Kim, K. Nakahira, and D. H. Hwang, "Fatty acids modulate toll-like receptor 4 activation through regulation of receptor dimerization and recruitment into lipid rafts in a reactive oxygen species-dependent manner," *Journal of Biological Chemistry*, vol. 284, no. 40, pp. 27384–27392, 2009.

[63] A. B. Lentsch and P. A. Ward, "Regulation of experimental lung inflammation," *Respiration Physiology*, vol. 128, no. 1, pp. 17–22, 2001.

[64] C.-C. Tsai, M.-T. Lin, J.-J. Wang, J.-F. Liao, and W.-T. Huang, "The antipyretic effects of baicalin in lipopolysaccharide-evoked fever in rabbits," *Neuropharmacology*, vol. 51, no. 4, pp. 709–717, 2006.

[65] B. A. Mizock, "The multiple organ dysfunction syndrome," *Disease-a-Month*, vol. 55, no. 8, pp. 476–526, 2009.

[66] O. S. Ali, L. Adamu, F. F. J. Abdullah et al., "Alterations in interleukin-1β and interleukin-6 in mice inoculated through the oral routes using graded doses of p. multocida type b: 2 and its lipopolysaccharide," *American Journal of Animal and Veterinary Sciences*, vol. 10, no. 1, pp. 1–8, 2015.

[67] F. Yan, W. Li, H. Jono et al., "Reactive oxygen species regulate Pseudomonas aeruginosa lipopolysaccharide-induced MUC5AC mucin expression via PKC-NADPH oxidase-ROS-TGF-α signaling pathways in human airway epithelial cells," *Biochemical and Biophysical Research Communications*, vol. 366, no. 2, pp. 513–519, 2008.

[68] P.-R. Burgel, E. Escudier, A. Coste et al., "Relation of epidermal growth factor receptor expression to goblet cell hyperplasia in nasal polyps," *Journal of Allergy and Clinical Immunology*, vol. 106, no. 4, pp. 705–712, 2000.

[69] K. Takeyama, J. V. Fahy, and J. A. Nadel, "Relationship of epidermal growth factor receptors to goblet cell production in human bronchi," *American Journal of Respiratory and Critical Care Medicine*, vol. 163, no. 2, pp. 511–516, 2001.

[70] J. H. Kim, S. Y. Lee, S. M. Bak et al., "Effects of matrix metalloproteinase inhibitor on LPS-induced goblet cell metaplasia,"

American Journal of Physiology—Lung Cellular and Molecular Physiology, vol. 287, no. 1, pp. L127–L133, 2004.

[71] W. Li, F. Yan, H. Zhou et al., "P. aeruginosa lipopolysaccharide-induced MUC5AC and CLCA3 expression is partly through Duox1 in vitro and in vivo," *PLoS ONE*, vol. 8, no. 5, Article ID e63945, 2013.

[72] C. D. Bingle, K. Wilson, H. Lunn et al., "Human LPLUNC1 is a secreted product of goblet cells and minor glands of the respiratory and upper aerodigestive tracts," *Histochemistry and Cell Biology*, vol. 133, no. 5, pp. 505–515, 2010.

[73] L. Bingle and C. D. Bingle, "Distribution of human PLUNC/BPI fold-containing (BPIF) proteins," *Biochemical Society Transactions*, vol. 39, no. 4, pp. 1023–1027, 2011.

[74] J. A. Bartlett, B. J. Hicks, J. M. Schlomann, S. Ramachandran, W. M. Nauseef, and P. B. McCray, "PLUNC is a secreted product of neutrophil granules," *Journal of Leukocyte Biology*, vol. 83, no. 5, pp. 1201–1206, 2008.

[75] B. Ghafouri, E. Kihlström, C. Tagesson, and M. Lindahl, "PLUNC in human nasal lavage fluid: multiple isoforms that bind to lipopolysaccharide," *Biochimica et Biophysica Acta*, vol. 1699, no. 1-2, pp. 57–63, 2004.

6

Systemic *Candida parapsilosis* Infection Model in Immunosuppressed ICR Mice and Assessing the Antifungal Efficiency of Fluconazole

Yu'e Wu,[1] Fangui Min,[1] Jinchun Pan,[1] Jing Wang,[1] Wen Yuan,[1] Yu Zhang,[1] Ren Huang,[1] and Lixin Zhang[2]

[1] *Guangdong Laboratory Animals Monitoring Institute, Guangdong Provincial Key Laboratory of Laboratory Animals, Guangzhou 510663, China*
[2] *Institute of Microbiology, Chinese Academy of Sciences, Beijing 100080, China*

Correspondence should be addressed to Yu Zhang; zhangyugzh@hotmail.com, Ren Huang; labking@sohu.com, and Lixin Zhang; lzhang03@gmail.com

Academic Editor: William Ravis

This study was to establish a systemic *C. parapsilosis* infection model in immunosuppressed ICR mice induced by cyclophosphamide and evaluate the antifungal efficiency of fluconazole. Three experiments were set to confirm the optimal infectious dose of *C. parapsilosis*, outcomes of infectious model, and antifungal efficiency of fluconazole in vivo, respectively. In the first experiment, comparisons of survival proportions between different infectious doses treated groups showed that the optimal inoculum for *C. parapsilosis* was 0.9×10^5 CFU per mouse. The following experiment was set to observe the outcomes of infection at a dose of 0.9×10^5 CFU *C. parapsilosis*. Postmortem and histopathological examinations presented fugal-specific lesions in multiorgans, especially in kidneys, characterized by inflammation, numerous microabscesses, and fungal infiltration. The CFU counts were consistent with the histopathological changes in tissues. Th1/Th2 cytokine imbalance was observed with increases of proinflammatory cytokines and no responses of anti-inflammatory cytokines in sera and kidneys. In the last experiment, model based evaluation of fluconazole indicated that there were ideal antifungal activities for fluconazole at dosages of 10–50 mg/kg/d. Data demonstrates that the research team has established a systemic *C. parapsilosis* infection model in immunosuppressed ICR mice, affording opportunities for increasing our understanding of fungal pathogenesis and treatment.

1. Introduction

Candida, usually kept as harmless commensals in healthy individuals, may become opportunistic pathogens in susceptible hosts, especially in severely drug-immunosuppressed or immunodeficient patients [1–3]. During the past two decades, the candidemia causative agent has changed from *C. albicans* to non-*C. albicans*, and the patients infected with the non-*C. albicans* were gradually increased. *Candida* infections have accounted for about 8 to 9 percent of hospital-acquired infections and become the fourth most common cause of such infections [4, 5]. *C. parapsilosis,* a typical commensal of human skin, has emerged notoriously for its capacity to grow in total parenteral nutrition and to form biofilms on catheters

and other implanted devices [6, 7]. During the last decade, the incidence of *C. parapsilosis* has dramatically increased and become the second most commonly isolated *Candida* species from blood cultures.

Given the incidence of disease and the unacceptably high mortality associated with *C. parapsilosis*, there is an urgent need of more effective preventive, diagnostic, and therapeutic strategies. Experimental animal models are a critical component of understanding the pathogenesis and host resistance to infection and to development of more efficacious antifungal therapies. Previously, an immunocompromised mouse model of *C. parapsilosis* established by us has been used to evaluate microbial metabolites as combination agents for the treatment of fungal infections [8]. After further optimization for establishment procedures, the animal model was more stable and presented outcomes of systemic infection. The present paper will describe in detail the outcomes of the systemic mouse *C. parapsilosis* model, including mortality, tissues fungal burdens, histopathology, serum and renal cytokines, and the usage of the model for evaluation of fluconazole.

2. Materials and Methods

2.1. Animals and Ethics Statement. SPF female ICR mice aged from 4 to 6 weeks and weighed 20 to 22 g were used in this study. Animals were purchased from SLAC Laboratory Animal Centre Co., Shanghai, and had never been used for any experimental procedures previously. After arrival, animals were acclimated for 3 days before the experiments.

Animal use protocols were reviewed and approved by IACUC of Guangdong Laboratory Animal Monitoring Institute in accordance with the *Guide for the Care and Use of Laboratory Animals* [9]. Animals were bred in negative pressure isolation cages in an animal negative pressure facility with an approval of and oversight by the Local Provincial Institutional Environmental Health and Safety Office.

2.2. Fungal Strain and Inoculum Preparation. *C. parapsilosis* ATCC22019 normally stored at $-86°C$ was used in this study. Stock inoculum suspensions of *C. parapsilosis* were obtained from >20 h cultures in RPMI medium 1640 incubated at 30°C with shaking at 150 rpm. And >95% of *C. parapsilosis* cells should be blastoconidia by microscopic examination.

2.3. Cyclophosphamide Induced Immunosuppression. Ten mice were intraperitoneally injected with cyclophosphamide (CY) (100 mg/kg weight/d) for continuous 3 days. Blood samples (0.20 mL) were collected via fossa orbitalis vein daily from 0 to 6 days after the injection of CY. Then, total leukocyte counts were performed by the *Sysmex XT-2000iv* automatic hematology analyzer. Another 10 mice receiving normal saline were set as controls.

2.4. Study Design. The first experiment was set to confirm the infectious dose. The immunosuppressed mice receiving CY were inoculated with 0.1 mL *C. parapsilosis* suspension via tail vein at doses of 1×10^2 CFU, 0.9×10^5 CFU, 5.0×10^5 CFU, and 8×10^5 CFU, respectively. The control mice receiving normal saline were inoculated with 0.1 mL normal saline via tail vein. According to the results of survival curves, the optimal infectious dose would be confirmed.

In the second experiment, another immunosuppressed group inoculated with optimal infectious dose of *C. parapsilosis* was set to observe the outcomes of infection. At days 1, 4, and 6 postinfection, 3 mice were euthanized, sera were collected, and target organs (heart, liver, spleen, lung, kidney, and brain) were excised for tissue fungal burdens, pathological examination, and cytokine measurement.

The third experiment was designed to evaluate fluconazole (Sigma). Four groups of infected mice were treated intraperitoneally with fluconazole at the dosages of 0, 0.5, 10, and 50 mg/kg/d of body weight 1 h postinfection for 7

consecutive days. Survival rates and tissue fungal burdens were used to evaluate the antifungal efficacy of fluconazole.

2.5. Clinical Assessment. Animals were observed daily throughout the study for alterations in behavior, appetite, and mortality.

2.6. Postmortem and Histopathological Examinations. The mice were sacrificed by CO_2 inhalation. Heart, liver, spleen, lung, kidney, brain, stomach, and bladder were removed immediately and preserved in 10% formalin. After paraffin embedding and sectioning, standard 5 μm sections were cut and stained with hematoxylin and eosin (H&E) and periodic acid-Schiff (PAS).

2.7. Tissue Fungal Burdens. Half of the target organs were homogenized in 1.0 mL of sterile normal saline. Tissue homogenates from individual mice were serially diluted on SDA plates and incubated for 48 h at 35°C. Results are expressed as CFU $\log_{10}$ per organ.

2.8. Cytokine Measurement. IL-1α, IL-1β, IL-2, IL-4, IL-5, IL-6, IL-10, IL-17, IL-23, GM-CSF, IFN-γ, and TNF-α in serial sera and renal samples of control and infected mice were measured by cytometric bead array.

2.9. Data Analysis. All data was expressed as mean ± SD. Between-group differences of quantitative data were analyzed by *t*-tests. While the between-group differences of survival cures were performed by *Log-rank (Mantel-Cox) Test*. Significance was judged at the 0.05 level.

3. Results

3.1. CY Induced Immunosuppression. No significant changes were found in total leukocyte counts for the control mice injected with saline. However, the mice receiving CY showed a time corresponding decrease from days 1 to 4. At day 4, the total leukocyte counts of mice receiving CY reached the lowest levels followed by a gradual increase to basal levels till day 14 (Figure 1). The results indicate that the optimal infection time points are days 3 to 6 after CY administration.

3.2. Confirmation of Infectious Dose by Survival Proportions. In the first study, every immunosuppressed group presented death of animals postinfection. All except 1×10^2 CFU group died out from days 1 to 15 postinfection. For 1×10^2 CFU group, 92% of animals survived until 12 days postinfection for necropsy.

The survival curves were shown in Figure 2. 0.9×10^5 CFU group showed significant differences with the other groups (*Log-rank Test*, $P < 0.05$). The median survival times of 0.9×10^5 CFU, 5.0×10^5 CFU, and 8.0×10^5 CFU groups are 5.5 days, 2 days, and 2.5 days, respectively. These data indicated that the optimal inoculum for *C. parapsilosis* was 0.9×10^5 CFU per mouse in immunosuppressed mice.

3.3. Clinical Signs of the Model. The clinical symptoms of distress, such as that decreased movement, decreased food

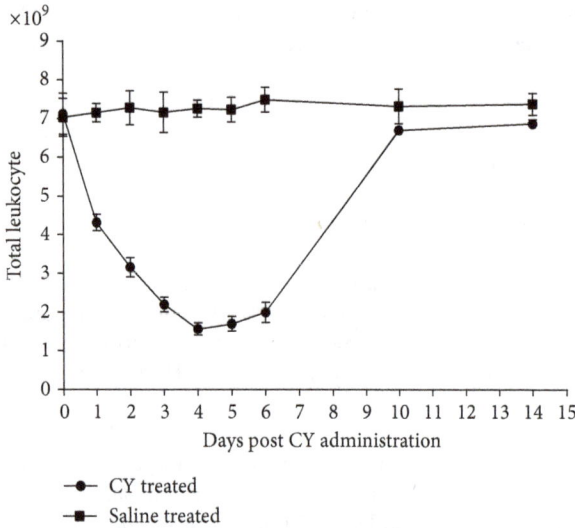

FIGURE 1: Total leukocyte counts. A time corresponding decrease was found in CY treated mice from days 1 to 4. The lowest data emerged at day 4 ($n = 10$).

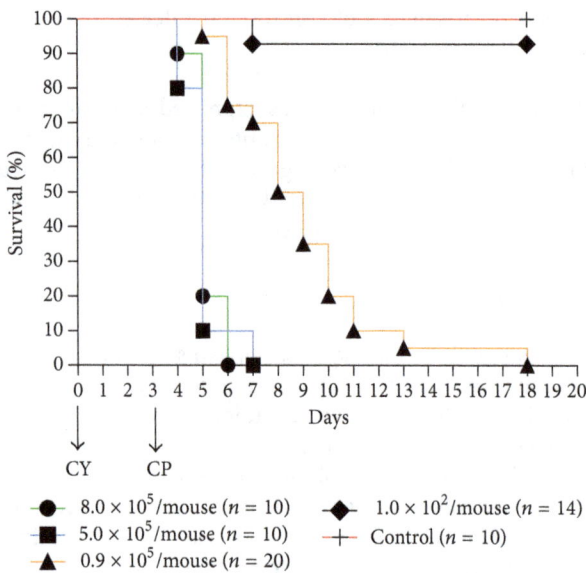

FIGURE 2: Survival curves. The mortality showed positive associations with infectious dose. And the optimal inoculum for *C. parapsilosis* was 0.9×10^5 CFU per immunosuppressed mouse.

and water consumption, weight loss, self-imposed isolation, and difficult breathing, were conspicuous in most infected animals 2 days postinfection. Each infected group presented death of animals during the infection period. Before death, most of them exhibited severe neurologic disorders, including opisthotonus, torticollis, and ataxia.

3.4. Gross Observation of the Model. At necropsy, swollen kidneys covered with white foci were observed in all infected mice (Figure 3). Some cases showed petechiae and petechial bleeding on the surface of the lung lobes and brains. Besides,

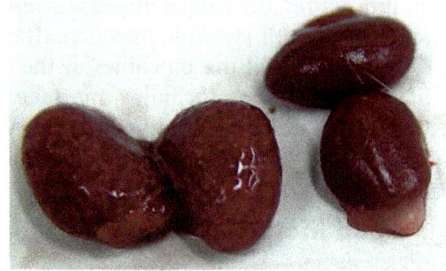

FIGURE 3: Gross observation of kidneys. The right two kidneys were the normal controls and the left swollen kidneys covered with petechiae were from infected mice.

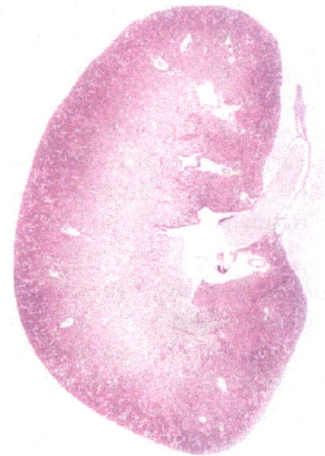

(a)

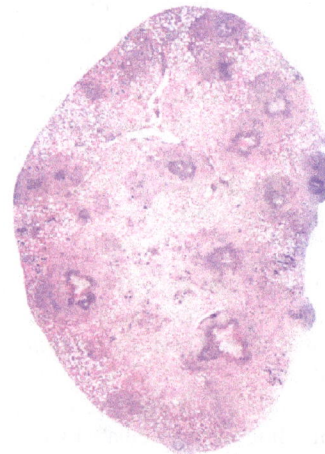

(b)

FIGURE 4: Histopathological changes in kidneys. Figure 4(a) was the control mouse showing no observed lesions. Figure 4(b) was the infected mouse presenting numerous granulomas in tissue section of the kidney.

moderate enlargements of the spleens were observed in most animals. No specific gross lesions were found in other organs.

3.5. Histological Analysis of the Model. At day 1, the lesions in all organs were relatively temperate, characterized by inflammation and slightly fungal infiltration of kidney tissues.

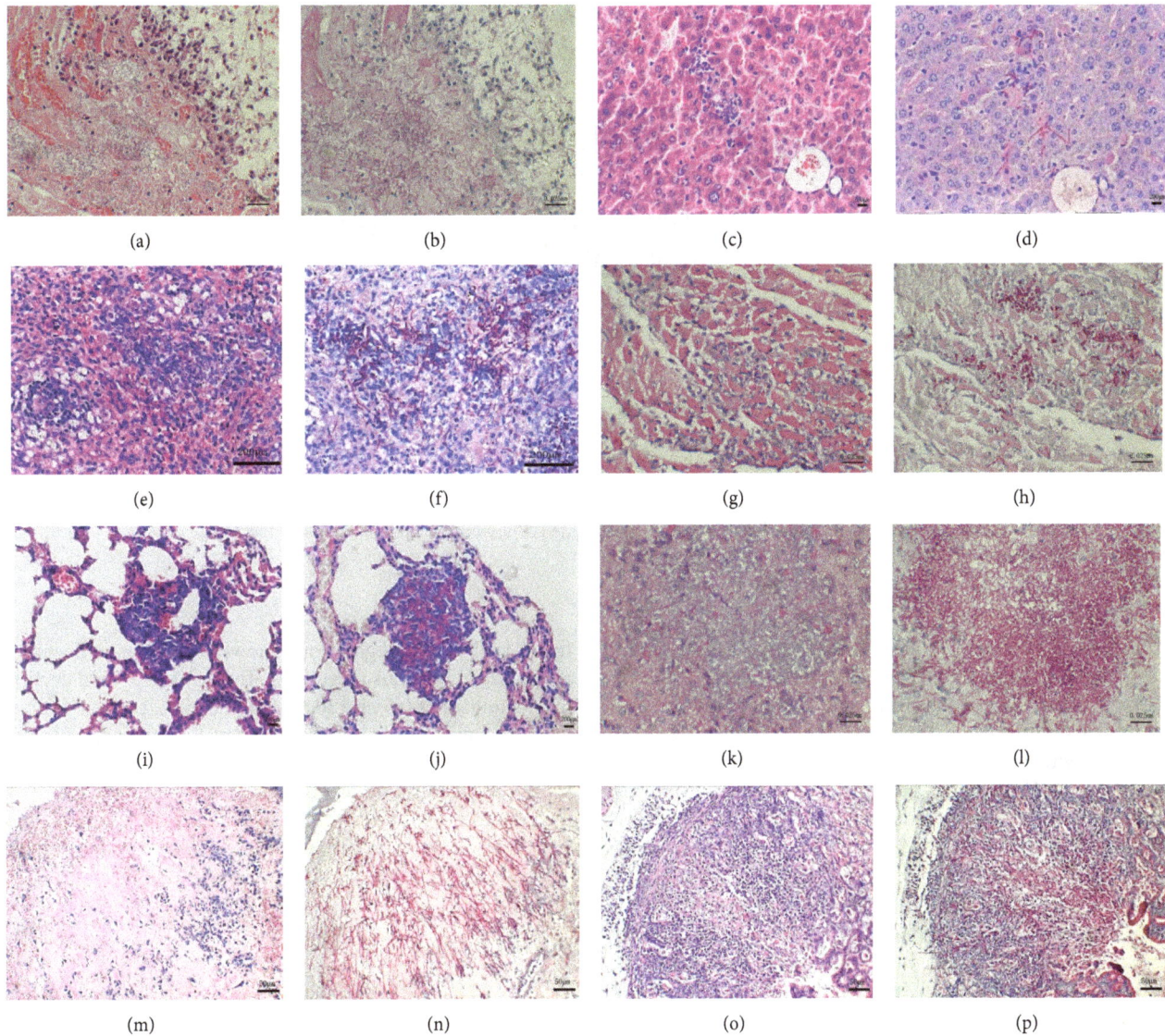

FIGURE 5: Histological findings of infected immunosuppressed mice. Figures 5(a), (c), (e), (g), (i), (k), (m), and (o) were H&E stained sections displaying the representative lesions in kidney, liver, spleen, heart, lung, brain, stomach, and bladder walls, respectively. Figures 5(b), (d), (f), (h), (j), (l), (n), and (p) stained by PAS showed fungal mycelia infiltration in kidney, liver, spleen, heart, lung, brain, stomach, and bladder walls, respectively.

At s 4 and 6, representative lesions could be observed in most organs. The kidney suffered the most severe lesions compared to the other organs or tissues. Numerous granulomas were diffused in renal cortex and medulla (Figure 4). Microscopic examination revealed that all granulomas contained fungal mycelia, blastospores, and chlamydospore-like structures (Figures 5(a) and 5(b)). The liver only experienced minor lesions, presenting periportal infiltration with a few polymorphonuclear leukocytes and fungal elements (Figures 5(c) and 5(d)). The spleen demonstrated the nonspecific lesion of the decrease of lymphocytes in white pulp and infiltration of a few PAS-positive fungal elements (Figures 5(e) and 5(f)). A certain number of granulomas or focal necrosis could be observed in the cardiac muscles, which were always composed by a necrotic center, infiltration of leukocytes,

mycelia, blastospores, and PAS-positive components (Figures 5(g) and 5(h)). Some certain focal necroses infiltrated by erythrocytes, lymphocyte-like cells, PAS-positive mycelia, blastospores, and chlamydospore-like structures were found in lung interstitium (Figures 5(i) and 5(j)). The lesions in brains were relatively more severe than the other organs, except kidneys. Focal liquefactive necrosis with abundant invading fungal pseudohyphae disrupted much of the forebrain (Figures 5(k) and 5(l)). Multifocal to coalescent necrosis and fungal invasions were observed in the gastric wall, which destroyed the deep structures of gastric wall including lamina propria, lamina muscularis, and stratum subvascular (Figures 5(m) and 5(n)). Similar lesions and extensive fungal invasion to gastric wall were also present within the bladder wall (Figures 5(o) and 5(p)).

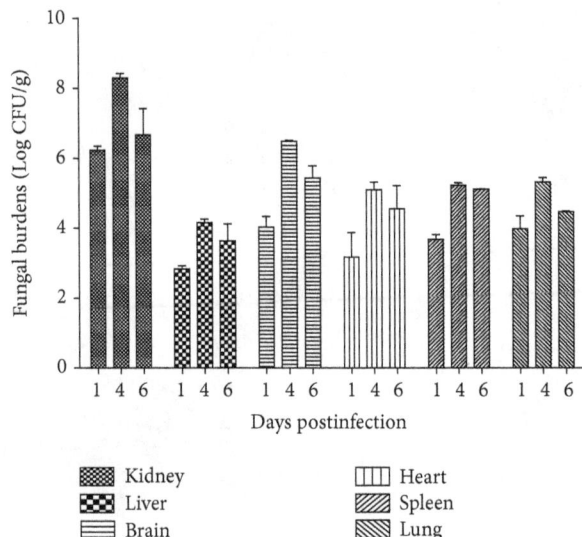

FIGURE 6: Dynamic changes of tissue fungal burdens. Tissue fungal burdens showed a transient increase during the infection period. And the kidney suffered the highest CFU scores.

3.6. Tissue Fungal Burdens of the Model.

C. parapsilosis could be detected out from the kidney, liver, brain, heart, spleen, and lung tissue suspension from day 1 postinfection. The dynamic changes of fungal burdens were the same in these organs, showing a transient increase with a brief peak at day 4 postinfection (Figure 6). The kidneys presented with much higher CFU scores compared with the other organs of the same time (t-test, $P < 0.05$).

3.7. Cytokine Levels of the Model.

For the CY group, all the detected serum and renal cytokines showed no significant changes all the time. Unlike the CY group, the *C. parapsilosis* infected mice presented different dynamic changes in serum and renal cytokines (Figure 7). Serum IL-6 and TNF-α showed a transient increase and reached the highest points at day 4, followed by the increase of serum IFN-γ. The other serum cytokines (IL-2, IL-4, IL-5, IL-10, IL-17, IL-23, GM-CSF, IL-1α, and IL-1β) showed no specific changes. Renal IL-6, TNF-α, IFN-γ, IL-1α, and IL-1β presented significant increases from days 4 to 6 postinfection. However, the other renal cytokines (IL-2, IL-4, IL-5, IL-10, IL-17, IL-23, and GM-CSF) presented no specific changes.

3.8. Model Based Evaluation of Antifungal Activity of Fluconazole.

Four groups of infectious models were used to evaluate the antifungal efficiency of fluconazole by administrating different dosages of fluconazole. During the experiment period, all animals of 50 mg/kg/d group survived, while mortalities of 100%, 80%, and 40% were observed in 0, 0.5, and 10 mg/kg/d groups, respectively. Survival curves were generated and compared between each 2 groups (Figure 8). Significant differences were found between 50 mg/kg/d group and the other groups (*Log-rank Test*, $P < 0.05$). There were also significant differences between 10 mg/kg/d group and the others. No significant differences were shown between 0.5 mg/kg/d group and the control. After receiving

fluconazole, 50 mg/kg/d group showed a significant decline of renal fungal burdens (Figure 9). Though there were declines in mortalities of 0.5 and 10 mg/kg/d groups, the renal fungal burdens significantly increased at day 4 postinfection (t-test, $P < 0.05$) (Figure 9). When compared with the control, renal fungal burdens of both 50 and 10 mg/kg/d groups at days 4 and 6 were significantly lower than the control (t-test, $P < 0.05$). Results indicated that there were ideal antifungal activities for fluconazole at dosages of 10–50 mg/kg/d.

4. Discussion

C. albicans has been kept as the major species associated with human *Candida* infections for decades. And the majority of experimental animal models for *Candida* species have focused on *C. albicans* too. Though many kinds of animals have been used to study *Candida* infections, the rodent infection models occupied the majority for economic reasons, easy handling, and the availability of genetic modification [10]. In this paper, we will try to introduce an ideal *C. parapsilosis* infection model based on immunosuppressed ICR mice.

Many regents have been used to obtain the immunosuppressed mice, for example, cortisone acetate and hydrocortisone succinate [11]. Here, we used CY to induce immunosuppression in ICR mice. Mice presented a time transient decrease of the total leukocyte counts and reached the lowest point at day 4 after receiving CY for 3 consecutive days at a dosage of 100 mg/kg body weight. Result demonstrated that days 3 to 6 after CY administration were the optimal infection time points. And the day 4 was chosen to infect mice in this study.

To assure the infectious dose of *C. parapsilosis*, immunosuppressed mice were infected with 4 dosages, respectively. According to the results of survival curves, the dosage of 0.9×10^5 CFU *C. parapsilosis* was the optimal infectious dose in immunosuppressed ICR mice. The morphology

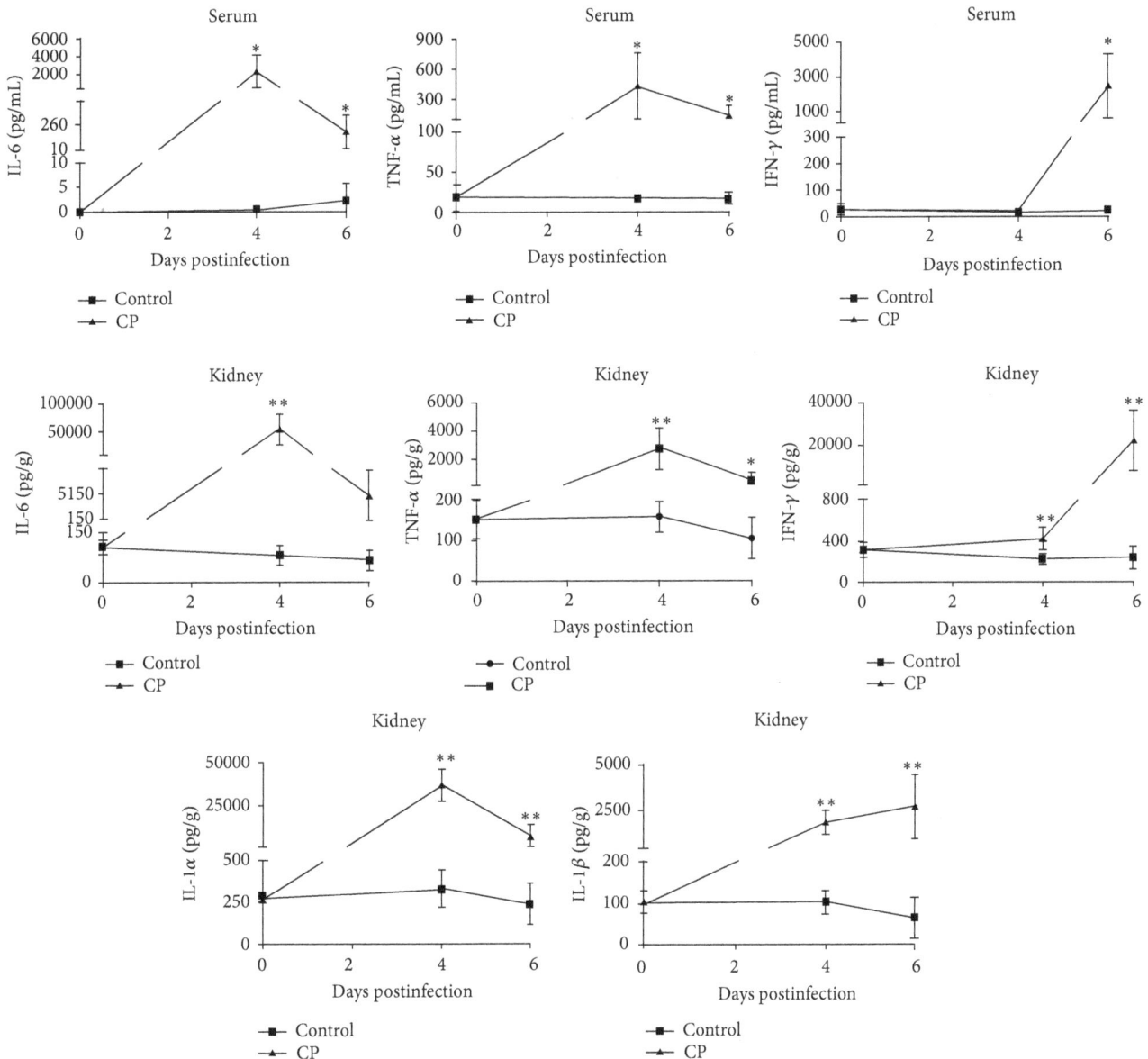

FIGURE 7: Dynamic changes of serum and renal cytokines. Serum IL-6, TNF-α, and IFN-γ and renal IL-6, TNF-α, IFN-γ, IL-1α, and IL-1β presented significant increases during the infection period.

of *Candida* species was important to animal models. Our previous experiments showed that mycelium *C. parapsilosis* has more virulence than fungal spores. And the inoculums containing >95% fungal spores were used in this study.

The infection model based on 0.9×10^5 CFU *C. parapsilosis* presented a median survival time of 5.5 days, which was long enough to satisfy researches on antifungal agents. Histopathology and tissues fungal burdens revealed the model to be a systemic infection one, and the kidneys suffered the most severe lesions, indicating that kidney could be a suitable target organ for screening antifungal agents. The fungal burdens showed a transient increase with a brief peak at day 4 postinfection in multiple organs, demonstrating that day 4 postinfection was an optimal time point to assess the fungal burdens for research or evaluation of antifungal

agents, which were further identified by using the infectious model in evaluation of antifungal activity of fluconazole. Some serum and renal proinflammatory cytokines were induced and consistent with the tissue fungal burdens, while anti-inflammatory cytokines showed no significant increase. Th1/Th2 cytokine imbalance might result in high mortality of infected mice.

This project established a systemic *C. parapsilosis* infection model in immunosuppressed ICR mice. In this model, multiorgans, including kidneys, liver, lungs, spleen, brains, and bladder wall, represented numerous microabscesses, which demonstrated congestion, hemorrhages, tubular degeneration, and heterophilic infiltration. This model affords opportunities for increasing our understanding of fungal pathogenesis and treatment.

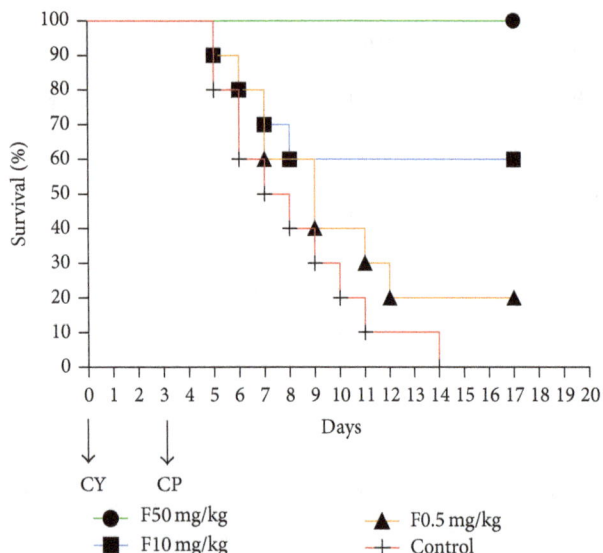

FIGURE 8: Survival curves of fluconazole treated mice ($n = 10$ per group). Comparisons between each two groups except 0.5 and 10 mg/kg/d groups that showed significant differences (Log-rank Test, $P < 0.05$).

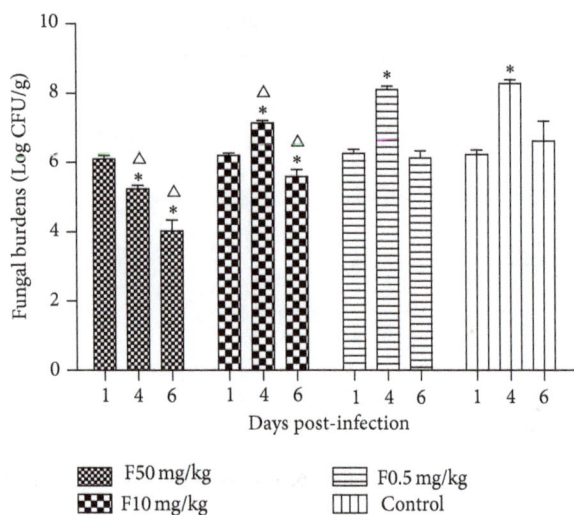

FIGURE 9: Renal fungal burdens of fluconazole treated mice ($n = 5$ per day). 50 mg/kg/d group showed a significant decline of renal fungal burdens, while, the other groups showed a transient increase during the experiment period. $^*P < 0.05$, t-test, versus that of day 1. $^\triangle P < 0.05$, t-test, versus that of control of the same time point.

Conflict of Interests

The authors declare that there is no conflict of interests regarding the publication of this paper.

Authors' Contribution

Yu'e Wu and Fangui Min are co-first authors. Yu'e Wu, Fangui Min, Yu Zhang, and Ren Huang conceived and designed the study. The first five coauthors performed the experiments.

Lixin Zhang provided the fungal strain and gave constructive advices. All coauthors read and approved the final paper.

Acknowledgment

This work was supported by Grants 2010B060500019 and 2014A010107018 of Guangdong Provincial Science and Technology Project.

References

[1] J. Marchena-Gomez, T. Saez-Guzman, M. Hemmersbach-Miller et al., "Candida isolation in patients hospitalized on a surgical ward: significance and mortality-related factors," *World Journal of Surgery*, vol. 33, no. 9, pp. 1822–1829, 2009.

[2] T. Nakamura and H. Takahashi, "Epidemiological study of *Candida* infections in blood: susceptibilities of *Candida* spp. to antifungal agents, and clinical features associated with the candidemia," *Journal of Infection and Chemotherapy*, vol. 12, no. 3, pp. 132–138, 2006.

[3] S.-Y. Ruan and P.-R. Hsueh, "Invasive candidiasis: an overview from Taiwan," *Journal of the Formosan Medical Association*, vol. 108, no. 6, pp. 443–451, 2009.

[4] A. M. Tortorano, G. Dho, A. Prigitano et al., "Invasive fungal infections in the intensive care unit: a multicentre, prospective, observational study in Italy (2006–2008)," *Mycoses*, vol. 55, no. 1, pp. 73–79, 2012.

[5] H. Wisplinghoff, H. Seifert, R. P. Wenzel, and M. B. Edmond, "Current trends in the epidemiology of nosocomial bloodstream infections in patients with hematological malignancies and solid neoplasms in hospitals in the United States," *Clinical Infectious Diseases*, vol. 36, no. 9, pp. 1103–1110, 2003.

[6] R. Saha, S. Das Das, A. Kumar, and I. R. Kaur, "Pattern of Candida isolates in hospitalized children," *Indian Journal of Pediatrics*, vol. 75, no. 8, pp. 858–860, 2008.

[7] Z. Y. Zhang, K. C. Qian, and S. L. Chen, "Distribution of Candidemia and antifungal drugs assay in our hospital from 2005–2008," *Modern Medicine & Health*, vol. 25, pp. 3411–3412, 2009.

[8] L. X. Zhang, K. Z. Yan, Y. Zhang et al., "High-throughput synergy screening identifies microbial metabolites as combination agents for the treatment of fungal infections," *Proceedings of the National Academy of Sciences of the United States of America*, vol. 104, no. 11, pp. 4606–4611, 2007.

[9] National Research Council, *Guide for the Care and Use of Laboratory Animals*, National Academy Press, Washington, DC, USA, 2011.

[10] F. de Bernardis, L. Morelli, T. Ceddia, R. Lorenzini, and A. Cassone, "Experimental pathogenicity and acid proteinase secretion of vaginal isolates of *Candida parapsilosis*," *Journal of Medical and Veterinary Mycology*, vol. 28, no. 2, pp. 125–137, 1990.

[11] G. M. Chaves, M. A. de Q Cavalcanti, A. M. A. Carneiro-Leão, and S. L. Lopes, "Model of experimental infection in healthy and immunosuppressed Swiss albino mice (*Mus musculus*) using *Candida albicans* strains with different patterns of enzymatic activity," *Brazilian Journal of Microbiology*, vol. 35, no. 4, pp. 324–329, 2004.

7

Prevalence of Dog Erythrocyte Antigens 1, 4, and 7 in Podenco Ibicenco (Ibizan Hounds) from Ibiza Island

Eva Spada,[1] Daniela Proverbio,[1] Luis Miguel Viñals Flórez,[2]
Blanca Serra Gómez de la Serna,[3] Maria del Rosario Perlado Chamizo,[4]
Luciana Baggiani,[1] and Roberta Perego[1]

[1] Veterinary Transfusion Unit (REV), Department of Health, Animal Science and Food Safety (VESPA),
 University of Milan, Via G. Celoria 10, 20133 Milan, Italy
[2] Centro de Transfusión Veterinario (CTV), Arturo Soria 267, 28033 Madrid, Spain
[3] Clinical Veterinary Hospital, CEU Cardenal Herrera University, Alfara del Patriarca, 46115 Valencia, Spain
[4] Laboratorio de Análisis Clínico, Hospital Clínico Veterinario, Universidad Alfonso X el Sabio, Avenida de la Universidad,
 Villanueva de la Cañada, 28691 Madrid, Spain

Correspondence should be addressed to Eva Spada; eva.spada@unimi.it

Academic Editor: Remo Lobetti

The aims of this study were to evaluate the prevalence of Dog Erythrocyte Antigens (DEA) 1, 4, and 7 in Ibizan hounds, to compare the results with the prevalence of DEA in Spanish greyhounds, and to determine the risk of sensitization following the first transfusion of blood not typed for DEA 1 and the probability of an acute hemolytic reaction following a second incompatible transfusion using untyped DEA 1 blood. DEA 1, 4, and 7 status was determined in 92 Ibizan hounds. Results were compared with the previously reported prevalence in Spanish greyhounds. The risks of sensitization and of a hemolytic transfusion reaction were determined amongst Ibizan hounds and between Ibizan hounds and Spanish greyhounds. The prevalence of DEA 1, 4, and 7 was 75%, 98.9%, and 25%, respectively. There was a significantly higher expression of DEA 1 and 7 in Ibizan hounds than in Spanish greyhounds. The probability of sensitization of a recipient dog to DEA 1 with transfusions amongst Ibizan hounds was 18.5% and between Ibizan hounds and Spanish greyhounds was 13.7%. The probability of an acute hemolytic reaction in each group was 3.5% and 1.9%, respectively. There is a higher prevalence of DEA 1 and 7 in Ibizan hounds than in other sighthounds.

1. Introduction

There is international standardization of seven canine blood groups as categorized by presence of Dog Erythrocyte Antigen (DEA) 1, 3, 4, 5, 6, 7, and 8 [1]. Other antigen systems have been reported, such as the recently described Dal blood type [2], but none of these systems have been standardized. A donor may express more than one blood group and canine red blood cells can be negative or positive for any given blood type [3].

DEA 1 and 7 are the most important blood types with regard to canine blood transfusions. DEA 1 antigen has recently been classified as a unique DEA epitope with variable surface expression (rather than the expression of different alleles, DEA 1.1, DEA 1.2, and DEA 1.3, as is previously thought) [4] and is present in approximately half the canine population [5–11]. There are no naturally occurring antibodies to DEA 1 in dogs. DEA 1 negative dogs exposed to DEA 1 positive RBCs will become "sensitized" within 9 days by production of anti-DEA 1 antibodies [12, 13]. Anti-DEA 1 antibodies have been reported to cause acute hemolytic transfusion reactions in previously sensitized DEA 1 negative dogs [14].

DEA 7 antigens are reported to occur naturally in between 40 and 72% of the canine population [8, 9, 13, 15, 16]. Between 10 and 40% of dogs negative for these antigens have naturally occurring antibodies to DEA 7 [3, 17] and delayed RBC survival is thought to occur in antigen negative dogs receiving DEA 7 positive blood [15].

There is also a high prevalence of DEA 4 antigens (98–100%) in the canine population [3, 8, 9, 16] and a hemolytic transfusion reaction due to DEA 4 alloantibodies has been reported in a dog [18].

An ideal blood donor does not have blood antigens of types that commonly cause reactions in unmatched recipients. There is no universally agreed definition of a universal canine donor. The most restrictive definition of the universal canine donor would be a dog negative for DEA 1, DEA 3, DEA 5, and DEA 7 and positive for DEA 4. Since 98% of dogs are positive for DEA 4, the rarity of DEA 4 negative dogs means that this antigen is unlikely to influence donor selection. Some transfusion specialists do not exclude DEA 7 positive dogs from the donor pool. In fact the concept of the universal donor in dogs has long been debated since the tests for DEA 3 and DEA 5 antigens are often not available and the quality of these tests is variable; currently typing sera are available only for DEA 1, 4, and 7 antigens. As previously proposed [14], universal donors are therefore often considered to be dogs that are DEA 1 and 7 negative. Point-of-care tests are currently only available for DEA 1, although, in specialized laboratories, polyclonal antisera are available for DEA 4 and DEA 7 typing.

Ibizan hounds are medium-size sighthounds originating from the island of Ibiza. They are traditionally used in the Balearic Islands (and less so in Spain and France) to hunt rabbits and other small game. In recent times this breed has been disseminated worldwide through a variety of adoption programs. The Ibizan hound is classified by the Fédération Cynologique Internationale (FCI) in Group 5 (spitz and primitive types) and in section primitive type-hunting dogs. This dog is a typical and robust representative of one of the oldest breeds still in existence (http://www.fci.be/en/nomenclature/IBIZAN-PODENCO-89.html).

The aims of this study were threefold: (1) to evaluate the prevalence of DEA 1, DEA 4, and DEA 7 blood type in Ibizan hounds; (2) to compare the results with the previously published prevalence of DEAs in other sighthounds (i.e., Spanish greyhound); (3) to determine the risk of recipient sensitization following the first transfusion of blood not typed for DEA 1 and the probability an acute hemolytic reaction following a second incompatible transfusion of blood untyped for DEA 1 both amongst Ibizan hounds and between Ibizan hounds and Spanish greyhounds.

2. Material and Methods

2.1. Samples. In this prospective study EDTA-anticoagulated blood samples were collected from 92 healthy owned Ibizan hounds in January 2015. Dogs were between 1-year and 3-year old, 89 were female (96.7%) and 3 were male (3.3%), and all were living on Ibiza Island, Spain.

With the owners' consent cephalic blood samples were collected with a 23 G needle (Sterican Braun®, B. Braun Melsungen AG, Melsungen, Germany) connected to a 2 mL syringe (Injekt Braun®, B. Braun Melsungen AG,

Melsungen, Germany). They were transferred to a 1 mL EDTA-anticoagulated tube and were stored between 4 and 5°C. All blood samples were collected as part of a study to determine the distribution of blood groups in this breed. This study was conducted according to European legislation (2010/63/EU). In all samples blood typing was performed as described below.

2.2. DEA 1 Blood Typing. DEA 1 status was determined using a commercially available card agglutination technique (RapidVet-H, Canine DEA 1.1, Agrolabo SpA, Scarmagno, Turin, Italy) according to the manufacturer's instructions and as previously described [19, 20]. The principle of this card-based agglutination test is a visible hemagglutination reaction resulting from the binding of the DEA 1 RBC surface antigen to a murine monoclonal antibody that is lyophilized on the card test.

2.3. DEA 4 and DEA 7 Blood Typing. Analysis for DEA 4 and 7 antigens was performed by gel column agglutination within microtubes (ID-CARD NaCl, Enzyme Test and Cold Agglutinins, DiaMed, Cressier FR, Switzerland) as previously described [21] using polyclonal anti-DEA antibodies produced by Animal Blood Resources International (ABRINT, Stockbridge, MI, USA).

Anti-DEA 4 and 7 antibodies were imported and used in this study with the authorization of Italian Health Minister (protocol authorization number 0021278-15/10/2014-DGSAF-DGSAF-P). Blood-typing was performed at the Veterinary Transfusion Unit (REV) of the University of Milan, Milan, Italy.

Briefly 25 μL of a 0.8% RBC suspension made by suspending 10 μL of the RBC pellet in 1 mL of low ionic strength solution (LISS, ID-DILUENT 2, modified LISS solution, DiaMed, Cressier FR, Switzerland) was mixed with 25 μL of DEA 7 antibodies or with 15 μL of DEA 4 antibodies in the reaction chamber of saline gel columns. For all samples a negative control column with saline solution was included. The gel columns were incubated at 4°C for 30 minutes and were then centrifuged in a special gel column card centrifuge (ID-CENTRIFUGE 24 S, DiaMed-ID Micro Typing System, Cressier sur Morat, Switzerland) at 80 × g for 10 minutes. Finally the gel column cards were evaluated for presence and strength of agglutination. Only results validated by negative controls were included in analysis.

The cards were visually interpreted as follows: (0) negative, when all RBCs were at the bottom of the column; 1+, when very few RBC agglutinates were dispersed in the lower part of the gel, with most RBCs at the bottom of the tube; 2+, when all RBCs were agglutinated and dispersed in the gel; 3+, when some RBC agglutinates were dispersed in the upper part of the gel and most of the RBCs formed a red line on the surface of the gel; and 4+, when all RBCs formed a red line on top of the gel. Results were interpreted as negative if no agglutination or 1+ agglutination was present, whereas ≥2+ agglutination reactions were considered positive.

2.4. Sensitization and Transfusion Risk Analysis for DEA 1. The probability of an Ibizan hound becoming sensitized following the first transfusion of blood that was neither cross-matched nor typed for DEA 1 was calculated using the following formula [5, 10]:

$$\left[\frac{(\% \text{ DEA 1 negative} \times \% \text{ DEA 1 positive})}{100} \right]. \quad (1)$$

The probability of the same dog developing an acute hemolytic reaction with a second incompatible transfusion using untyped blood from any other dog was calculated using the following formula [10]:

$$\frac{\left[(\% \text{ DEA 1 negative} \times \% \text{ DEA 1 positive}) \times \% \text{ sensitization for the first transfusion} \right]}{10,000}. \quad (2)$$

2.5. Statistical Analysis. Results were analysed by absolute prevalence analysis. Using contingency tables or Fisher's exact test the prevalence of DEA 1, 4, and 7 and universal donors in Ibizan hounds calculated in this study was compared with a population of 205 Spanish greyhounds (galgo) in which the prevalence of DEA 1, 4, and 7 and universal donors (i.e., DEA 1 and 7 negative and DEA 4 positive) was 54.6%, 100%, 8%, and 46.7%, respectively [22].

All statistical analysis was performed using statistical software (Medcalc software version 14.10.2, Mariakerke, Belgium) with significance set at $P < 0.05$.

3. Results

3.1. DEA 1, DEA 4, and DEA 7 Prevalence. For DEA 1 blood type, 69 (75%) dogs tested positive and 23 (25%) tested negative. For DEA 4 blood type, 91 (98.9%) dogs tested positive (all showed 4+ agglutination) and 1 (1.1%) dog tested negative. For DEA 7 blood type, 23 (25%) dogs tested positive (16 samples showed 3+ agglutination and 7 samples showed 2+ agglutination) and 69 (75%) were negative (no samples showed agglutination). Of the 92 dogs, 16 (17.4%) were DEA 4 positive only (universal donors) and 1 (1.1%) dog was negative for all DEA. All control samples in the gel columns tested negative (absence of agglutination).

3.2. Comparison of DEA 1, 4, and 7 Prevalence with Spanish Greyhounds. Ibizan hounds had a significantly higher prevalence of DEA 1 and DEA 7 positivity than Spanish greyhounds ($P = 0.005$ and $P = 0.002$, resp.). The prevalence of universal donors (DEA 1 and DEA 7 negative and DEA 4 positive or negative) was lower in Ibizan hounds ($P = 0.000008$) than in Spanish greyhounds. There was no significant difference in DEA 4 prevalence between the 2 breeds.

3.3. Risk of Sensitization for DEA 1 and a Hemolytic Acute Reaction in an Untyped Recipient. The probability of an Ibizan hound recipient becoming sensitized following the first transfusion of blood from an Ibizan hound donor that was not cross-matched nor typed for DEA 1 was approximately 1 in 5 (18.8%). The probability of the same dog developing an acute hemolytic reaction with a second incompatible transfusion using blood untyped for DEA 1 from any other Ibizan hound was 3.5%.

The probability of a recipient Ibizan hound becoming sensitized following the first transfusion of blood from a Spanish greyhound that was not cross-matched nor typed for DEA 1 was approximately 1 in 7 (13.7%). The probability of the same dog developing an acute hemolytic reaction with a second incompatible transfusion using untyped DEA 1 blood from Spanish greyhound was 1.9%.

4. Discussion

There are breed and geographical differences in the prevalence of different blood group antigens [8, 15]. It is essential to type donor blood in order to select compatible canine blood donors. The prevalence of positivity to antigens in a potential donor population can be used to calculate the likelihood that such an antigen will cause an adverse transfusion reaction and therefore the risk associated with any transfusion can be assessed.

In this study the prevalence of DEA 1 expression in Ibizan hounds was 75%, which is higher than previously reported in other pure breeds [7–9, 15, 16] and in cross-breed dogs [6]. The prevalence of DEA 1 in Ibizan hounds was also much higher than previously reported in other sighthounds, such as Greyhounds and Spanish greyhounds, in which the prevalence of DEA 1 has been reported to be 13.1% [16] and 51.7% [11], respectively. The prevalence of DEA 1 was statistically significantly higher in Ibizan hounds than in a population of Spanish greyhounds tested for DEA 1 [22].

All 92 Ibizan hounds were blood typed and only one was DEA 4 negative. This prevalence of DEA 4 expression (98.9%) is in agreement with the prevalence in the general canine population [6, 7, 9, 16, 21].

The prevalence of DEA 7-positive dogs in the study population (25%) was similar to that reported in Golden Retrievers in USA and Brazil (25% and 27% resp.) [7, 9] but higher than the prevalence reported in cross-breeds (11%) and German Shepherd dogs (8%) in Brazil [6] and lower than in Greyhounds in USA (29.1%) [16] and Turkish Kangal dogs (71.1%) [8]. The prevalence of DEA 7 expression in Ibizan hounds was statistically significantly higher than in a population of Spanish greyhounds previously tested by the authors for DEA 7 [22]. These results confirm that as for other canine blood types, the prevalence of DEA 7 differs between populations.

The prevalence of universal or "ideal" donors, that is, dogs positive only for DEA 4 or negative for all DEA, in our population of Ibizan hounds, was 18.5%. This is lower than the prevalence of 57.3% found in greyhounds [16] and in a population of Spanish greyhounds previously blood typed, in which prevalence of universal donors was 46.7% [22].

In this study the probability of a recipient becoming sensitized and produced antibodies against DEA 1 following the first transfusion of blood that was neither cross-matched nor typed for DEA 1 was 18.8% (1 in 5) amongst Ibizan hounds and 13.7% (1 in 7) between Ibizan hounds and Spanish Greyhounds. These probabilities were lower than previously reported in dogs from Portugal [10], in Spanish greyhounds in Spain [11] and in dogs in Brazil [5] in which probabilities were 24.5%, 22.9%, and 24.9%, respectively. The risk of a hemolytic transfusion reaction was also lower than the 6% reported in a previous study [10] since there was a higher prevalence of DEA 1 positivity in the Ibizan hounds (so these dogs could receive either DEA 1 negative or DEA 1 positive blood at first transfusion without transfusion reactions).

The gel agglutination technique has been used for decades. This test is sensitive for the detection of DEA 1 and is suited for screening blood donors in a blood bank program [19, 20]. This study used, for only the third time in the canine blood typing, column gel agglutination with polyclonal antibodies for DEA 4 and DEA 7 [21, 22]. The column gel agglutination test is simple to perform, does not require washing of RBC, requires only small sample and reagent volumes, and yields results that are simple to read and stable over time (for up to three days). The study that validated this technique with polyclonal antibodies for DEA 4 and 7 demonstrated that the test was not 100% sensitive for identification of DEA 7 [21]. In fact, when gel agglutination was compared with tube agglutination (considered the gold standard), there were 12 discordant results for DEA 7 (concordance of 84%). The gel agglutination test had a specificity of 100% and a sensitivity of 53% for identification of the DEA 7 positive samples when compared with tube agglutination [21]. This may represent a limitation of our study as the true prevalence of DEA 7 positive dogs may have been higher than detected using this test.

Another limitation of this study was that the study population of Ibizan hounds was almost exclusively female, mirroring the environment in which Ibizan hounds live. Hunters run these dogs in mostly female packs, as the female is considered the better hunter. In addition we did not know how closely related the dogs used in this study were. It is possible that a closed population of closely related individuals could bias the prevalence of blood types. Finally DEA 3, DEA 5, and Dal blood types were not tested since relevant antisera were unavailable at the time the study was performed.

5. Conclusion

The population of Ibizan hounds studied here showed a different prevalence for DEA 1 and 7 with respect to previous reports of other sighthounds. Although the risk of sensitization and an acute transfusion reaction following incompatible blood transfusion is low, it remains best practice to blood type and cross-match recipients before transfusion.

Ethical Approval

All applicable international, national, and/or institutional guidelines for the care and use of animals were followed.

Conflict of Interests

The authors declare that there is no conflict of interests regarding the publication of this paper.

References

[1] R. W. Bull, "Animal blood groups," in *American Association of Blood Banks Technical Workshop on Veterinary Transfusion Medicine*, J. S. Smith and R. G. Westphal, Eds., pp. 1–2, American Association of Blood Banks, Bethesda, Md, USA, 1989.

[2] M.-C. Blais, L. Berman, D. A. Oakley, and U. Giger, "Canine Dal blood type: a red cell antigen lacking in some Dalmatians," *Journal of Veterinary Internal Medicine*, vol. 21, no. 2, pp. 281–286, 2007.

[3] A. Hale, "Canine blood groups and blood typing," in *BSAVA Manual of Canine and Feline Haematology and Transfusion Medicine*, M. J. Day and B. Kohn, Eds., pp. 280–283, British Small Animal Veterinary Association, Gloucester, UK, 2nd edition, 2012.

[4] M. M. Acierno, K. Raj, and U. Giger, "DEA 1 expression on dog erythrocytes analyzed by immunochromatographic and flow cytometric techniques," *Journal of Veterinary Internal Medicine*, vol. 28, no. 2, pp. 592–598, 2014.

[5] A. A. Novais, A. E. Santana, and L. A. Vicentin, "Prevalence of DEA 1 canine blood group system in dogs (*Canis familiaris*, Linnaeus, 1758) reared in Brazil," *Brazilian Journal of Veterinary Research and Animal Science*, vol. 36, no. 1, pp. 23–27, 1999.

[6] A. A. Novais, J. J. Fagliari, and A. E. Santana, "Prevalência dos antígenos eritrocitários caninos (DEA- dog erythrocyte antigen) em cães domésticos (Canis familiaris) craidos no Brasil. [DEA prevalence in domestic dogs (Canis familiaris) reared in Brazil]," *Ars Veterinaria*, vol. 20, no. 2, pp. 212–218, 2004.

[7] A. S. Hale, J. Werfelmann, M. Lemmons, B. Smiler, and J. Gerlach, "An evaluation of 9,570 dogs by breed and dog erythrocyte antigen typing," *Journal of Veterinary Internal Medicine*, vol. 22, article 740, 2008.

[8] S. Arikan, M. Guzel, N. Mamak, and Y. Z. Ograk, "Frequency of blood types DEA 1.1, 3, 4, 5 and 7 in Kangal dog," *Revue in Médicine Véterinarie*, vol. 160, no. 4, pp. 180–183, 2009.

[9] V. Sinnott Esteve, L. de Almeida Lacerda, C. S. Lasta, V. Pedralli, and F. H. D. González, "Frequencies of DEA blood types in a purebred canine blood donor population in Porto Alegre, RS, Brazil," *Pesquisa Veterinária Brasileira*, vol. 31, no. 2, pp. 178–181, 2011.

[10] R. R. F. Ferreira, R. R. Gopegui, and A. J. F. Matos, "Frequency of dog erythrocyte antigen 1.1 expression in dogs from Portugal," *Veterinary Clinical Pathology*, vol. 40, no. 2, pp. 198–201, 2011.

[11] I. Mesa-Sánchez, R. Ruiz de Gopegui-Fernández, M. M. Granados-Machuca, and A. Galan-Rodriguez, "Prevalence of dog erythrocyte antigen 1.1 in galgos (Spanish greyhounds)," *Veterinary Record*, vol. 174, no. 14, p. 351, 2014.

[12] S. N. Swisher, L. E. Young, and N. Trabold, "*In vitro* and *in vivo* studies of the behavior of canine erythrocyte-isoantibody systems," *Annals of the New York Academy of Sciences*, vol. 97, no. 1, pp. 15–25, 1962.

[13] C. D. De Wit, N. A. Coenegracht, P. H. A. Poll, and J. D. van der Linde, "The practical importance of blood groups in dogs," *Journal of Small Animal Practice*, vol. 8, no. 5, pp. 285–289, 1967.

[14] U. Giger, C. J. Gelens, M. B. Callan, and D. A. Oakley, "An acute hemolytic transfusion reaction caused by dog erythrocyte antigen 1.1 incompatibility in a previously sensitized dog," *Journal of the American Veterinary Medical Association*, vol. 206, no. 9, pp. 1358–1362, 1995.

[15] A. S. Hale, "Canine blood groups and their importance in veterinary transfusion medicine," *The Veterinary Clinics of North America: Small Animal Practice*, vol. 25, no. 6, pp. 1323–1332, 1995.

[16] M. C. Iazbik, M. O'Donnell, L. Marin, S. Zaldivar, D. Hudson, and C. G. Couto, "Prevalence of dog erythrocyte antigens in retired racing Greyhounds," *Veterinary Clinical Pathology*, vol. 39, no. 4, pp. 433–435, 2010.

[17] A. S. Hale and J. Werfelmann, "Incidence of canine serum antibody to known dog erythrocyte antigens in potential donor population," *Journal of Veterinary Internal Medicine*, vol. 20, supplement, pp. 768–769, 2006.

[18] K. J. Melzer, K. J. Wardrop, A. S. Hale, and V. M. Wong, "A hemolytic transfusion reaction due to DEA 4 alloantibodies in a dog," *Journal of Veterinary Internal Medicine*, vol. 17, no. 6, pp. 931–933, 2003.

[19] U. Giger, K. Stieger, and H. Palos, "Comparison of various canine blood-typing methods," *American Journal of Veterinary Research*, vol. 66, no. 8, pp. 1386–1392, 2005.

[20] M. Seth, K. V. Jackson, S. Winzelberg, and U. Giger, "Comparison of gel column, card, and cartridge techniques for dog erythrocyte antigen 1.1 blood typing," *American Journal of Veterinary Research*, vol. 73, no. 2, pp. 213–219, 2012.

[21] R. J. Kessler, J. Reese, D. Chang, M. Seth, A. S. Hale, and U. Giger, "Dog erythrocyte antigens 1.1, 1.2, 3, 4, 7, and Dal blood typing and cross-matching by gel column technique," *Veterinary Clinical Pathology*, vol. 39, no. 3, pp. 306–316, 2010.

[22] E. Spada, D. Proverbio, L. M. Viñals Flórez et al., "Prevalence of dog erythrocyte antigens 1, 4, and 7 in galgos (Spanish Greyhounds)," *Journal of Veterinary Diagnostic Investigation*, vol. 27, no. 4, pp. 558–561, 2015.

8

Blood Pressure, Serum Glucose, Cholesterol, and Triglycerides in Dogs with Different Body Scores

Mauro José Lahm Cardoso,[1] **Rafael Fagnani,**[2] **Carolina Zaghi Cavalcante,**[3]
Marcelo de Souza Zanutto,[1] **Ademir Zacarias Júnior,**[4]
Luciane Holsback da Silveira Fertonani,[4] **Jéssica Ragazzi Calesso,**[5] **Maíra Melussi,**[5]
Helena Pinheiro Costa,[4] **and Eduardo Yudi Hashizume**[1]

[1]*Department of Veterinary Clinics, State University of Londrina, Londrina, PR, Brazil*
[2]*Northern Paraná State University, Londrina, PR, Brazil*
[3]*Pontifical Catholic University of Paraná, Curitiba, PR, Brazil*
[4]*Northern Paraná University, Bandeirantes, PR, Brazil*
[5]*Veterinary Space Life, Londrina, PR, Brazil*

Correspondence should be addressed to Mauro José Lahm Cardoso; maurolahm@gmail.com

Academic Editor: Remo Lobetti

The objective of this research was to determine the frequency for the occurrence of MS in dogs, using the criteria determined, and to correlate the criteria of dogs that would characterize the MS with different body condition score (BCS). 271 dogs with different body scores were studied, with 101 dogs with BCS 4-5; 101 dogs with BCS 6-7; and 69 dogs with BCS 8-9. Among the dogs studied, 62 (22,87%) had two or more inclusion criteria for MS. Of these, 28 had BCS 6-7, while 34 dogs had BCS 8-9. Therefore, 27,72% of overweight dogs had inclusion criteria for MS and 49,27% of obese ones had two or more inclusion criteria for MS. When only overweight and obese dogs were considered as a total population, it was observed that 36,47% got inclusion criteria for the MS. No dog with BCS 4-5 showed two or more inclusion criteria for MS. The metabolic syndrome, according to the parameters for inclusion defined in the literature, was observed in 22,87% of the animals studied and in 36% of dogs overweight or obese. Furthermore, MS was most common in obese (49%) compared to overweight dogs (27%).

1. Introduction

Metabolic syndrome (MS) gained attention in human medicine because of the association with the development of *diabetes mellitus* and cardiovascular disease [1]. To characterize this MS is necessary for the presence of visceral (central) obesity in conjunction with dyslipidemia including the increase of triglyceride and decrease of HDL-cholesterol, hypertension, and glucose intolerance. In veterinary medicine MS in equines is well described and known to be a risk factor for the development of laminitis and other diseases [2]. Obese dogs may develop some components of the MS, including insulin resistance, hyperlipidemia, and mild hypertension, which improve with weight loss [3–5].

The consensus statement that defines the inclusion of the human patient as having MS [6] includes the presence of at least three to five of the following: triglycerides >150 mg/dL (>1,7 mmol/L); HDL-cholesterol <40 mg/dL (<1,3 mmol/L) in men or 50 mg/dL (<1,29 mmol/L) in women; arterial systolic pressure >135/85 mmHg; plasma glucose >100 mg/dL (5,6 mmol/L); increased waist circumference [6]. The first criteria suggested for the classification of MS in naturally obese dogs were BCS 7–9/9 points and two of the following of these criteria: triglycerides >200 mg/dL (2,3 mmol/L); total cholesterol >300 mg/dL (7,8 mmol/L); systolic blood pressure >160 mmHg; plasma glucose >100 mg/dL (5,6 mmol/L); previous diagnosis of *diabetes mellitus* type 2 [7].

The objective of this research was to determine the frequency for the occurrence of MS in dogs, using the criteria determined by Tvarijonaviciute et al. [7], and to correlate the criteria of dogs that would characterize the MS with different BCS.

2. Material and Methods

Between January 2013 and October 2014, 271 healthy dogs attended in Veterinary Hospitals of the Universidade Estadual do Norte do Paraná (Bandeirantes, Paraná State) and Universidade Estadual de Londrina (Londrina, Paraná State) and the Espaço Vida Veterinária (Londrina, Paraná State) were selected, to participate in this research. All owners signed an informed consent to participate in this research. This study was approved by ethics board of the animal experiments, State University of Northern Paraná, School of Veterinary Medicine, Department of Production and Veterinary Medicine, Bandeirantes, Paraná, Brazil, and is in accordance with the ethical principles of animal experimentation.

The animals remained fasting for 12 hours prior to the collection of blood samples. The dogs were weighed and had their body condition score (BCS) determined using the system of 9 points proposed by Laflamme [8] and distributed in these groups: control group (BCS 4-5/9), overweight group (BCS 6-7/9), and obese group (BCS 8-9/9). An initial screening to evaluate the overall health was performed including history, physical exam, blood count, serum chemistry profile, total thyroxin (TT4), free thyroxin (FT4), thyroid stimulating hormone (TSH), and suppression test low dose of dexamethasone (performed only in dogs over or equal to the BCS 6).

The animals with endocrine, liver, kidney and/or heart disease, heart failure congestive, and pancreatitis and those receiving glucocorticoids systemically or topically, anticonvulsant, and hypotensive drugs were excluded from the study. To exclude dogs with hypothyroidism FT4, TT4, and TSH tests were performed. Dogs that showed a decrease in TT4 concentration were excluded, even with no increase in TSH. To exclude dogs with Cushing's disease suppression test was performed with low dose of dexamethasone. The blood count, urinalysis, serum chemistry profile, and abdominal ultrasonography were used to rule out kidneys, liver, and pancreas diseases. The electrocardiography, echocardiography, and thoracic radiography were used to rule out heart diseases.

Definition of metabolic syndrome is as follows: (1) body score 7-9/9 points and two of the following criteria: (2) triglycerides >200 mg/dL (2,3 mmol/L); (3) total cholesterol >300 mg/dL (7,8 mmol/L); (4) systolic blood pressure >160 mmHg; (5) plasma glucose >100 mg/dL (5,6 mmol/L); (6) previous diagnosis of *diabetes mellitus* type 2.

2.1. Systolic Blood Pressure. Systolic blood pressure (SBP) was obtained by noninvasive method using Doppler flowmeter (Doppler Vascular DV 610, Medmega Industry Medical Equipment) as described previously [9]. SBP in five different measurements was obtained and the average was calculated, discarding the lowest and the highest. All dogs were in sternal recumbency and cuffs were selected according to the right forelimb diameter (40% of the circumference of the limb).

2.2. Sample Collection. Blood samples were collected by jugular venipuncture after 12 hours fasting in tubes containing clot activator and gel bottles containing sodium fluoride. The samples were centrifuged at 2000 G/minute for 10 minutes up to one hour after collection. After obtaining serum and plasma, the samples were stored in a freezer at −70°C. Serum cholesterol, triglycerides, and plasma concentrations of glucose were performed on automated chemistry analyzer (Catalyst One Chemistry Analyzer, IDEXX Laboratories, USA) using commercial kits and using the methodology recommended by the manufacturer, with a coefficient of variation within and between-run <2% for all analyses. Serum cortisol measurements (Total T4 RIA 125 kit, Siemens Healthcare Diagnostics, Tarrytown, NY), FT4 (Free T4, Two-Step, 125 I RIA Kit, DiaSorin, Stillwater, MN), and TSH (Canine TSH IRMA; Diagnostic Products Corp., Los Angeles, CA) were performed according to manufacturer's recommendations.

2.3. Statistical Analysis. The retrospective study evaluated a population of 6,729 dogs, where 2,557 were overweight and obese, and of these 271 (10.6%) met the inclusion and exclusion criteria.

The animals were classified into four groups: three according to the BCS: BCS 4-5 (ideal weight or control group), BCS 6-7 (overweight group), and BCS 8-9 (obese group); and the fourth group were the dogs with two or more inclusion criteria for MS. The inclusion of animals in the fourth group did not exclude groups based on BCS. The experimental design was completely randomized and considered any differences on serum levels of cholesterol, triglycerides, glucose, blood pressure, and age among the four groups. Variables not normal and equality by the Kolmogorov-Smirnov test and Liliefors test ($p < 0,05$). Thus, the differences between groups were assessed by Kruskal-Wallis test ($p < 0,05$). The percentage of dogs with hypercholesterolemia (>300 mg/dL), hypertriglyceridemia (>200 mg/dL), hyperglycemia (>100 mg/dL), and pressure (>160 mg/hg) was compared among the four groups tested by Chi-square test ($p < 0,05$). The occurrence of neutered dogs and ratio male/female was also compared among the four groups by Chi-square test ($p < 0,05$). The likelihood of these events occurring among the four groups was calculated using the odds ratio of the formula: $(p/(1 - p))/(q/(1-q))$, where p is the probability that an event occurs; q is the probability that the second event occurs. Within the group of dogs with two or more MS criteria the BCS with serum levels of cholesterol, triglycerides, glucose, and blood pressure were correlated by nonlinear Spearman correlation.

3. Results

The dogs were 2–14 years old, with 95 between 2 and 6 years old, 127 between 6 and 10 years old, and 49 between 10 and 14 years old. Crossbred dogs (102) were included as well as Beagle (6), Border Collie (8), Boxer (9), Chow-Chow (1),

TABLE 1: Median, minimum, and maximum values and number of observations (N) in 271 dogs grouped according to the BCS and inclusion criteria for metabolic syndrome.

		BCS 4-5 N = 101	BCS 6-7 N = 101	BCS 8-9 N = 69	MS N = 62
Cholesterol (mg/dL)	Average	196[a]	229[ab]	276[b]	418[c]
	Min–max	93–827	113–1055	131–827	175–1055
Triglycerides (mg/dL)	Average	124[a]	148[ab]	175.5[b]	299[c]
	Min–max	44–935	54–1005	74–1314	93–1314
Glucose (mg/dL)	Average	91[a]	94[ab]	97[bc]	108.5[c]
	Min–max	65–156	76–159	80–133	78–159
SH (mm/Hg)	Average	131[a]	135[a]	142[b]	144[b]
	Min–max	120–181	93–223	114–256	114–256
Age (years old)	Average	6[a]	8[b]	9[b]	8[b]
	Min–max	1–15	1–14	3–14	3–13

Medians followed by different letters in the same line showed differences ($p < 0.05$) according to the Kruskal-Wallis test. BCS: body condition scale and MS: metabolic syndrome.

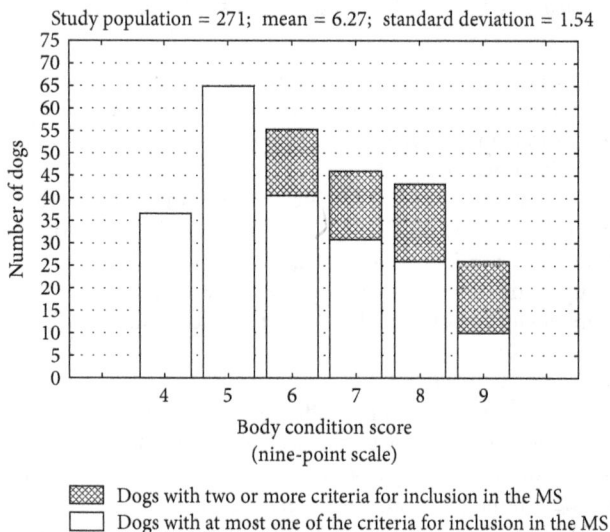

FIGURE 1: Absolute frequency of 271 dogs grouped according to the BCS and separated according to the number of criteria used for inclusion in the metabolic syndrome (MS).

Cocker Spaniel (8), Fila Brasileiro (1), Golden Retriever (3), Labrador Retriever (12), Lhasa Apso (16), Maltese (2), English Mastiff (1), German Shepherd (1), Pekingese (1), American Pit Bull Terrier (16), Poodle (23), Pug (3), Rottweiler (7), Schnauzer (8), Shih-Tzu (7), German Spitz (7), Dachshund (16), Brazilian Terrier (1), and Yorkshire Terrier (12).

Of the 271 dogs studied 62 (22,87%) had two or more MS inclusion criteria. Of these, 28 had BCS 6-7, while 34 dogs had BCS 8-9. Therefore, 27,72% of overweight dogs had MS inclusion criteria and 49,27% of obese had two or more MS inclusion criteria (Figure 1). This difference in proportion was considered significant in Chi-square test. No dog with BCS 4-5 showed two or more MS inclusion criteria.

Table 1 shows the distribution of cholesterol, blood glucose, triglycerides levels, and the BCS. For dogs in the group with two or more inclusion criteria for MS, fasting blood glucose was above 100 mg/dL in 39 (62,90%), hypertriglyceridemia in 57 (91,94%), hypercholesterolemia in 51 (82,26%), and systolic hypertension (SH) in 24 (38,71%). In these animals, 19 had higher triglycerides 400 mg/dL (moderate hypertriglyceridemia) and only two dogs had values greater than 1000 mg/dL (severe hypertriglyceridemia). In 20 dogs serum cholesterol concentration greater than 500 mg/dL (moderate hypercholesterolemia) was detected and eight dogs had values above 750 mg/dL (severe hypercholesterolemia). Of the 62 dogs in the MS group, 14 had moderate increase in the systolic hypertension (160–179 mmHg) and 10 had severe increase (>180 mmHg).

The breed distribution of the 62 dogs with MS was American Pit Bull Terrier (4/16), Beagle (4/6), Boxer (1/9), Cocker Spaniel (2/8), Labrador (2/12) Lhasa Apso (3/16), Maltese (1/2), Poodle (6/23), Pug (2/3), Rottweiler (1/7), Schnauzer (5/8), Shih-Tzu (2/7), Spitz German (1/7), Dachshund (1/16), Brazilian Terrier (1/1), Yorkshire Terrier (7/12), and crossbreed dogs (19/102).

The majority correlations occurring in the 62 dogs with MS were weak (Table 2), and only moderate association between serum concentrations of glucose and triglyceride (0,39), cholesterol and age (12 : 31), and BCS and SBP (0,38) occurred. The correlation between these variables is represented by polynomials expressed in Tables 2 and 3.

Table 3 shows that the frequency of hyperglycemia in dogs with BCS 4-5 was lower than other groups. The probability of a dog with MS to present hyperglycemia (37,09%) is the same as compared with BCS 6-7 and BCS 8-9. With regard to dogs with BCS 4-5 the ratio was statistically different and decreased to 14,85% the likelihood of a dog with these scores developing hyperglycemia. The chance of dogs with BCS >5 or MS present hyperglycemia was on average 2,91 times higher when compared to BCS 4-5.

Dogs with MS are 17,9% more likely to develop hypercholesterolemia than other groups (increased from 29,52% to 79,03%). In this group, the chance of animals having hypertriglyceridemia increases by 28,04 times compared to the group BCS 4-5.

TABLE 2: Spearman rank order correlations pairwise matrix from 62 dogs with two or more inclusion criteria for MS.

	Glucose	TG	COL	SBP	BCS	Age
Glucose		0.392171*	0.078798	0.034454	0.041343	−0.170240
TG	0.392171*		0.137775	−0.006817	0.072856	−0.198283
COL	0.078798	0.137775		−0.181512	0.016145	0.313763*
SBP	0.034454	−0.006817	−0.181512		0.385798*	−0.076325
BCS	0.041343	0.072856	0.016145	0.385798*		0.285910*
Age	−0.170240	−0.198283	0.313763*	−0.076325	0.285910*	

*Marked correlations are significant at $p < 0.05$. TG: triglycerides, COL: cholesterol, SBP: systolic blood pressure, MS: metabolic syndrome, and BCS: body condition score.

TABLE 3: Absolute frequency and relative hyperglycemia (>100 mg/dL), hypercholesterolemia (>300 mg/dL), hypertriglyceridemia (>200 mg/dL), hypertension (>160 mmHg), castration, and sex in 271 dogs grouped according to body condition and inclusion criteria for MS.

		BCS 4-5	BCS 6-7	BCS 8-9	MS
Hyperglycemia	Yes/no	15/86[a]	28/73[b]	25/44[b]	23/39[b]
	%	14.85	27.72	36.23	37.09
Hypercholesterolemia	Yes/no	18/83[a]	29/72[abc]	29/40[b]	49/13[d]
	%	17.82	28.71	42.03	79.03
Hypertriglyceridemia	Yes/no	16/85[a]	28/73[b]	30/39[c]	57/5[d]
	%	15.84	27.72	43.48	91.94
SH	Yes/no	1/100[a]	13/88[b]	19/50[c]	24/38[c]
	%	0.09	12.87	27.54	38.71
Spayed	Yes/no	40/61[a]	57/44[bc]	49/20[cd]	49/13[d]
	%	39.61	56.44	71.01	79.03
Sex	F/M	57/44[a]	66/35[a]	46/26[a]	38/24[a]
	%	56.44	65.35	62.32	61.29

Followed proportions of different letters in the same line differed in the Chi-square test ($p < 0.05$). SH: systolic hypertension, MS: metabolic syndrome, and BCS: body condition score.

The frequency of hypertension was higher in groups with BCS 8-9 and MS with values of 27,54% and 38,71%, respectively, and without difference when compared. But when compared to dogs of other groups there is statistical difference ($p < 0,05$). However, when comparing BCS 8-9 and MS group with others, the chance of developing hypertension decreases by 8,33 times (odds ratio) in BCS 4-5 and 6-7 group.

Neutering was associated with the BCS and the dogs with MS. In the MS group the probability of a dog being neutered was 79,03%, presenting 4,09 more chances (odds ratio) of having neutered dogs with MS than neutered dogs with BCS 4-5 and BCS 6-7. The proportion of females and males did not differ between groups according to the BCS and MS inclusion criteria.

4. Discussion

101 dogs (37,27%) had ideal weight, 101 (37,27%) were overweight, and 69 (25,46%) were obese and therefore 62,73% of the studied population was overweight, with results higher than previous studies [10, 11]. Nevertheless, the results do not reveal the prevalence of obesity in all three veterinary centers where the survey was conducted. In these places, the frequency of dogs overweight and obese was 47% in unpublished data.

The inclusion criteria in the MS group were found in Pugs (66%), Schnauzers (62,5%), Beagles (66%), Labradors (17%), and Yorkshire Terriers (58%) overweight and obese, admittedly breeds with higher risk for obesity [10, 11]. However, due to the small number of dogs of each breed in MS group multivariate linear regression could not be performed to assess whether it was adiposity, breed, or metabolic factors that influenced the development of the changes in the MS. The dogs that met the criteria for metabolic syndrome were of different races and sizes, and 28 of 62 dogs (45%) weighed even 10 kg of live weight. The findings suggest that small dogs have higher adiposity than medium or large dogs. However, more than 50% of the study population consisted of small dogs.

Elevation of cholesterol and triglycerides with the increases in the BCS can indicate that the degree of fat has influence on these substances, though the median values of cholesterol and triglycerides of MS group have slight increase. Serum triglyceride concentrations in dogs with BCS 8-9 and dogs with MS are similar in other studies [7, 12, 13] and higher in others [14, 15]. The median values of cholesterol in the BCS 8-9 group were similar to described previously [14, 15] but in the MS group were higher when compared to these same studies. Pancreatitis, hepatobiliary disease, atherosclerosis, eye damage [12], insulin resistance [16], and seizures are complications associated with hyperlipidemia, but none of the animals had these complications. In dogs overweight and obese 27 with triglycerides above 445 mg/dL and 19 (70,37%) dogs from MS group were observed. According to Verkest et al. [5], plasma concentrations above 445 mg/dL have been associated with increased immunoreactive lipase activity in the risk of developing pancreatitis.

The glucose values were higher ($p < 0,05$) in the MS group, probably due to insulin resistance. In dogs with BCS 6-7/8-9 and 9/9 median glucose was below 100 mg/dL, and similar results were described in which the average blood glucose level was lower than 100 mg/dL or 5,55 mol/L [15, 17, 18]. Only in MS group the median was greater than 100 mg/dL, indicating hyperglycemia according to the inclusion criteria described by Tvarijonaviciute et al. [7]. More studies are needed to define the cutoff point for the classification of hypoglycemic or normoglycemic animals [19], as well as the blood glucose cutoff point to cause insulin resistance. However, in this study the serum insulin and insulin resistance has not been evaluated. The comparison of induced obesity studies and spontaneous obesity studies can be misleading, because in spontaneous obesity it is not possible to accurately determine the time of fat mass accumulation and it can determine the development of insulin resistance.

The high SBP was the less common of the criteria among the four groups. However, the median values of the four groups were within normal values, which are values at low risk of developing lesions in target organs such as kidneys, retina, heart, and brain, worsening morbidity and mortality [20, 21]. Similar results were observed in 19 dogs with BCS 7-9/9 and 19 animals with BCS 5/9 [20].

Dogs can develop many of the components of the MSN: obesity [3, 4, 7, 17, 22, 23], insulin resistance [24], increased blood pressure [20, 24, 25], and hyperlipidemia [7, 13], and these changes were observed in 22% of the animals studied and in nearly 50% of dogs with BCS 8-9, with statistically significant difference from the other groups of this study.

In 22,87% dogs two or more inclusion criteria to MS group were observed, similar to another study that found 20% of 35 dogs with MS criteria [7]. Among the 69 dogs with BCS 8-9/9, 49,28% (34) had two or more inclusion criteria to MS group, while only 27,72% (28 of 101) of overweight dogs had it. Apparently the degree and duration of fatness and visceral/central adiposity have contributed to the dogs being classified in MS. However, further research is needed to develop a method of measuring central obesity that may contribute to the understanding of the metabolic changes of obesity.

Of the 62 dogs the fasting blood glucose was higher than 100 mg/dL in 39 patients (62,9%), hypertriglyceridemia was present in 57 (91,94%), hypercholesterolemia in 51 (82,26%), and SBP in 24 (38,71%) of dogs. However, Tvarijonaviciute et al. [7] observed elevated blood glucose in 31,43%, serum triglycerides in 8,57%, cholesterol in 14,43%, and SBP in 28,57% of dogs included in the MS group, differing from our findings. The reasons for these differences have not been determined, but the variation in collection time and the objectives of the studies (effects of weight loss versus epidemiological study) may have contributed to the results obtained. Hyperglycemia has been reported in previous studies, but the cutoff point is a factor that differs largely

[13, 17–19, 26], but was not present in other studies [5, 27]. In 39 dogs that had blood glucose levels above 100 mg/dL, 13 had values between 120 and 159 mg/dL. According to criteria adopted in this study fasting hyperglycemia was observed.

Dogs from MS group were 2,91 times more likely to develop hyperglycemia when compared to dogs with BCS 4-5. It is demonstrated that the adiposity increases the risk of elevated blood glucose or hyperglycemia, as previous studies [12, 13, 17, 18, 26, 27].

The occurrence of spontaneous hypercholesterolemia, hypertriglyceridemia, and obesity [2, 7, 14, 15, 28] as the induced obesity [3] has been described. Our results differ from these studies because, between the dogs with inclusion criteria for MS, 20 had moderate hypercholesterolemia and eight severe hypercholesterolemia. However, most obese dogs presented cholesterol values below (>750 mg/dL) the risk limits for the development of atherogenic disease [4, 16, 29] while 12,95% of 69 dogs had cholesterol in the risk range for the development of atherosclerosis. In 19 dogs for MS group only two dogs had severe hypertriglyceridemia, as described in obese dogs [13, 18, 26, 29]. There are rare reports of obese dogs with values above 1000 mg/dL and in this study, only two dogs had increased values.

Occurrence of hypercholesterolemia was like other studies [7, 12, 18, 28, 29]. The hypertriglyceridemia (43,48%) was present in dogs with BCS 8-9, higher than observed for Brunetto et al. [29]. However, it was not possible to assess whether this is due to the inclusion in the MS group or the influence of adiposity, but the risk of developing hypertriglyceridemia was lower than 10 times in obese animals than in those with normal weight and overweight.

The frequency of hypertension was higher in groups with score 8-9 and MS (27,54% and 38,71%, resp.) without difference when compared. This value is higher than that described by other authors [20, 24]. Rocchini et al. [30] found that weight gain caused an increase in SBP, while other researchers found no correlation between obesity and SBP [25]. Contributing to the claims of the latter authors, a recent study found that 10 of 35 dogs had SBP higher than 160 mmHg and with the weight loss eight dogs remained with the SBP at the same levels [10]. The differences could be due to population differences, breed, age, and time of adiposity in dogs, as well as the absence of comorbidities in this group. Also, obesity may be a risk factor in the development of hypertension. When comparing the dogs of BCS 8-9 and MS group with others, the chance of developing hypertension decreases in 8:33 times (odds ratio) in the BCS 4-5 and BCS 6-7 groups. The fact that the dogs with MS brings more risks in the development of hypertension may be important in obese dogs with other comorbidities that predispose to hypertension, as endocrine and kidney diseases. This fact justifies the importance of adopting a metabolic classification as proposed by Tvarijonaviciute et al. [7]. It is important to conduct further studies in dogs with comorbidities and to define inclusion criteria for MS.

In obese dogs, hypertension can occur by different mechanisms including the activation of the renin-angiotensin-aldosterone axis [31], hyperadrenergic activation and insulin resistance causing hyperadrenergic activation [32], and increased production of angiotensin and proinflammatory cytokines [17, 31, 33]. The moderate to severe increase associated with other changes in the MS group such as dyslipidemia and elevated blood glucose, and probably resistance insulin, may contribute to the development of complications associated with hypertension including stroke (CVA), retinopathy, choroidopathy, ventricular hypertrophy, albuminuria/microalbuminuria, and nephropathy [12, 17].

Previous studies have found a few animals with severe metabolic parameters [10, 14, 18]. It was not possible in this study to indicate the causes of these differences, but the fatness can contribute to higher levels of metabolic parameters. The highest number of animals studied and less time collecting samples compared to that performed may be one of the causes of these differences, which pointed out that these authors aimed to compare the MS parameters before and after loss weight.

Schnauzer dogs may have primary dyslipidemia. Therefore, the inclusion of this breed in this study on the prevalence of MS may be debatable. However, the authors chose to include them, since all the criteria for MS were met, so the dogs of this breed had to have hypertension, blood glucose >100 mg/dL, hypertriglyceridemia, and hypercholesterolemia. The five dogs of this breed in the study had all the criteria of MS but have a previous diagnosis of *diabetes mellitus* and moreover were aged between 3 and 8 years.

In MS group the probability of a dog being neutered was 79,03%, with 4,09 likely (odds ratio) to have neutered dogs with MS compared to neutered dogs with scores 4-5 and 6-7. This result is similar to those described, because castration increases the risk of obesity and probably also increases the risk of the development of the factors leading MS [18].

Age at MS group showed the same behavior described earlier in obese dogs; in other words, it was more common in older dogs (over 6 years of age). Apparently, age seems to influence the development of alterations compatible with MS, probably due to longer adiposity.

Some problems were detected in this study, such as the inability to determine the risk factors for the inclusion of the 62 dogs in the MS group because when it held the division into categories by breed, age, sex, neutered or not spayed, type of feed, or level of physical activity each category had a small number of animals. Another problem was the nonquantification of fat by dual-energy X-ray absorptiometry (DEXA) and its influence on severe increases in SBP, serum concentrations of cholesterol and triglycerides in the MS group dogs, and determining the time of adiposity of animals included in the study. The absence of serum insulin and HOMA test to identify impaired glucose tolerance and/or insulin resistance is another deficiency in this study. However, it is well established that animals overweight and obese may have hyperinsulinemia [5, 13, 18, 26, 27].

According to the criteria defined it was determined that significant portion (about 22%) of overweight and obese dogs have metabolic abnormalities consistent with MS. However, a longitudinal study of this population makes it possible to detect whether these animals are at risk of developing complications such as *diabetes mellitus*, atherosclerosis, heart attack, and stroke [25], which are described as complications of MS in humans, but the occurrence is questionable in dogs [19].

Based on the results we can say that the long-term changes may bring clinical changes. Therefore, we disagree with other authors who claim that this classification for the MS is unnecessary. There are currently not well-defined values cut to the serum concentration of triglycerides, cholesterol, and glucose levels as we have for the SBP, but it is important to try to set them on the basis of normal values. Future studies are needed to identify why some dogs develop metabolic changes (hyperglycemia, insulin resistance, hyperlipidemia, and hypertension) associated with obesity and others do not. The reasons dogs apparently do not develop the consequences of MS from other species like type II diabetes, atherosclerosis, and stroke also require confirmation as they are currently not known.

5. Conclusions

It follows that the metabolic syndrome according to the parameters defined in the literature for inclusion was observed in 22,87% of the animals studied and in 36% of dogs overweight or obese. Furthermore, the MS was most common in obese (49%) compared to overweight dogs (27%).

Competing Interests

The authors disclose no conflict of interests.

Acknowledgments

The authors acknowledge Araucaria Foundation for project financing (931/13) and the granting of Scientific Initiation Scholarships.

References

[1] D. Leroith, "Pathophysiology of the metabolic syndrome: implications for the cardiometabolic risks associated with type 2 diabetes," *American Journal of the Medical Sciences*, vol. 343, no. 1, pp. 13–16, 2012.

[2] N. Frank, "Equine metabolic syndrome," *Journal of Equine Veterinary Science*, vol. 29, no. 5, pp. 259–267, 2009.

[3] I. C. Jeusette, E. T. Lhoest, L. P. Istasse, and M. O. Diez, "Influence of obesity on plasma lipid and lipoprotein concentrations in dogs," *American Journal of Veterinary Research*, vol. 66, no. 1, pp. 81–86, 2005.

[4] K. Kawasumi, T. Suzuki, M. Fujiwara, N. Mori, I. Yamamoto, and T. Arai, "New criteria for canine metabolic syndrome in Japan," *Journal of Animal and Veterinary Advances*, vol. 11, no. 21, pp. 4005–4007, 2012.

[5] K. R. Verkest, L. M. Fleeman, J. M. Morton, K. Ishioka, and J. S. Rand, "Compensation for obesity-induced insulin resistance in dogs: assessment of the effects of leptin, adiponectin, and glucagon-like peptide-1 using path analysis," *Domestic Animal Endocrinology*, vol. 41, no. 1, pp. 24–34, 2011.

[6] P. Zimmet, E. J. Boyko, G. R. Collier, and M. D. Courten, "Etiology of the metabolic syndrome: potential role of insulin resistance, leptin resistance, and other players," *Annals New York Academy Sciences*, vol. 18, pp. 25–44, 1999.

[7] A. Tvarijonaviciute, J. J. Ceron, S. L. Holden et al., "Obesity-related metabolic dysfunction in dogs: a comparison with human metabolic syndrome," *BMC Veterinary Research*, vol. 8, pp. 147–154, 2012.

[8] D. P. Laflamme, "Development and validation of a body condition score system for dogs," *Canine Practice*, vol. 22, pp. 10–15, 1997.

[9] R. A. Henik, M. K. Dolson, and L. J. Wenholz, "How to obtain a blood pressure measurement," *Clinical Techniques in Small Animal Practice*, vol. 20, no. 3, pp. 144–150, 2005.

[10] K. P. Aptekmann, W. G. Suhett, A. F. M. Junior et al., "Nutritional and environment aspects of canine obesity," *Ciencia Rural*, vol. 44, no. 11, pp. 2039–2044, 2014.

[11] E. A. Courcier, R. M. Thomson, D. J. Mellor, and P. S. Yam, "An epidemiological study of environmental factors associated with canine obesity," *Journal of Small Animal Practice*, vol. 51, no. 7, pp. 362–367, 2010.

[12] N. Mori, P. Lee, K. Kondo, T. Kido, T. Saito, and T. Arai, "Potential use of cholesterol lipoprotein profile to confirm obesity status in dogs," *Veterinary Research Communications*, vol. 35, no. 4, pp. 223–235, 2011.

[13] K. R. Verkest, L. M. Fleeman, J. S. Rand, and J. M. Morton, "Evaluation of beta-cell sensitivity to glucose and first-phase insulin secretion in obese dogs," *American Journal of Veterinary Research*, vol. 72, no. 3, pp. 357–366, 2011.

[14] H.-J. Park, S.-E. Lee, J.-H. Oh, K.-W. Seo, and K.-H. Song, "Leptin, adiponectin and serotonin levels in lean and obese dogs," *BMC Veterinary Research*, vol. 10, article no. 113, 2014.

[15] R. M. Yamka, K. G. Friesen, and N. Z. Frantz, "Identification of canine markers related to obesity and the effects of weight loss on the markers of interest," *International Journal Applied Research Veterinary Medicine*, vol. 4, pp. 282–292, 2006.

[16] J. D. Chiu, C. M. Kolka, J. M. Richey et al., "Experimental hyperlipidemia dramatically reduces access of insulin to canine skeletal muscle," *Obesity*, vol. 17, no. 8, pp. 1486–1492, 2009.

[17] A. J. German, M. Hervera, L. Hunter et al., "Improvement in insulin resistance and reduction in plasma inflammatory adipokines after weight loss in obese dogs," *Domestic Animal Endocrinology*, vol. 37, no. 4, pp. 214–226, 2009.

[18] G. B. Li, P. Lee, N. Mori et al., "Supplementing five-point body condition score with body fat percentage increases the sensitivity for assessing overweight status of small to medium sized dogs," *Veterinary Medicine: Research and Reports*, vol. 3, pp. 71–78, 2012.

[19] K. R. Verkest, "Is the metabolic syndrome a useful clinical concept in dogs? A review of the evidence," *Veterinary Journal*, vol. 199, no. 1, pp. 24–30, 2014.

[20] E. Mehlman, M. J. Bright, C. Porsche, D. N. R. Veeramachaneni, and M. Frye, "Echocardiographic evidence of left ventricular hypertrophy in obese dogs," *Journal Veterinary Internal Medicine*, vol. 27, no. 1, pp. 62–68, 2013.

[21] G. B. P. Neto, M. A. Brunetto, M. G. Sousa, A. C. Carciofi, and A. A. Camacho, "Effects of weight loss on the cardiac parameters of obese dogs," *Pesquisa Veterinária Brasileira*, vol. 30, no. 2, pp. 167–171, 2010.

[22] N. Thengchaisri, W. Theerapun, S. Kaewmokul, and A. Sastravaha, "Abdominal obesity is associated with heart disease in dogs," *BMC Veterinary Research*, vol. 10, article no. 131, 2014.

[23] K. R. Verkest, L. M. Fleeman, J. M. Morton et al., "Association of postprandial serum triglyceride concentration and serum canine pancreatic lipase immunoreactivity in overweight and obese dogs," *Journal of Veterinary Internal Medicine*, vol. 26, no. 1, pp. 46–53, 2012.

[24] A. P. Pérez-Sánchez, J. Del-Angel-Caraza, I. A. Quijano-Hernández, and M. A. Barbosa-Mireles, "Obesity-hypertension and its relation to other diseases in dogs," *Veterinary Research Communications*, vol. 39, no. 1, pp. 45–51, 2015.

[25] A. R. Bodey and A. R. Michell, "Epidemiological study of blood pressure in domestic dogs," *Journal of Small Animal Practice*, vol. 37, no. 3, pp. 116–125, 1996.

[26] K. R. Verkest, J. S. Rand, L. M. Fleeman, and J. M. Morton, "Spontaneously obese dogs exhibit greater postprandial glucose, triglyceride, and insulin concentrations than lean dogs," *Domestic Animal Endocrinology*, vol. 42, no. 2, pp. 103–112, 2012.

[27] K. R. Verkest, L. M. Fleeman, J. S. Rand, and J. M. Morton, "Basal measures of insulin sensitivity and insulin secretion and simplified glucose tolerance tests in dogs," *Domestic Animal Endocrinology*, vol. 39, no. 3, pp. 194–204, 2010.

[28] M. M. Jericó, F. C. De Chiquito, K. Kajihara et al., "Chromatographic analysis of lipid fractions in healthy dogs and dogs with obesity or hyperadrenocorticism," *Journal of Veterinary Diagnostic Investigation*, vol. 21, no. 2, pp. 203–207, 2009.

[29] M. A. Brunetto, S. Nogueira, F. C. Sá, M. Peixoto Ricardo Souza Vasconcellos, A. J. Ferraudo, and A. C. Carciofi, "Correspondence between obesity and hyperlipidemia in dogs," *Ciencia Rural*, vol. 41, no. 2, pp. 266–271, 2011.

[30] A. P. Rocchini, C. P. Moorehead, S. DeRemer, and D. Bondie, "Pathogenesis of weight-related changes in blood pressure in dogs," *Hypertension*, vol. 13, no. 6, pp. 922–928, 1989.

[31] K. Rahmouni, M. L. G. Correia, W. G. Haynes, and A. L. Mark, "Obesity-associated hypertension: new insights into mechanisms," *Hypertension*, vol. 45, no. 1, pp. 9–14, 2005.

[32] J. E. Hall, "Pathophysiology of obesity hypertension," *Current Hypertension Reports*, vol. 2, no. 2, pp. 139–147, 2000.

[33] A. Tvarijonaviciute, F. Tecles, S. Martínez-Subiela, and J. J. Cerón, "Effect of weight loss on inflammatory biomarkers in obese dogs," *The Veterinary Journal*, vol. 193, no. 2, pp. 570–572, 2012.

9

Respiratory Support for Pharmacologically Induced Hypoxia in Neonatal Calves

C. G. Donnelly,[1] C. T. Quinn,[2] S. G. Nielsen,[3] and S. L. Raidal[2]

[1]*Cornell University College of Veterinary Medicine, Ithaca, NY 14850, USA*
[2]*School of Animal and Veterinary Sciences, Charles Sturt University, Wagga Wagga, NSW 2650, Australia*
[3]*Quantitative Consulting Unit, Research Office, Charles Sturt University, Wagga Wagga, NSW 2650, Australia*

Correspondence should be addressed to S. L. Raidal; sraidal@csu.edu.au

Academic Editor: Yoshiaki Hikasa

Practical methods to provide respiratory support to bovine neonates in a field setting are poorly characterised. This study evaluated the response of healthy neonatal calves with pharmacologically induced respiratory suppression to nasal oxygen insufflation and to continuous positive airway pressure (CPAP) delivered via an off-the-shelf device. Ten calves were randomised to receive either nasal oxygen insufflation (Group 1, $n = 5$) or CPAP (Group 2, $n = 5$) as a first treatment after induction of respiratory depression by intravenous administration of xylazine, fentanyl, and diazepam. Calves received the alternate treatment after 10 minutes of breathing ambient air. Arterial blood gas samples were obtained prior to sedation, following sedation, following the first and second treatment, and after breathing ambient air before and after the second treatment. Oxygen insufflation significantly increased arterial oxygen partial pressure (PaO_2) but was also associated with significant hypercapnia. When used as the first treatment, CPAP was associated with significantly decreased arterial partial pressure of carbon dioxide but did not increase PaO_2. These results suggest that the use of CPAP may represent a practical method for correction of hypercapnia associated with inadequate ventilation in a field setting, and further research is required to characterise the use of CPAP with increased inspired oxygen concentrations.

1. Introduction

Respiratory dysfunction is recognised as a major source of mortality and morbidity in the bovine neonate [1, 2]. Prematurity, asphyxia, meconium aspiration, infection, and persistent pulmonary hypertension may play a role in the development of respiratory dysfunction and resultant hypoxaemia, hypercapnia, and acidosis [3]. Respiratory compromise can further contribute to an impaired ability to maintain homeostasis and thermogenesis, thereby reducing calf vitality [3, 4].

Respiratory disease in the bovine neonate has been reviewed previously [3, 5]. Conditions resulting from maladaption to the extrauterine environment are more likely to be seen in preterm neonates [6] and are primarily manifest as respiratory distress syndrome (RDS). The primary cause of RDS is a lack of surfactant; however, meconium aspiration and vascular shunting may contribute to respiratory dysfunction. The incidence of this syndrome has been estimated to be

as high as 66% in calves, with one-third of farms reporting at least one loss to the condition each year [7]. Calves with increased muscling and calves born after Caesarian section are at greater risk for development of RDS; hence the incidence of the condition may be higher in neonates of increased genetic or financial value [7–10].

There is little information available in the literature on respiratory support of neonatal cattle, as well as an overall deficiency of evidence for respiratory support techniques in large animal neonatology other than in foals [11]. Treatment of respiratory dysfunction in the bovine neonate is poorly documented and seldom practiced due to the lack of supervision at birth and the limited availability of equipment and expertise to treat bovine neonates. The application of intranasal oxygen insufflation, although not commonly used, has been reported for bovine neonates with respiratory compromise [3, 12–14]. However, there is evidence of detrimental effects of oxygen delivery on respiratory physiology and cerebral blood flow [15, 16] and treatment failure may occur due to vascular shunting [13], hypoventilation, prematurity, and decreased surfactant [14]. Synchronised intermittent mandatory ventilation has been used to mechanically ventilate calves that did not respond to oxygen insufflation [13, 17] in a dedicated research and specialist hospital facility, with modest survival to discharge. Pharmacological agents, such as doxapram and methylxanthines, have been used as respiratory stimulants [18] but have the potential to reduce cerebral blood flow and may result in negative long-term neurological complications.

Continuous positive airway pressure (CPAP) has been advocated in human neonatology and cardiopulmonary resuscitation. The use of the technique for ventilatory support of human patients was reported as early as the 1930s [19, 20], but use in neonates was not described until much later [21]. In combination with the administration of exogenous surfactant and preterm glucocorticoid administration, CPAP is now widely used for respiratory support of human neonates [22–24]. CPAP primarily improves ventilation but may also have a role in improving intrapulmonary perfusion by increasing transpulmonary pressure (as inspiratory and expiratory pressure are maintained higher than ambient pressure), resulting in an increased functional reserve capacity (FRC). Increased FRC has several follow-on effects including reduced work of breathing, redistribution of lung fluid, reduction in airway resistance, decreased intrapulmonary shunting, and improved surfactant function. Cumulatively these responses improve oxygenation and reduce the partial pressure of carbon dioxide. This is advantageous for neonatal respiratory support as these patients are subject to reduced FRC, atelectasis, and increased work of breathing. The technique is technically less demanding than true ventilatory techniques and is less invasive than mechanical ventilation. It is therefore more readily available and is not associated with complications such as bronchopulmonary dysplasia or tracheal necrosis.

To date there has been limited evaluation of CPAP for respiratory support of neonates in the veterinary literature. Use of the technique in preterm neonatal lambs resulted in a greater increase in lung compliance, volume, and FRC than mechanical ventilation or no treatment [6]. More broadly, Briganti et al. [25] demonstrated increased arterial oxygen partial pressure following CPAP treatment of sedated adult dogs, compared to oxygen insufflation alone. The technique has been used in anaesthetised adult horses [26–28].

The rise in advanced reproduction techniques including *in vitro* embryo production and cloning, combined with the increased economic value of these calves, suggests that the incidence and inclination to intervene in bovine neonatal respiratory disease will increase [13], and this warrants the development of appropriate therapies for respiratory support of newborn calves [29]. Investigations into improved methods of support must include scope for ease of treatment and cost of equipment and utility in a field setting. As CPAP is less demanding than ventilation, CPAP may present an appropriate technique for use in the bovine neonate. The adaptation of techniques utilising readily available portable compressor driven devices is particularly attractive as a field treatment for neonatal calves without the need for supplemental oxygen, advanced expertise, or more invasive ventilator support. The present study was undertaken as a pilot study to evaluate the effect of oxygen insufflation and a portable off-the-shelf CPAP device on arterial blood gas measurements in calves delivered by Caesarean section and following pharmacological induction of hypoxaemia.

2. Materials and Methods

2.1. Experimental Animals. Six male (BW 38 ± 7 kg) and six female (BW 37 ± 4.4 kg) Angus ($n = 10$) and Angus-Hereford cross ($n = 2$) calves were made available for inclusion in this study following elective Caesarean delivery (gestation day 275 ± 7). Surgeries occurred over two days with six calves delivered on each day. Cows were pretreated on gestation day 274 ± 7 with dexamethasone (0.44 mg/kg, Dexafort 3 mg/mL, Intervet, East Bendigo, Australia) and received preoperative procaine penicillin (Depocillin 300 mg/mL, MSD Animal Health, East Bendigo, Australia) (40 mg/kg by intramuscular injection) and clenbuterol (Planipart 30 μg/mL, Boehringer Ingelheim, North Ryde, Australia) (0.65 mg/kg by intramuscular injection). At delivery calves were suspended vertically by their hind legs for a period of 30 seconds. Neonatal viability was assessed at this time and again after five minutes using a modified Apgar score adapted from Born [30]. Calves were allowed to nurse from their dam, with time to stand and nurse recorded. Calves were considered suitable for inclusion in this experiment if they had an Apgar score ≥ 6 at five minutes postpartum and physical examination within normal limits at 20–24 hours of age. All procedures were undertaken at 20–24 hours postpartum and were approved by the Animal Care and Ethics Committee at Charles Sturt University (ACEC 12/037).

2.2. Experimental Method. Calves were restrained in left lateral recumbency on foam matting for the duration of the experiment. Calves were not sedated before restraint nor during preparation for sampling. The right jugular grove and left medial antebrachium were clipped and surgically prepared with chlorhexidine and alcohol. A 16-gauge two-and-a-half-inch catheter (Surflo catheter, Terumo, Tokyo, Japan) was placed in the right jugular vein and a 22-gauge one-inch catheter (Surflo catheter, Terumo, Tokyo, Japan) was placed in the left brachial artery. Catheters were secured with polyacrylamide adhesive and patency was maintained with heparinised saline (5 IU/L). Data collection began immediately following placement of these catheters (T0) with collection of both venous and arterial samples. Venous samples were collected into EDTA and serum vacutainers (BD Australia, North Ryde, Australia) for complete blood count and serum biochemistry. Arterial samples were collected anaerobically into preheparinised syringes (BD Preset Arterial Blood Gas Syringe, BD Australia, North Ryde, Australia) for blood gas analysis, as described below.

Respiratory depression was induced by treatment with diazepam (Pamlin 5 mg/mL, Parnell, Alexandria, Australia) (0.1 mg/kg IV), xylazine hydrochloride (Xylazil 10 mg/mL, Troy Laboratories, Glendenning, Australia) (0.01 mg/kg IV), and fentanyl (fentanyl 50 μg/mL, DBL Hospira, Melbourne, Australia) (3 μg/kg IV). At this time and throughout the course of the experiment calves were monitored with an oxygen saturation probe (Masimo Radical, Masimo Australia, Frenchs Forest, Australia). Arterial samples were collected anaerobically as follows:

T0: baseline—before tranquilization with calves breathing ambient air.

T1: ten minutes after administration of sedation, calves breathing ambient air.

T2: ten minutes after initiation of respiratory support (CPAP or oxygen insufflation).

T3: rest—ten minutes following discontinuation of initial respiratory support, breathing ambient air.

T4: ten minutes after initiation of alternate respiratory support (oxygen insufflation or CPAP).

T5: recovery—ten minutes following discontinuation of second respiratory intervention, breathing ambient air.

Heart rate, rectal temperature, and oxygen saturation data were also collected at each time point. Oxygen saturation was determined by pulse oximetry (Masimo Radical, Masimo Australia, Frenchs Forest, Australia), with the probe attached to the lip (nonpigmented animals) or tongue. At the conclusion of the experiment calves were administered with an equipotent dose of atipamezole (Antisedan 5 mg/mL, Pfizer Animal Health, West Ryde, Australia) (0.01 mg/kg IM) to reverse the effects of xylazine.

2.3. Respiratory Support.

Both CPAP and oxygen insufflation were delivered via a standard canine anaesthesia mask following validation of mask fit and pressure maintenance using a pressure manometer during CPAP in pilot cadaver studies. Mask dead space was approximately 250 millilitres, measured by water displacement. The mask used to provide CPAP was modified to accommodate exhaust gases by drilling a series of holes into the upper portion of the mask to allow for the escape of gas during expiration and thereby prevent mask seal failure. CPAP was provided using a titrated off-the-shelf constant pressure generator (Resmed 8, ResMed Inc., Bella Vista, Australia). The machine generated a positive pressure via compressor, delivering room air at 10 cm H_2O. Air delivered via the CPAP apparatus was not humidified and did not include a ramp. Humidified oxygen was delivered through standard oxygen tubing to the mask at a rate of 5 L/min.

2.4. Blood Gas Analysis.

Samples obtained anaerobically from the brachial artery catheter into preheparinised syringes were immediately placed on ice and processed within 4 hours of collection [31]. Samples were processed in order of collection. Arterial blood pH, partial pressure of oxygen (PaO_2), partial pressure of carbon dioxide ($PaCO_2$), lactate, bicarbonate (HCO_3^-), and oxygen saturation were determined using a bench-top analyser (GEM Premier 3500, Instrumentation Laboratory, Brisbane, Australia), with values adjusted for contemporaneous rectal temperature.

2.5. Experimental Design and Statistical Analysis.

A randomised block design was utilised with first treatment (oxygen insufflation or CPAP) assigned by random number generation. Pairs of calves were considered one replicate, with each calf of a replicate pair receiving a different first treatment. For analysis, Group 1 calves received oxygen supplementation (5 L/min) at T2, followed by CPAP at T4; Group 2 calves received CPAP at T2 and oxygen insufflation at T4. Analysis of covariance (ANCOVA) was performed using the statistical software R (GNU Operating Systems, MIT, Cambridge, USA) with time and treatment (oxygen supplementation or CPAP) as fixed effects and calf and replicate as covariates. Data distribution was tested for normality using Levine's test. Weighted analysis was performed on nonnormal data. *Post hoc* evaluation was performed using Tukey's test to verify independence, with differences considered significant for $P \leq 0.05$. Respiratory support (oxygen insufflation and CPAP) and treatment order were further evaluated by two-way repeated measures analysis of variance with time (T2 and T4) and treatment (O_2 and CPAP) as factors. Unless otherwise stated, data are presented as mean $\pm$ standard deviation.

3. Results

3.1. Clinical Observations.

Twelve calves were available for inclusion in the experiment. One calf was excluded at the beginning of the experiment because a patent arterial cannulation could not be established. A second calf was excluded due to an umbilical infection, detected at the preexperiment physical exam. Data is presented from the remaining five male (BW 39.7 $\pm$ 7 kg) and five female calves (38.1 $\pm$ 3.7 kg). Birth weight (39.4 $\pm$ 6.6) for Group 1 calves (receiving oxygen at T2 and CPAP at T4) was not significantly different to that recorded for Group 2 calves (35.6 $\pm$ 4.8) ($P = 0.11$). The Apgar score was greater at five minutes postpartum (7.5 $\pm$ 0.7) than immediately after birth (5.6 $\pm$ 1.2), but this difference was not significant ($P \geq 0.05$). All calves met the inclusion criterion of an Apgar score ≥ 6 at five minutes postpartum. Mean score for Group 1 calves (4.8 $\pm$ 0.8) was significantly less than that of Group 2 calves (6.6 $\pm$ 0.9) immediately after birth ($P = 0.01$), but differences were not significant by 5 minutes postpartum (7.8 $\pm$ 0.4, Group 1; 7.0 $\pm$ 0.7, Group 2; $P = 0.07$).

Both mask insufflation and mask delivered CPAP were well tolerated. No adverse response to the placement of the mask, or to the sound of the machine, was observed during this experiment and no attempt was made by calves to remove the mask. Mask seal failure during CPAP, recognised as machine alerts, was observed infrequently, and all failures were immediately rectified by adjustment of the mask position. Subjectively, the expiratory effort of calves was mildly increased during CPAP treatment when compared to efforts observed during oxygen insufflation or between treatments whilst breathing ambient air. No complications attributable to treatment with CPAP or oxygen were encountered during the experiment.

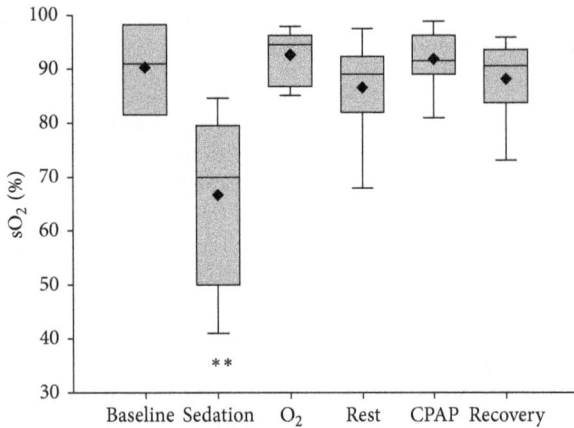

FIGURE 1: Haemaglobin saturation determined by pulse oximetry following sedation and respiratory support by oxygen insufflation or continuous positive airway pressure (CPAP). Values are shown as median (horizontal line), mean (diamond), quartiles, and range immediately after catheter placement (T0, baseline), 10 minutes following sedation (T1, sedation), following 10 minutes of oxygen supplementation (O_2), following 10 minutes of CPAP, and after 10 minutes of breathing ambient air following respiratory support (T3, rest, and T5, recovery). Order of respiratory support (O_2 supplementation or CPAP) was randomly assigned to replicate groups of paired calves and administered at T2 (5 calves) or T4 (5 calves); treatment order had no significant effect on response to O_2 supplementation or CPAP. Values obtained following sedation were significantly less than at all other times ($**P < 0.001$).

Calves were markedly affected by the sedation protocol, which consistently produced recumbency and obtunded mentation. Oxygen saturation (sO_2) was significantly reduced following sedation ($P < 0.01$, Figure 1) and was increased following respiratory support. Treatment order (CPAP or O_2 insufflation as first treatment) did not have a significant effect on the observed response. Recovery following reversal was variable between calves, with most regaining ambulation within four hours. Two calves did not regain ambulation for more than four hours, with one of these calves treated with intravenous fluids and naloxone. Both calves were able to maintain sternal recumbency following reversal, and by 24 hours after the experiment all calves demonstrated no residual effects. At one week of age calves included in the experiment had gained equivalent amounts of weight to calves that were delivered at the same time and not included in the experiment.

3.2. Blood Gas Analysis. Time of sampling had a significant effect ($P = 0.001$) on PaO_2, and there was a significant time and treatment interaction ($P = 0.000$). Sedation decreased PaO_2 values from 57.8 ± 16.9 mmHg at T0 to 31.5 ± 11.9 mmHg, although this difference was not significant (Figure 2). Oxygen insufflation, but not CPAP, caused increased PaO_2 relative to postsedation values. This effect was significant at both T2 and T4 and although values obtained at T2 (102.4 ± 61.5 mmHg) were less than those obtained at T4 (146.6 ± 91.0 mmHg), this difference was not significantly

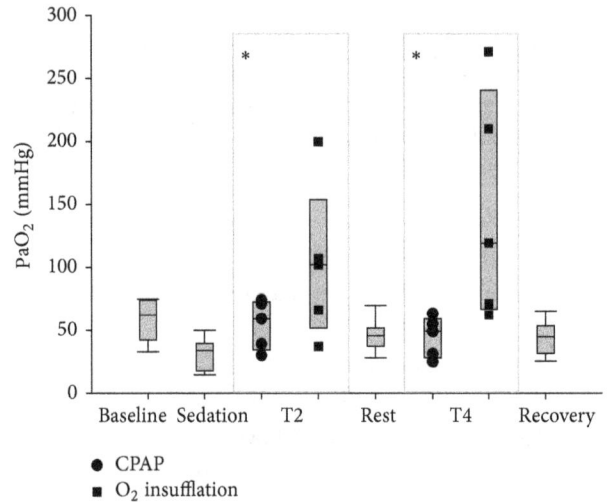

● CPAP
■ O_2 insufflation

FIGURE 2: Arterial partial pressure of oxygen (PaO_2) following respiratory support by oxygen insufflation or continuous positive airway pressure (CPAP). Values are shown as median (horizontal line) and quartiles and range immediately after catheter placement (T0, baseline), 10 minutes following sedation (T1, sedation), following 10 minutes of oxygen supplementation (O_2), following 10 minutes of CPAP, and after 10 minutes of breathing ambient air following respiratory support (T3, rest, and T5, recovery). Individual results following respiratory support (CPAP or O_2 insufflation) are shown at T2 and T4. Order of respiratory support at T2 (CPAP or O_2 insufflation) was randomly assigned to replicate groups of paired calves. The alternate treatment (O_2 insufflation or CPAP) was administered at T4. Values obtained following O_2 insufflation were significantly greater than values obtained following sedation ($P < 0.05$). Treatment order had no significant effect on response to O_2 supplementation or CPAP.

different. There was no apparent effect on PaO_2 attributable to CPAP at T2 (54.6 ± 19.4 mmHg) or T4 (44.6 ± 16.1 mmHg), although values obtained were greater than was observed following sedation (31.5 ± 11.9 mmHg).

Significant time ($P = 0.009$) and treatment ($P = 0.012$) effects were observed on arterial $PaCO_2$, although treatment and time interactions were not significant. Arterial CO_2 partial pressure was increased following sedation (64.5 ± 3.5 mmHg, mean $\pm$ sd) compared with baseline values (55.7 ± 7.2 mmHg), and oxygen insufflation was associated with a further increase in $PaCO_2$ (69.3 ± 9.4 mmHg, Figure 3). This trend was more marked in calves receiving oxygen insufflation at T2, 10 minutes following sedation. When order of treatment was taken into account, CPAP resulted in significantly lower $PaCO_2$ levels if it was used as a first treatment (T2) than was observed following oxygen supplementation at this time ($P < 0.05$).

Blood pH was significantly affected by treatment ($P = 0.050$) and time ($P = 0.007$). Consistent with changes in $PaCO_2$, pH was decreased following sedation (7.31 ± 0.03) and after oxygen treatment (7.27 ± 0.06), when compared to baseline results (7.37 ± 0.04) (Figure 4). There was no significant interaction between treatment and time, and order of treatment had no effect on plasma pH ($P > 0.05$).

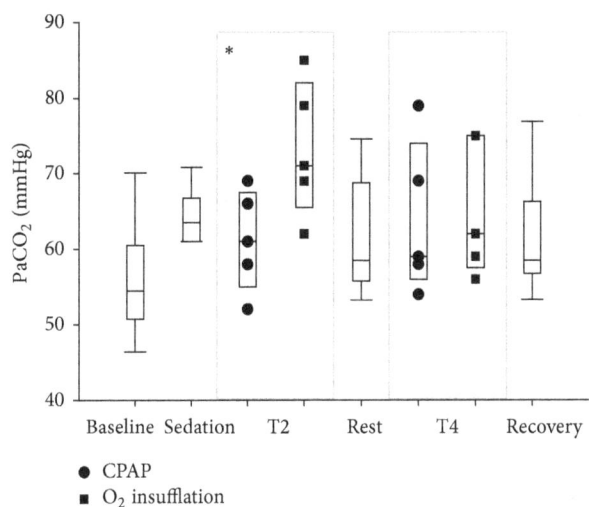

FIGURE 3: Arterial partial pressure of carbon dioxide ($PaCO_2$) following respiratory support by oxygen insufflation or continuous positive airway pressure (CPAP). Values are shown as median (horizontal line) and quartiles and range immediately after catheter placement (T0, baseline), 10 minutes following sedation (T1, sedation), following 10 minutes of oxygen supplementation (O_2), following 10 minutes of CPAP, and after 10 minutes of breathing ambient air following respiratory support (T3, rest, and T5, recovery). Individual results following respiratory support (CPAP or O_2 insufflation) are shown at T2 and T4. Order of respiratory support at T2 (CPAP or O_2 insufflation) was randomly assigned to replicate groups of paired calves. The alternate treatment (O_2 insufflation or CPAP) was administered at T4. CPAP was associated with significantly lower $PaCO_2$ values than was evident following O_2 insufflation at T2 ($^*P < 0.05$).

A significant time ($P = 0.001$) effect was observed on blood lactate concentrations (Figure 5). Lactate concentrations were significantly ($P < 0.001$) lower in all samples obtained after sedation than in the baseline sample. Order of treatment did not have a significant effect on measured lactate concentrations and an interaction between treatment and time was not detected. Neither oxygen supplementation nor CPAP affected ($P > 0.05$) arterial blood bicarbonate concentrations, and there was no significant effect of time or time-treatment interaction detected for this analyte (data not shown).

4. Discussion

Consistent with previous reports [12], the current study demonstrated that oxygen insufflation effectively increased PaO_2 in hypoxaemic calves. All calves in the current study showed significantly higher PaO_2 levels immediately after treatment with oxygen insufflation delivered through a mask. Other studies have suggested that the positive response to oxygen insufflation may not be apparent in all treated calves, particularly those with incomplete transition from foetal circulation and resultant left to right shunting [13]. Further, in neonates with RDS, especially preterm neonates, atelectasis due to a relative or absolute deficiency in surfactant may

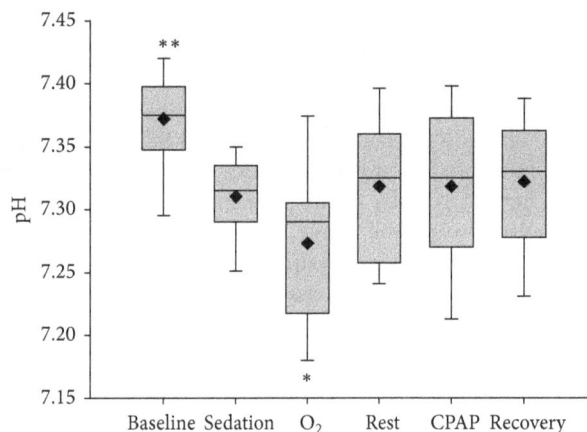

FIGURE 4: Arterial blood pH following sedation and respiratory support by oxygen insufflation or continuous positive airway pressure (CPAP). Values are shown as median (horizontal line) and mean (diamond) and quartiles and range immediately after catheter placement (T0, baseline), 10 minutes following sedation (T1, sedation), following 10 minutes of oxygen supplementation (O_2), following 10 minutes of CPAP, and after 10 minutes of breathing ambient air following respiratory support (T3, rest, and T5, recovery). Order of respiratory support (O_2 supplementation or CPAP) was randomly assigned to replicate groups of paired calves and administered at T2 (5 calves) or T4 (5 calves); treatment order had no significant effect on response to O_2 supplementation or CPAP. Baseline results were significantly higher than results obtained at all other times ($^{**}P < 0.001$), and results obtained following O_2 supplementation were significantly lower than all other results ($^*P < 0.005$).

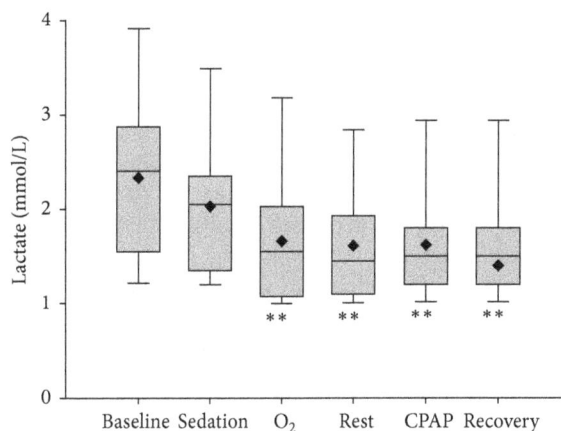

FIGURE 5: Arterial blood lactate concentration following respiratory support by oxygen insufflation or continuous positive airway pressure (CPAP). Values are shown as median (horizontal line) and mean (diamond) and quartiles and range immediately after catheter placement (T0, baseline), 10 minutes following sedation (T1, sedation), following 10 minutes of oxygen supplementation (O_2), following 10 minutes of CPAP, and after 10 minutes of breathing ambient air following respiratory support (T3, rest, and T5, recovery). A significant time effect was observed, as results obtained after sedation were significantly less than baseline ($^{**}P < 0.001$). Order of respiratory support (O_2 supplementation or CPAP) was randomly assigned and had no significant effect on response to O_2 supplementation or CPAP.

compromise the ability to ventilate and hence limit response to oxygen supplementation [14]. Calves in the current study were born at term or close to term and had antenatal exposure to exogenous glucocorticoids. It is unlikely, therefore, that an absolute or relative deficiency of surfactant had a significant impact on respiratory measures in this study. Arterial blood gases following oxygen insufflation in many calves in the current study were well above physiological requirements. Supraphysiologic oxygen partial pressure may potentiate oxidative stress and be deleterious in neonates [15, 32] due to reflex vasoconstriction of arteriolar smooth muscle and consequent reduced blood flow to the brain, heart, and kidney [16].

Minor increases in PaO_2 were observed in most calves following treatment with CPAP, although observed differences were not significant. Power analysis of data from this study suggested that inclusion of an increased number of animals ($n = 7$) would demonstrate a significant treatment effect ($\alpha = 0.05$, 0.80) if these findings are reproducible. As CPAP provides constant pressure throughout the respiratory cycle it prevents the collapse of small airways and alveoli, increasing the FRC. Intrinsically CPAP maintains and to an extent increases the surface area of exchange barriers, potentially allowing increased PaO_2 by reducing ventilation deficits rather than by increasing the oxygen gradient. Thus the increased PaO_2 observed in the current study associated with CPAP delivered room air, whilst small, may indicate the prevention of atelectasis.

Oxygen insufflation was associated with a significant increase in $PaCO_2$ in the current study, and this effect was more pronounced when oxygen was used as a first treatment. Although expired gas measurements were not taken in the current experiment, it was speculated that hypercapnia resulted from a reduced respiratory drive with a consequent decrease in minute ventilation and resultant increased alveolar partial pressure of CO_2. Alternatively (or additionally), the administration of supplementary oxygen may increase metabolic rate and hence carbon dioxide production [33].

In contrast to findings subsequent to oxygen supplementation, $PaCO_2$ was decreased following CPAP treatment, relative to values obtained following sedation or oxygen insufflation, and this effect was significant when CPAP was used as the first treatment. Hypercapnia has a direct effect on acid-base balance. In the current study, the induction of respiratory depression and treatment with oxygen insufflation resulted in significantly decreased pH, and this effect was prevented or corrected by CPAP. As CPAP prevents alveolar collapse during expiration, the ability for carbon dioxide to diffuse across the pulmonary membrane is increased. The major benefit of CPAP may therefore derive from improved CO_2 exchange without more invasive ventilatory support.

The experimental model used in the current study was designed to replicate the physiological consequences of respiratory distress via a reversible model of respiratory compromise with limited welfare cost to experimental subjects. However, care must be taken in extrapolating the effects observed in these, otherwise healthy, calves, to individuals with inadequate surfactant production or other respiratory pathology. The respiratory depressant effects of fentanyl and cardiac depressant effect of xylazine are well known in other veterinary species [34–36] but have not been reported in the bovine neonate. The increased $PaCO_2$ measurements observed following administration of these agents may be due to synergistic negative effects on respiratory function. Hypoxia and hypercapnia associated with xylazine sedation are primarily from a peripherally mediated increase in the shunt fraction (Q_s/Q_t) and not from hypoventilation or postural changes [36]. In contrast fentanyl produces direct depression of respiration through a centrally mediated reduction in inspiratory effort and frequency. In humans the effect of fentanyl is dose limiting; however, in animal species examined it is dose dependent and plateaus and is considered mild [35].

Lateral recumbency may affect blood gas pressure [37, 38]. Calves included in this study were slightly hypercapnic at inclusion, relative to previously published values for calves of this age [12, 13]. In light of the relatively normal PaO_2 levels at this time, the higher $PaCO_2$ results were attributed to a mild left to right shunt or possibly due to positioning in lateral recumbency. Hence, it is possible that calves in the current study had a degree of respiratory dysfunction beyond that induced pharmacologically. However inclusion criteria ensured that they were not affected by overt primary respiratory dysfunction and, as such, the largest effect on the experimental respiratory depression and observed PaO_2 and $PaCO_2$ was the administration of pharmacologic agents. This implies that PaO_2 and $PaCO_2$ would likely improve as the pharmacologic agents were eliminated, a consideration supported by the stronger treatment effects observed at T2 than T4. In the current study, such considerations were controlled for by inclusion of alternate pairs of calves (rather than individuals) as the experimental unit, as well as by randomisation of the first treatment. This ensured that bias was not introduced by additive treatment effects or from the waning action of pharmacological agents employed.

The results of the present study demonstrate that whilst oxygen supplementation alone may address hypoxia, this technique may be insufficient for calves with inadequate surfactant and/or hypoventilation. Our results suggest that CPAP may address hypercapnia and therefore be a useful adjunctive treatment for the management of respiratory distress in bovine neonates. Calves used in the current study were a convenience sample of healthy animals, and further studies with larger populations and evaluating spontaneous disease are warranted.

The CPAP methodology used in the current study shows promise as a field treatment for respiratory depression in calves as it maintained or improved PaO_2 at levels comparable with untreated calves and was not associated with hypercapnia. However, in order to optimise the treatment, investigations into CPAP with an increased inspired oxygen content/concentration (or partial pressure) are warranted. An off-the-shelf at home compressor driven device was evaluated as a simple, readily available, noninvasive, and inexpensive method of respiratory support. Whilst this form of CPAP did not cause harm to the animals, some inadequacies were identified. Increased expiratory effort was observed, likely due to the generation of a constant airflow, with titrated inspiratory and expiratory pressure. In calves, the initial phase of expiration is passive recoil, followed by an active component. An increase in the active component of respiration may lead to fatigue of the muscles involved in respiration [32]. To avoid this, human neonatal systems generally use fluidic flow devices to produce the distending pressure. In addition they also have an expiratory limb similar to that used in a circle anaesthesia circuits. This results in the flow reversing by the Coanda effect during expiration, whilst maintaining airway pressure, and therefore does not lead to an exaggerated expiratory effort [32] and would negate the need for venting of expired gases through the mask.

5. Conclusion

The institution of mask delivered CPAP was well tolerated by subjects and did not result in adverse outcomes in the current experiment. Improvements in blood gas parameters were modest and suggested that CPAP may be of primary benefit in preserving eucapnia. Whilst the use of oxygen insufflation in hypoxaemic calves effectively increased arterial oxygen tensions to supraphysiologic levels, this treatment was associated with increased arterial carbon dioxide concentrations and decreased pH, presumably due to reduced respiratory drive. The pharmacologically induced hypoxaemia, hypercapnia, and acidaemia in this experiment model the physiological consequences of respiratory insufficiency well and, as such, provide a platform for further investigations aimed at optimising CPAP delivery. However, the pharmacological induction of respiratory compromise does not replicate spontaneous disease, and the results of the current study justify further investigation into the use of CPAP in naturally occurring disease.

Conflict of Interests

The authors declare that there is no conflict of interests regarding the publication of this paper.

Acknowledgments

The authors thank Paula Ellul, Andrea Barnard, John Bromfield, Tony Hobson, Dr. Jennifer Clulow, James Dawson, John Campbell, and Jannah Pye for assistance with data collection. This study was funded by an Honours Scholarship from the E. H. Graham Centre for Agricultural Innovation.

References

[1] R. A. Bellows, D. J. Patterson, P. J. Burfening, and D. A. Phelps, "Occurrence of neonatal and postnatal mortality in range beef cattle. II. Factors contributing to calf death," *Theriogenology*, vol. 28, no. 5, pp. 573–586, 1987.

[2] J. M. Nix, J. C. Spitzer, L. W. Grimes, G. L. Burns, and B. B. Plyler, "A retrospective analysis of factors contributing to calf mortality and dystocia in beef cattle," *Theriogenology*, vol. 49, no. 8, pp. 1515–1523, 1998.

[3] U. Bleul, "Respiratory distress syndrome in calves," *Veterinary Clinics of North America—Food Animal Practice*, vol. 25, no. 1, pp. 179–193, 2009.

[4] P. G. Murray and M. J. Stewart, "Use of nasal continuous positive airway pressure during retrieval of neonates with acute respiratory distress," *Pediatrics*, vol. 121, no. 4, pp. E754–E758, 2008.

[5] K. P. Poulsen and S. M. McGuirk, "Respiratory disease of the bovine neonate," *Veterinary Clinics of North America—Food Animal Practice*, vol. 25, no. 1, pp. 121–137, 2009.

[6] A. H. Jobe, B. W. Kramer, T. J. Moss, J. P. Newnham, and M. Ikegami, "Decreased indicators of lung injury with continuous positive expiratory pressure in preterm lambs," *Pediatric Research*, vol. 52, no. 3, pp. 387–392, 2002.

[7] F. Rollin, F. Danlois, H. Aliaoui, and H. H. Guyot, "Respiratory distress syndrome in full-term newborn calves," in *Proceedings of the European Meeting of the French Buiatrics Society*, European College of Bovine Health Management, Paris, France, 1998.

[8] D. E. Noakes, "Dystocia in cattle," *The Veterinary Journal*, vol. 153, no. 2, pp. 123–124, 1997.

[9] C. Uyspruyst, J. Coghe, T. H. Dorts et al., "Effect of three resuscitation procedures on respiratory and metabolic adaptation to extra uterine life in newborn calves," *Veterinary Journal*, vol. 163, no. 1, pp. 30–44, 2002.

[10] C. Uyspruyst, J. Coghe, T. Dorts et al., "Optimal timing of elective caesarean section in Belgian White and Blue breed of cattle: the calf's point of view," *Veterinary Journal*, vol. 163, no. 3, pp. 267–282, 2002.

[11] J. E. Palmer, "Ventilatory support of the critically ill foal," *Veterinary Clinics of North America: Equine Practice*, vol. 21, no. 2, pp. 457–486, 2005.

[12] U. T. Bleul, B. M. Bircher, and W. K. Kähn, "Effect of intranasal oxygen administration on blood gas variables and outcome in neonatal calves with respiratory distress syndrome: 20 cases (2004–2006)," *Journal of the American Veterinary Medical Association*, vol. 233, no. 2, pp. 289–293, 2008.

[13] A.-C. Brisville, G. Fecteau, S. Boysen et al., "Respiratory disease in neonatal cloned calves," *Journal of Veterinary Internal Medicine*, vol. 25, no. 2, pp. 373–379, 2011.

[14] T. Karapinar and M. Dabak, "Treatment of premature calves with clinically diagnosed respiratory distress syndrome," *Journal of Veterinary Internal Medicine*, vol. 22, no. 2, pp. 462–466, 2008.

[15] A. Tan, A. Schulze, C. O'Donnell, and P. Davis, "Air versus oxygen for resuscitation of infants at birth," *Cochrane Database of Systematic Reviews*, no. 1, pp. 1–22, 2009.

[16] S. Iscoe, R. Beasley, and J. A. Fisher, "Supplementary oxygen for nonhypoxemic patients: O_2 much of a good thing?" *Critical Care*, vol. 15, article 305, 2011.

[17] S. Buczinski, S. R. Boysen, and G. Fecteau, "Mechanical ventilation of a cloned calf in respiratory failure," *Journal of Veterinary Emergency and Critical Care*, vol. 17, no. 2, pp. 179–183, 2007.

[18] U. Bleul, B. Bircher, R. S. Jud, and A. P. N. Kutter, "Respiratory and cardiovascular effects of doxapram and theophylline for the treatment of asphyxia in neonatal calves," *Theriogenology*, vol. 73, no. 5, pp. 612–619, 2010.

[19] E. Poulton and D. Oxon, "Left sided heart failure with pulmonary edema: its treatment with the pulmonary plus pressure machine," *The Lancet*, vol. 228, no. 5904, pp. 981–983, 1936.

[20] A. Barach, J. Martin, and M. Eckman, "Positive pressure respiration and its application to the treatment of acute pulmonary oedema and respiratory obstruction," in *Proceedings of the 29th Annual Meeting of the American Society for Clinical Investigation*, Atlantic City, NJ, USA, 1937.

[21] G. A. Gregory, J. A. Kitterman, R. H. Phibbs, W. H. Tooley, and W. K. Hamilton, "Treatment of the idiopathic respiratory-distress syndrome with continuous positive airway pressure," *The New England Journal of Medicine*, vol. 284, no. 24, pp. 1333–1340, 1971.

[22] A. G. DePaoli, P. G. Davis, B. Faber, and C. J. Morley, "Devices and pressure sources for administration of nasal continuous positive airway pressure (NCPAP) in preterm neonates," *The Cochrane Collaboration*, vol. 32, no. 1, Article ID CD002977, 2008.

[23] J. Ho, D. Henderson-Smart, and P. Davis, "Continuous distending pressure for respiratory distress syndrome in preterm infants," *Cochrane Database of Systematic Reviews*, no. 4, pp. 1–34, 2008.

[24] P. Subramaniam, D. Henderson-Smart, and P. Davis, "Prophylactic nasal continuous positive airways pressure for preventing morbidity and mortality in preterm infants," *The Cochrane Collaboration*, no. 1, pp. 1–19, 2009.

[25] A. Briganti, P. Melanie, D. Portela, G. Breghi, and K. Mama, "Continuous positive airway pressure administered via face mask in tranquilized dogs," *Journal of Veterinary Emergency and Critical Care*, vol. 20, no. 5, pp. 503–508, 2010.

[26] P. D. MacFarlane and M. Mosing, "Early experience with continuous positive airway pressure (CPAP) in 5 horses—a case series," *Canadian Veterinary Journal*, vol. 53, no. 4, pp. 426–429, 2012.

[27] M. Mosing and S. Junat, "Use of continuous positive airway pressure (CRAP) in a horse with diaphragmatic hernia," *Pferdeheilkunde*, vol. 27, no. 1, pp. 66–69, 2011.

[28] M. Mosing, M. Rysnik, D. Bardell, P. J. Cripps, and P. MacFarlane, "Use of Continuous Positive Airway Pressure (CPAP) to optimise oxygenation in anaesthetised horses—a clinical study," *Equine Veterinary Journal*, vol. 45, no. 4, pp. 414–418, 2013.

[29] F. V. Meirelles, E. H. Birgel Jr., F. Perecin, and L. C. G. Silva, "Delivery of cloned offspring: experience in Zebu cattle (*Bos indicus*)," *Reproduction, Fertility and Development*, vol. 22, no. 1, pp. 88–97, 2010.

[30] E. Born, "Bei 57 termingerecht geborenen Kalbern wurde 20 bis 30 Minuten," *Reproduction in Domestic Animals*, vol. 16, no. 5, pp. 227–234, 1981.

[31] O. Szenci and T. Besser, "Changes in blood gas and acid-base values of bovine venous blood during storage," *Journal of the American Veterinary Medical Association*, vol. 197, no. 4, pp. 471–474, 1990.

[32] J. P. Goldsmith and E. Karotkin, *Assisted Ventilation of the Neonate: Expert Consult*, Saunders Elsevier, St. Louis, Mo, USA, 5th edition, 2011.

[33] J. P. Mortola, P. B. Frappell, A. Dotta et al., "Ventilatory and metabolic responses to acute hyperoxia in newborns," *American Review of Respiratory Disease*, vol. 146, no. 1, pp. 11–15, 1992.

[34] S. A. Greene and J. C. Thurmon, "Xylazine—a review of its pharmacology and use in veterinary medicine," *Journal of Veterinary Pharmacology and Therapeutics*, vol. 11, no. 4, pp. 295–313, 1988.

[35] B. Kukanich and T. P. Clark, "The history and pharmacology of fentanyl: relevance to a novel, long-acting transdermal fentanyl solution newly approved for use in dogs," *Journal of Veterinary Pharmacology and Therapeutics*, vol. 35, supplement 2, pp. 3–19, 2012.

[36] E. Rioja, C. L. Kerr, S. S. Enouri, and W. N. McDonell, "Sedative and cardiopulmonary effects of medetomidine hydrochloride and xylazine hydrochloride and their reversal with atipamezole hydrochloride in calves," *American Journal of Veterinary Research*, vol. 69, no. 3, pp. 319–329, 2008.

[37] M. W. McMillan, K. E. Whitaker, D. Hughes, D. C. Brodbelt, and A. K. Boag, "Effect of body position on the arterial partial pressures of oxygen and carbon dioxide in spontaneously breathing, conscious dogs in an intensive care unit," *Journal of Veterinary Emergency and Critical Care*, vol. 19, no. 6, pp. 564–570, 2009.

[38] M. R. Paradis, *Equine Neonatal Medicine: A Case-Based Approach*, Saunders Elsevier, St. Louis, Mo, USA, 2006.

10

Prevalence and Risk Factors Associated with Faecal Shedding of *Cryptosporidium* Oocysts in Dogs in the Federal Capital Territory, Abuja, Nigeria

Gbemisola Magaret Olabanji, Beatty Viv Maikai, and Gbeminiyi Richard Otolorin

Department of Veterinary Public Health and Preventive Medicine, Faculty of Veterinary Medicine, Ahmadu Bello University, Zaria, Kaduna State, Nigeria

Correspondence should be addressed to Gbemisola Magaret Olabanji; golabanji@yahoo.com

Academic Editor: Cynthia C. Powell

Cryptosporidium is one of the causes of diarrhoeal illness in man and animals worldwide. The aim of the study was to determine the prevalence and risk factors associated with faecal shedding of *Cryptosporidium* oocysts in dogs in FCT Abuja, Nigeria. A total of 276 dog faecal samples were examined using Modified Acid Fast (MAF) technique and Enzyme Linked Immunosorbent Assay (ELISA). Fifteen (5.4%) and 51 (18.5%) out of the 276 dog faecal samples examined were positive for *Cryptosporidium* oocysts and coproantigens, respectively. There was a fair agreement (0.371) between the two tests used in this study. The prevalence of *Cryptosporidium* infection was highest in 4 dogs (21.0%) between 3 and 9 months of age. Ten diarrhoeic dogs (30.3%) and 31 dogs from rural settlements were more infected (22.46%) with *Cryptosporidium* oocysts. There was statistical association between prevalence of *Cryptosporidium* and confinement of dogs (OR = 0.41; 95% CI on OR: 0.21 < OR < 0.80). However, there was no statistical association (*P* > 0.05) between prevalence of *Cryptosporidium* and age, diarrhoeic status of the dogs, sex, breed, and location. A total of 62.7% respondents did not have prior knowledge about dogs harbouring organisms that can infect humans. The finding of this research is of public health significance.

1. Introduction

Cryptosporidium is an obligate intracellular, protozoan parasite of great public health significance that causes cryptosporidiosis in animals and humans [1]. Due to unrestricted movement of dogs across major cities across the nations, dogs are exposed to both the endemic and nonendemic intestinal protozoan infections in Nigeria [2]. It has been suggested for some time that dogs can be a significant source of human cryptosporidiosis [3]. *Cryptosporidium parvum* and *Cryptosporidium hominis* are the two most common species found in humans and account for more than 90% of humans cases in the world. Other species and genotypes of *Cryptosporidium* have occasionally been recorded in humans including *Cryptosporidium canis* [4, 5]. It is speculated that humans may acquire infection from naturally infected dogs [6]. Zoonotic transmission from a dog was suspected in one case when a veterinary student working in a ward where an infected dog was being cared for developed acute self-limiting diarrhoea and *Cryptosporidium* oocysts were identified in her feces [6].

Dogs can be naturally infected with *Cryptosporidium canis*, *Cryptosporidium parvum*, and *Cryptosporidium meleagridis* [7, 8]. *Cryptosporidium canis* is reported to be the most frequently identified species of *Cryptosporidium* in dogs. In addition, small numbers of zoonotic *C. parvum*, *C. muris*, and *C. meleagridis* have also been detected in dogs. *Cryptosporidium canis* infections in dogs are usually asymptomatic but may cause severe diarrhoea, malabsorption, and weight loss [9]. Recent molecular study indicates that dogs may transmit the cattle genotype, which is known to be pathogenic to humans [10]. Dogs are the most commonly domesticated pet animals primarily used for security purposes in Nigeria, making their population density high in major cities including Abuja; however there is no readily available data on canine cryptosporidiosis as an emerging zoonoses in Abuja, on the potential hazard these oocysts from dogs poses to public health in Abuja, Nigeria, and in general, therefore making it necessary to investigate the prevalence of canine cryptosporidiosis and also understand the risk factors that lead to the transmission and possible spread of infection in animals in Abuja, Nigeria.

2. Materials and Methods

2.1. Study Area and Study Design. The Federal Capital Territory is the home of Abuja, the capital of Nigeria. A cross-sectional study was used. Three (3) area councils in Abuja were selected using convenience sampling method. One area council, namely, Abuja municipal, was selected as a representative of major urban settlement with the highest population of dogs in the territory, while the remaining two were Abaji and Kwali, both representing the rural setting in the territory.

2.2. Sample Collection. A total of 276 faecal samples were collected. 138 faecal samples were collected from Abuja municipal area council (23 samples each from Central area, Garki, Wuse, Maitama, Asokoro, and Gwarimpa districts) while 69 faecal samples each were collected from Abaji (23 samples each from Abaji, Toto, Nasarawa, and Kotokarfe) and Kwali (23 samples each from Kwali, Lambata, and Kwaita towns) area councils, respectively. Convenience sampling technique was used to select houses in districts and wards of each area council for the selection of individual dog-owning households in the study areas. Sampling was done between July and September 2014. Faecal sample was collected from the rectum of each animal by means of a disposable plastic bag and emptied into a wide-mouthed disposable plastic container [11]. Faecal samples collected were stored in 10% formalin prior to transportation to the Parasitic Zoonoses Laboratory of the Department of Veterinary Public Health and Preventive Medicine, Ahmadu Bello University, Zaria, for processing.

2.3. Administration of Questionnaires. Prior to sample collection, structured questionnaires were used to obtain information for each dog from which faecal sample was collected and also to obtain information that may help identify risk factors for the faecal shedding of *Cryptosporidium* in dogs. The questionnaire consisted of two sections: *Section A* contained biodata of respondents and questions relating to transmission of the disease; *Section B* contained questions on age, sex, breed, confinement of dogs, source of drinking water, and presence of diarrhoea or loose faeces.

2.4. Sample Processing and Laboratory Procedure Using Modified Acid Fast Technique and ELISA. The faecal samples were treated using formol-ether concentration method and stained using Modified Acid Fast (MAF) [12]. Each faecal sample collected was correspondingly examined for the presence of *Cryptosporidium* spp. antigens by ELISA using a commercial kit (*Copro*ELISA for detection of *Cryptosporidium* antigen in faeces, Savyon Diagnostics Limited, Israel). Samples with optical density (OD) higher than 0.5 were reported as positive

TABLE 1: Level of agreement between MAF and ELISA using Kappa's Statistic.

Type of test	Number positive	Specific rate (%)	κ-value
Modified Acid Fast[Ref]	15	5.4	
ELISA	51	18.5	0.371

Note: κ-value means Kappa value.
Kappa value within the range 0.21–0.40 indicates a fair agreement between the outcome of the two tests.
Note: Ref refers to reference category.

while those with OD less than 0.5 were reported as negative for *Cryptosporidium* coproantigens.

2.5. Data Analysis. The results obtained were presented using tables and charts (descriptive statistics). Using the Statistical Package for Social Science (SPSS) version 17.0 (SPSS Inc., Chicago, IL, USA), Chi-square and Fisher's exact tests were used to check for association between *Cryptosporidium* and factors studied. Odds ratio (OR) and 95% confidence intervals were calculated for dichotomous variables using EP1 INFO version 3.1. OR values greater than unity denote association and less than unity denote that the factor may have a protective effect. Values of $P < 0.05$ were considered statistically significant.

3. Results and Discussion

Out of the 276 dog faecal samples examined using Modified Acid Fast (MAF) staining, 15 (5.4%) samples were positive for *Cryptosporidium* oocysts, while 51 (18.5%) dog faecal samples were positive for *Cryptosporidium* coproantigens using Enzyme Linked Immunosorbent Assay (ELISA). The infection rates from this study were higher than that reported by Adejimi and Osayomi [2]. From this study it was observed that ELISA test was more sensitive than MAF. There was a fair agreement (κ-value: 0.371) between the two tests used in this research (Table 1), indicating a fair outcome between both tests because of the varied number of positives obtained between the two tests.

The presence of *Cryptosporidium* in household dogs may cause cryptosporidiosis in humans due to zoonotic transmission of the infection through close contact with dogs and other domestic animals [13–15]. Abuja is an urban area where dogs are freely kept by most households, usually for security purposes and as pets. Humans have close interactions with companion animals, sharing their living space, and consequently are exposed to microorganisms/parasites that may cause diseases [16]. *Cryptosporidium* spp. isolated in dogs have been found to infect healthy children and adults [4, 17]; hence its control in dogs and other domestic animals is very important.

Infection rates in dogs sampled were higher in dogs between 3 and 9 months of age (Table 2). This result is in contrast to other works where *Cryptosporidium* infection was highest in younger dogs [16, 18, 19]. The high proportion of *Cryptosporidium* infection in older dogs was probably due to the use of older dogs for security purposes thereby increasing

TABLE 2: Effect of age on the prevalence of *Cryptosporidium* infection in dogs using ELISA and MAF techniques in the FCT, Abuja.

Age group (months)	Number of dogs examined	Number positive (%)		Chi-square χ^2	P value & df
		*MAF	**ELISA		
<3	77	2 (2.60)	13 (16.88)	*2.010	0.366; 2
>3–9	100	9 (9.00)	21 (21.00)		
>9	99	4 (4.04)	17 (17.17)	**0.664	0.717; 2

*Chi-square χ^2 in reference to MAF.
**Chi-square χ^2 in reference to ELISA.

TABLE 3: Odds ratio and 95% confidence interval on effect of diarrhoea on the prevalence of *Cryptosporidium* infection in dogs using MAF and ELISA in the FCT, Abuja.

Diarrhoea	Number examined	Number positive	Specific rate (%)	Odds ratio (OR)	95% confidence interval on OR
MAF					
Present[Ref]	33	8	24.24	1.00	
Absent	243	7	2.88	10.79	3.21–36.74
ELISA					
Present[Ref]	33	10	30.30	1.00	
Absent	243	41	16.87	2.14	0.88–5.16

Note: Ref refers to reference category.

TABLE 4: Odds ratio and 95% confidence interval on effect of sex on the prevalence of *Cryptosporidium* infection in dogs using MAF and ELISA in the FCT, Abuja.

Sex	Number examined	Number positive	Specific rate (%)	Odds ratio (OR)	95% confidence interval on OR
MAF					
Male[Ref]	181	12	6.63	1.00	
Female	95	3	3.16	2.18	0.55–9.99
ELISA					
Male[Ref]	181	32	17.68	1.00	
Female	95	19	20.00	0.86	0.44–1.69

Note: Ref refers to reference category.

their tendency to move around more often and possibly getting infected with the *Cryptosporidium* oocysts.

Prevalence of *Cryptosporidium* infection was highest in 8 (24.24%) and 10 (30.30%) dogs with diarrhoea with the use of MAF and ELISA, respectively, as compared to 7 (2.88%) and 41 (16.87%) in the corresponding dogs without diarrhoea. There was statistical significance ($P < 0.05$) between prevalence of *Cryptosporidium* in the MAF (OR = 10.79; 95% CI on OR: 3.21 < OR < 36.74) (Table 3). The higher rate of infection in diarrhoeic dogs may probably be because some of the dogs tested were already manifesting the disease undetected as one of the clinical signs of cryptosporidiosis is diarrhoea [20]; various authors have reported higher rates of infection in dogs, humans, and other domestic animals with diarrhoea [13, 14, 21].

Prevalence of *Cryptosporidium* infection was more in females (20.0%) than males (17.68%) in samples examined using ELISA. There was no statistical significance between prevalence of *Cryptosporidium* in both the MAF (OR = 2.18; 95% CI on OR: 0.55 < OR < 9.99) and ELISA (OR = 0.86; 95% CI on OR: 0.44 < OR < 1.69) (Table 4). The higher rate of infection in females than in male dogs, examined with the use of ELISA, may be probably due to a reduced immunity at

certain periods in females physiologic cycle. A similar study conducted in China and Brazil reported similar findings [22].

Prevalence of *Cryptosporidium* infection was more in crossbreed of dogs (19.23%) compared to exotic and local breed of dogs in samples examined using ELISA. There was no statistical significant association between prevalence of *Cryptosporidium* in both the MAF ($\chi^2 = 0.379$, df = 2, and P value = 0.827) and ELISA ($\chi^2 = 0.052$, df = 2, and P value = 0.974) with the breed of the dog sampled (Table 5). This is in contrast with results gotten by Adejimi and Osayomi [2] who reported a higher prevalence of *Cryptosporidium* infection in local breed of dogs. Prevalence of *Cryptosporidium* infection was highest in 10 (7.25%) and 31 (22.46%) dogs in the rural area councils with the use of MAF and ELISA, respectively, as compared to 5 (3.62%) and 20 (14.49%) in the corresponding dogs in the urban area council. The high prevalence in household dogs from rural part of the study area is in agreement with work done by Adriana et al. [23]. This high prevalence can be correlated with the dogs living close to other domestic animals as cattle and sheep that may be infected and shedding the *Cryptosporidium* oocyst and also dogs in this area are prone to roam about and may easily be infected.

TABLE 5: Effect of breed and location on the prevalence of *Cryptosporidium* infection in dogs using ELISA and MAF in the FCT, Abuja.

Variable	Number of dogs examined: $n = 276$	Number positive (%)		Chi-square χ^2	P value & df
		*MAF	**ELISA		
Breed					
Exotic	150	9 (6.00)	27 (18.00)	*0.379	0.827; 2
Local	74	3 (4.05)	14 (18.92)		
Cross	52	3 (5.77)	10 (19.23)	**0.052	0.974; 2
Location					
Urban	138	5 (3.62)	20 (14.49)	*1.762	0.144; 1
Rural	138	10 (7.25)	31 (22.46)	**2.910	0.060; 1

*Chi-square χ^2 in reference to MAF.
**Chi-square χ^2 in reference to ELISA.

TABLE 6: Odds ratio and 95% confidence interval on effect of confinement on the prevalence of *Cryptosporidium* infection in dogs using MAF and ELISA in the FCT, Abuja.

Confinement	Number examined	Number positive	Specific rate (%)	Odds ratio (OR)	95% confidence interval on OR
MAF					
Yes[Ref]	201	8	3.98	1.00	
No	75	7	9.33	0.40	0.13–1.29
ELISA					
Yes[Ref]	201	29	14.42	1.00	
No	75	22	29.33	0.41	0.21–0.80

Note: Ref refers to reference category.

TABLE 7: Factors associated with the prevalence of *Cryptosporidium* infection in dogs within sampled households in the FCT, Abuja.

Variable	Frequency (%)	Number of ELISA positive samples (%)	Chi-square χ^2	P value & df
Close contact to dogs				
Yes	162 (58.7)	23		
No	114 (41.3)	28	4.771	0.029; 1
Knowledge about dogs harbouring organisms that can infect humans				
Yes	103 (37.3)	15		
No	173 (62.7)	36	1.672	0.196; 1
Housing of dogs within premises				
Specially constructed house/cage	181 (65.6)	32		
In-house passage way	48 (17.4)	7		
Anywhere in the premises	47 (17.0)	12	2.112	0.348; 2
Total	276			

Prevalence of *Cryptosporidium* infection was highest in 7 (9.33%) and 22 (29.33%) dogs that were not confined with the use of MAF and ELISA, respectively, as compared to 8 (3.98%) and 29 (14.42%) in the corresponding dogs that were confined. There was statistically significant association between the prevalence of *Cryptosporidium* in both the MAF (OR = 0.40; 95% CI on OR: 0.13 < OR < 1.29) and ELISA (OR = 0.41; 95% CI on OR: 0.21 < OR < 0.08) with dog confinement (Table 6). Dogs that were allowed to roam the neighbourhood by their owners had the highest rate of infection, as they are prone to exposure to *Cryptosporidium* oocysts as they move within the neighbourhood interacting with other animals and infectious material. Free-roaming dogs in urban areas constitute nuisance and promote indiscriminate shedding of parasitic organism in the environment and are an important public health issue; studies performed worldwide have demonstrated the presence of parasitic elements within samples of canine faecal material collected from public urban areas [24].

About 58.7% of the respondents said that they and other members of their households have close contact with the dogs in their premises. There was statistically significant association between prevalence of *Cryptosporidium* (χ^2 = 4.771, df = 1, and P value = 0.029) and humans contact with dogs (Table 7). A total of 62.7% respondents did not have knowledge about dogs harbouring organisms that can infect humans and there was no statistically significant association between prevalence of *Cryptosporidium* ($\chi^2 = 1.672$, df = 1, and *P* value = 0.196) and humans knowledge about dogs harbouring potentially harmful organisms to them. About 65.6% of the dogs were housed in specially constructed houses/cages while 17.4% and 17% of dogs in these households were housed on households' passage way and anywhere in the households, respectively. Individuals having close contact with pet animals have been shown to be a source of transmission of zoonotic infection between humans and animals, especially when humans are exposed to discharges and faeces of these animals [15]. Also most of the respondents did not have knowledge about dogs harbouring organisms that can infect humans and this poor knowledge recorded by the respondents may increase their exposure and interfere with the control of *Cryptosporidium* infection in the dogs in the study area.

4. Conclusion

This research was able to establish a higher sensitivity and specificity rate for ELISA in routine diagnosis of *Cryptosporidium* in dogs in comparison to MAF. The presence of *Cryptosporidium* infection in household dogs in the study area is of public health concern as infected dogs can serve as vehicle of transmission of the infection to humans. There was a fair agreement between the two tests used in this study. There was no statistical association between the prevalence of *Cryptosporidium* infection and age, sex, and breed in dogs sampled within the study area. Rate of infection was higher in diarrhoeic dogs and free-roaming dogs. A significant number of respondents in the households surveyed were unaware that dogs can shed organisms in their faeces that can be harmful to their health. Hence it is important that adequate public health programme is organized to educate dog owners about adequate protective measures to take to protect themselves. However the study has shown that associated risk factors such as dog confinement and their contact with man are of great significance.

Conflict of Interests

The authors declare that there is no conflict of interests regarding the publication of this paper.

References

[1] M. Mirzaei, "Epidemiological survey of *Cryptosporidium* spp. in companion and stray dogs in Kerman, Iran," *Veterinaria Italiana*, vol. 48, no. 3, pp. 291–296, 2012.

[2] J. O. Adejimi and J. O. Osayomi, "Prevalence of intestinal protozoan parasites of dogs in Ibadan, south western Nigeria," *Journal of Animal & Plant Sciences*, vol. 7, no. 2, pp. 783–788, 2010.

[3] L. Xiao and Y. Feng, "Zoonotic cryptosporidiosis," *FEMS Immunology & Medical Microbiology*, vol. 52, no. 3, pp. 309–323, 2008.

[4] L. Xiao, C. Bern, J. Limor et al., "Identification of 5 types of *Cryptosporidium* parasites in children in Lima, Peru," *Journal of Infectious Diseases*, vol. 183, no. 3, pp. 492–497, 2001.

[5] V. A. Cama, C. Bern, I. M. Sulaiman et al., "*Cryptosporidium* species andgenotypes in HIV-positive patients in Lima Peru," *Journal of Eukaryotic Microbiology*, vol. 50, pp. 531–533, 2003.

[6] C. E. Greene, G. J. Jacobs, and D. Prickett, "Intestinal malabsorption and cryptosporidiosis in an adult dog," *Journal of the American Veterinary Medical Association*, vol. 197, no. 3, pp. 365–367, 1990.

[7] R. Fayer, J. M. Trout, L. Xiao, U. M. Morgant, A. A. Lal, and J. P. Dubey, "*Cryptosporidium canis* n. sp. from domestic dogs," *Journal of Parasitology*, vol. 87, no. 6, pp. 1415–1422, 2001.

[8] O. Hajdušek, O. Ditrich, and J. Šlapeta, "Molecular identification of *Cryptosporidium* spp. in animal and human hosts from the Czech Republic," *Veterinary Parasitology*, vol. 122, no. 3, pp. 183–192, 2004.

[9] P. J. Irwin, "Companion animal parasitology: a clinical perspective," *International Journal for Parasitology*, vol. 32, no. 5, pp. 581–593, 2002.

[10] N. Abe, I. Kimata, and M. Iseki, "Identification of genotypes of *Cryptosporidium parvum* isolates from a patient and a dog in Japan," *Journal of Veterinary Medical Science*, vol. 64, no. 2, pp. 165–168, 2002.

[11] S. Jongwutiwes, R. Tiangtip, S. Yentakarm, and N. Chantachum, "Simple method for long-term copro-preservation of *Cryptosporidium oocysts* for morphometric and molecular analysis," *Tropical Medicine and International Health*, vol. 7, no. 3, pp. 257–264, 2002.

[12] WHO, *Basic Laboratory Methods in Medical Parasitology*, World Health Organization, Geneva, Switzerland, 1991.

[13] H. O. Tariuwa, I. Ajogi, C. L. Ejembi et al., "Incidence of *Cryptosporidium* infection in port-harcourt rivers state Nigeria based on regular contact with domestic animals," *Nigerian Veterinary Journal*, vol. 28, no. 3, 2007.

[14] B. V. Makai, J. U. Umoh, J. K. P. Kwaga, V. Maikai, and S. C. Egege, "Prevalence and risk factors associated with faecal sheding of *Cryptosporidium oocysts* in piglets, Kaduna state, Nigeria," *Journal of Parasitology and Vector Biology*, vol. 1, no. 1, pp. 001–004, 2009.

[15] F. Jian, F. Qi, X. He et al., "Occurrence and molecular characterization of *Cryptosporidium* in dogs in Henan Province, China," *BMC Veterinary Research*, vol. 10, article 26, 2014.

[16] N. E. Ramirez, L. A. Ward, and S. Sreevatsan, "A review of the biology and epidemiology of cryptosporidiosis in humans and animals," *Microbes and Infection*, vol. 6, no. 8, pp. 773–785, 2004.

[17] S. Pedraza-Diaz, C. Amar, A. M. Iversen, P. J. Stanley, and J. McLauchlin, "Unusual *Cryptosporidium* species recovered from human faeces: first description of *Cryptosporidium felis* and *Cryptosporidium* 'dog type' from patients in England," *Journal of Medical Microbiology*, vol. 50, no. 3, pp. 293–296, 2001.

[18] I. S. Hamnes, B. K. Gjerde, and L. J. Robertson, "A longitudinal study on the occurrence of *Cryptosporidium* and *Giardia* in dogs during their first year of life," *Acta Veterinaria Scandinavica*, vol. 49, no. 1, article 22, 2007.

[19] A. Titilincu, V. Mircean, D. Achelaritei, and V. Cozma, "Prevalence of *Cryptosporidium* spp. in asymptomatic dogs by ELISA and risk factors associated with infection," *Lucrări Stiinlifice Medicină Veterinară*, vol. 43, no. 1, 2010.

[20] R. C. Thompson, A. Armson, and U. M. Ryan, *Cryptosporidium: From Molecules to Disease*, Elsevier, 2003.

[21] A. O. Akinkuotu, B. O. Fagbemi, E. B. Otesile, M. A. Dipeolu, and A. B. Ayinmode, "*Cryptosporidium* infection in cattle in Ogun state, Nigeria," *Sokoto Journal of Veterinary Sciences*, vol. 12, article 2, 2014.

[22] J. Wang, P. Li, X. Xue et al., "Investigation on the infection situation of *Cryptosporidium* in dogs in hefei city," *Chinese Journal of Veterinary Parasitology*, vol. 16, no. 5, pp. 20–23, 2008 (Chinese).

[23] T. Adriana, M. Viorica, D. Achelaritei, and V. Cozma, "Prevalence of *Cryptosporidium* spp. Inasymptomatic dogs by elisa and risk factors associated with infection," *Lucrări Stiinlifice Medicină Veterinară*, vol. 13, no. 1, 2010.

[24] L. Rinaldi, M. P. Maurelli, V. Musella et al., "Giardia and *Cryptosporidium* in canine faecal samples contaminating an urban area," *Research in Veterinary Science*, vol. 84, no. 3, pp. 413–415, 2008.

11

Serological Survey of Foot-and-Mouth Disease Virus in Buffaloes (*Syncerus caffer*) in Zambia

T. K. W. Sikombe,[1,2] **A. S. Mweene,**[1] **John Muma,**[1] **C. Kasanga,**[3] **Y. Sinkala,**[1,4] **F. Banda,**[2] **M. Mulumba,**[5] **E. M. Fana,**[6] **C. Mundia,**[7] **and M. Simuunza**[1]

[1]*Department of Disease Control, School of Veterinary Medicine, University of Zambia, P.O. Box 32379, Lusaka, Zambia*
[2]*Central Veterinary Research Institute, P.O. Box 33980, Lusaka, Zambia*
[3]*Faculty of Veterinary Medicine, Sokoine University of Agriculture, P.O. Box 3021, Morogoro, Tanzania*
[4]*National Livestock Epidemiology and Information Centre, P.O. Box 30041, Lusaka, Zambia*
[5]*Southern African Development Community Secretariat, SADC House, Plot No. 54385, Central Business District, Private Bag 0095, Gaborone, Botswana*
[6]*Botswana Vaccine Institute, Private Bag 0031, Gaborone, Botswana*
[7]*Department of Veterinary Services, Southern African Development Community, Trans-Boundary Animal Disease Section, Ministry of Agriculture and Livestock, P.O. Box 50060, Lusaka, Zambia*

Correspondence should be addressed to T. K. W. Sikombe; tingiyasikombe@yahoo.com

Academic Editor: Timm C. Harder

A study was conducted to determine the serotypes of foot-and-mouth disease viruses (FMDV) circulating in African buffaloes (*Syncerus caffer*) from selected areas in Zambia. Sera and probang samples were collected between 2011 and 2012 and analysed for presence of antibodies against FMDV while probang samples were used to isolate the FMDV by observing cytopathic effect (CPE). Samples with CPE were further analysed using antigen ELISA. High FMD seroprevalence was observed and antibodies to all the three Southern African Territories (SAT) serotypes were detected in four study areas represented as follows: SAT2 was 72.7 percent; SAT1 was 62.6 percent; and SAT3 was 26.2 percent. Mixed infections accounted for 68.6 percent of those that were tested positive. For probang samples, CPE were observed in three of the samples, while the antigen ELISA results showed positivity and for SAT1 (*n* = 1) and SAT2 (*n* = 2). It is concluded that FMDV is highly prevalent in Zambian buffaloes which could play an important role in the epidemiology of the disease. Therefore livestock reared at interface with the game parks should be included in all routine FMDV vaccination programmes.

1. Introduction

Foot-and-mouth disease (FMD) is a highly infectious viral disease of domestic and wild cloven hoofed animals [1–3]. The disease is caused by the foot-and-mouth disease virus (FMDV) of the genus *Aphthovirus* belonging to the family Picornaviridae. The first report of FMD in Zambia dated from 1933 in Barotseland (now Western Province). Typing of the virus from Zambian FMD outbreaks began in 1948 when the Southern African Territories (SAT) immunological types of FMD virus were recognised [4]. Currently, FMD is endemic in some parts of Northern and Muchinga Provinces along areas bordering Tanzania and in southern border areas between Zambia and Zimbabwe, Botswana and Namibia and along the Kafue and Zambezi flood plains which are also bordered by parts of Kafue National Park. These areas are densely populated with domestic and game animals which are usually in contact for most part of the year. The FMD scenario in Zambia is complicated by the presence of a stable wildlife reservoir, the African buffaloes "*Syncerus caffer*," and traditional practice of transhumant grazing, where cattle farmers trek their animals to wildlife sanctuaries in search of water and pasture [5–7] and where there are several viruses with high sequence diversity due to the nature of

FMDV [8, 9]. African buffaloes are known to be carriers of FMDV and as such contact exposes cattle to the risk of being infected. It has also been reported that FMD may circulate undetected in vaccinated cattle herds and in some indigenous breeds reared in areas where FMD is endemic [10].

Zambia has continued to experience isolated outbreaks of FMD such as those that occurred in Namwala in 2005 [11] and in 2008 [12]; Itezhi-Tezhi in 2006 [13] and in 2008 [12]; and Monze and Mazabuka in 2007 [14] and in 2008 [12]. These outbreaks were considered as reoccurrences of the 2004 SAT1 outbreak (Yona Sinkala, personal communications, 2012). In December 2007, SAT2 FMDV outbreaks occurred in Sesheke district in Western Province and Kazungula district of Southern Province [12]. The disease spilled over in 2008 and spread to Senanga, Mongu, Shang'ombo, and Kalabo districts of Western Province [12]. In 2009, there was an outbreak in Mbala, Northern Province, where SAT1 was isolated [15]. In 2010, there was another outbreak in Mbala district, which spread to Chinsali district, and serotype O was isolated [16]. In 2012, Mbala district and Kazungula/Livingstone experienced further outbreaks, where SAT2 and SAT1 were isolated, respectively [17, 18].

FMD is endemic in Zambia and continues to impact negatively on the livestock industry development. Little understanding of the epidemiology of FMDV has led to the continuous occurrences of the disease in Zambia. Cattle movement and trade restrictions resulting from occurrence of this disease have led to severe negative impacts for pastoral and agropastoral families who are most reliant on livestock products for food and economic security [19]. In addition trade restrictions imposed by other countries mean that the country is not able to participate fully in trade of livestock and its byproducts regionally and internationally.

FMD vaccination campaigns are conducted biannually in most parts of Zambia, where the disease is endemic. Although vaccination offers a potential solution, there are questions surrounding the efficacy of the vaccines used since there are many different serotypes (SAT1, SAT2, and SAT3, type O and type A) of FMD viruses reported to be circulating in Zambia [4, 20]. Due to this the vaccines used may not sufficiently match the field strains circulating that often even their homologous potency is unknown and the cold chain crucial for the success of any FMD vaccination is difficult to maintain. Trivalent vaccines (SAT1, SAT2, and SAT3) were used annually in Southern, Central, and Western Provinces of Zambia before 2006. After 2006, bivalent vaccines (SAT1 and SAT2) were used in Southern, Central, and Western Provinces of Zambia where our study was based, while bivalent vaccines (SAT1 and SAT2 or SAT1 and type A or SAT1 and type O) have been used in Northern and Muchinga Provinces of Zambia, bordering Tanzania; unfortunately this area was not covered by our study. This study therefore was conducted to determine the infection status and FMD virus (FMDV) serotypes circulating in buffaloes in Zambia. Thus the epidemiological situation of FMDV will be discussed.

2. Material and Methods

2.1. Study Area. The study was carried out in areas located in National Parks (NP) and Game Management Areas

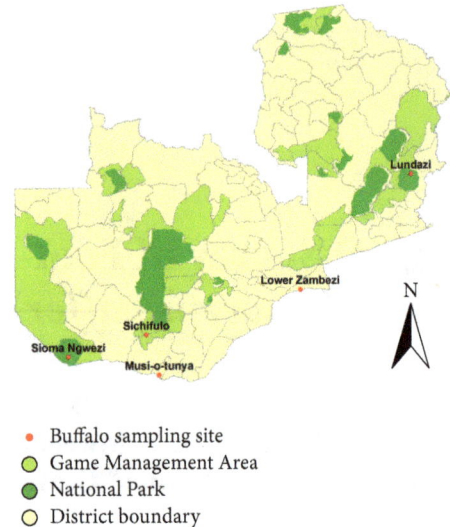

- • Buffalo sampling site
- ◯ Game Management Area
- ● National Park
- ◯ District boundary

FIGURE 1: Map of Zambia with sampling sites in Game Management Areas (GMA) and National Parks (NP).

(GMA) in Zambia (Figure 1). Five locations were selected for this study which included Mosi-oa-tunya (S: 17°52.370'; E: 025°50053'), Sichifulo (S: 16°49.470'; E: 025°29.482'), Lower Zambezi (S: 15°38.384'; E: 029°36.756'), Lundazi (S: 12°17.157'; E: 033°10.836'), and Sioma (S: 17°08.8900'; E: 23°65.3367'). These areas were purposively selected because of the presence of interactions between cattle and wildlife resulting from the transhumant cattle husbandry practice where traditional cattle farmers bring their livestock for grazing into wildlife habitats in search of greener pastures and water. These areas are among the major ecosystems of buffaloes in Zambia. Luangwa National Park has the highest density of buffaloes in Zambia (Chuma Simukonda, personal communications, 2011). However, cattle-wildlife interactions are more pronounced in the Kafue flats where FMD outbreaks occur frequently [5].

2.2. Study Design. This was a cross-sectional survey carried out from 2011 to 2012 under a special research licence provided by the Zambia Wildlife Authority (ZAWA). It was part of a wider survey undertaken by the Southern African Development Community Transboundary Animal Diseases (SADC TADs) disease surveillance programme. The licence approved sampling of 25 buffaloes from each of the five study areas (Mosi-oa-tunya, Sichifulo, Lower Zambezi, Lundazi, and Sioma) (DVLD/3/22/1: National Parks, Game Reserves and Wildlife). Therefore, we targeted to sample 125 animals.

2.3. Sample Collection. Targeted animals were buffaloes aged between six months and six years. This was done to exclude young animals that still had maternal antibodies and those older animals that were no longer prone to infection. The age range of the buffalo was determined by the protrusions of the horns based on aerial view first and before sampling the age range was determined by checking the horns and dentition [21]. Animals were first immobilised through remotely injecting chemical anaesthetic agent, etorphine hydrochloride (M99, Immobilon; Novartis, South Africa).

From the immobilised animals, about 8 mL of blood was collected from all the 99 buffaloes through the jugular vein puncture using a sterile vacutainer needle into plain vacutainer tubes. The blood was left to clot overnight at room temperature and then centrifuged at 2500 rpm for 5 minutes to separate the serum. Sera were stored at −20°C until needed for laboratory analysis.

Probang samples were collected from 49 buffaloes using probang cups as recommended in the OIE Terrestrial Manual [22]. The collected probang samples were mixed with FMDV transport media (composed of 0.08 M phosphate buffer containing 0.01% bovine serum albumin, 0.002% phenol red, 1000 units/mL penicillin, 100 units/mL mycostatin, 100 units neomycin, and 50 units/mL polymyxin and adjusted to pH 7.2) [22] in the ratio of 1 : 3 in a conical tube after which the mixture was transferred into a cryotube. The cryotube containing probang sample was then put into a liquid nitrogen tank. Probang cups were disinfected using citric acid (0.2%, wt/vol) and rinsed three times in water and then in PBS between samplings. Probang samples were stored in liquid nitrogen or in the freezer at −70°C in the laboratory awaiting treating and passaging. Furthermore, information on age and sex was recorded and latitude and longitude coordinates were collected with a handheld GPS device (nüvi 205 series; Garmin, USA).

After sampling, the immobilised buffaloes were revived by injection with diprenorphine (M5050, Revivon; Novartis, South Africa). All the samples were collected and processed following World Reference Laboratory (WRL) and World Organisation for Animal Health (Office International des Epizooties (OIE)) guidelines [10].

2.4. Sample Analysis. Detection of antibodies against FMDV in sera was done at Central Veterinary Research Institute (CVRI) in Lusaka and Botswana Vaccine Institute (BVI) using the liquid phase blocking ELISA (Institute for Animal Health, Pirbright Laboratory, UK) technique for the detection of antibodies against FMDV in sera as described by [23] and the PrioCHECK FMDV-NS test (Prionics Lelystad B.V., Netherlands), a blocking ELISA that can measure antibody level to 3ABC nonstructural proteins [24].

The probang samples were treated and passaged in RM monolayer cell cultures and then examined for cytopathic effect (CPE). If no CPE was detected after 48 hours, the cells were frozen and thawed, used to inoculate fresh cell cultures, and examined for CPE for another 48 hours. Some field viruses may require several passages before they become adapted [22]. In antigen ELISA (Institute for Animal Health, Pirbright Laboratory, UK) we tested the supernatants of CPE positive cell cultures inoculated with probang samples in order to confirm the specificity of the CPE and to serotype the isolate. The antigen ELISA kit was based on a standard indirect sandwich ELISA technique to determine the presence of FMDV antigens in samples as described by [22].

2.5. Data Analysis. Data was stored in basic Excel format for easy handling and storage. The data was transferred to SPSS 16.0 for statistical analysis. Proportion of positive

sera, with the 95% confidence intervals (CI) on both LPBE and PrioCHECK FMDV-NS test, were estimated. The associations between categorical variables and the ELISA tests results were evaluated using Fisher's exact test, while Kappa test was used to evaluate the agreement between the LPBE and PrioCHECK FMDV-NS test cross-tabulation results. p values <0.05 were considered statistically significant. Spatial mapping of the distribution of FMD in the study areas was done using ArcView_GIS (Environmental Systems Resource Institute, 1992–1999 ArcView 3.2, Redlands, CA).

3. Results

3.1. Serology Results

3.1.1. LPBE Test. A total of 99 serum samples were tested and the results are shown in Table 1. The overall FMD prevalence based on LPBE SAT serotype results was 92.9 percent (95% CI = 87.8–98.0). The SAT1 prevalence was highest in Lower Zambezi and Lundazi (88.0%, 95% CI = 68.8–97.4), while no animals tested positive to SAT1 serotypes in Sioma National Park. There was a significant difference in SAT1 prevalence among the sampling sites (p = 0.001). SAT2 prevalence was highest in Lundazi where all animals tested positive (100%, 95% CI = 83.3–100), with no animals testing positive in Sioma. There was a significant difference in prevalence among the sampling sites (p = 0.001). SAT3 prevalence was highest in Sichifulo (50%, 95% CI = 27.2–72.8), with no animals testing positive in Sioma. There was a significant difference in SAT3 prevalence among the sampling sites (p = 0.001). All the buffaloes sampled (100%, 95% CI = 83.3–100) from Lower Zambezi and Lundazi were positive to antibodies against FMDV on the LPBE test and all those from Lundazi were positive to at least (100%, 95% CI = 83.3–100) two serotypes.

The few calves (age ranging from six months to eight months) that were sampled were all from Sioma and were all negative for FMDV SAT antibodies. The highest prevalence according to age range was in the 1-2-year category of which all were positive for antibodies against FMDV. In the 3-4-year age category, 93.1% were positive for antibodies against FMDV, while, in the 5-6-year age category, all the samples were positive for FMDV antibodies. There was no significant difference in SAT serotypes prevalence between the different age groups (p > 0.05). Similarly, there was no significant difference in the prevalence of SAT serotypes between male and female buffaloes (p > 0.05).

3.1.2. PrioCHECK FMDV-NS Test. A total of 99 serum samples were tested on the assay. FMD overall prevalence, based on the PrioCHECK FMDV-NS ELISA test which detects antibodies to nonstructural viral proteins, was high, 84.8% (95% CI = 77.2–91.5). The prevalence according to area of sampling was as follows: Lower Zambezi (n = 25), 96% (95% CI = 88.3–103.7); Lundazi (n = 25), 100% (95% CI = 100–100); Mosi-oa-tunya (n = 25), 80% (95% CI = 64.3–95.7); and Sichifulo (n = 20), 75% (95% CI = 56.0–94.0). The few calves (age ranging from six months to eight months) that were sampled were all from Sioma and were all negative

TABLE 1: Seroprevalence of FMDV by LPBE SAT.

| Study area NP/GMA | Number tested | SAT serotype | | | Overall prevalence % | Mixed infection % |
		SAT1 %	SAT2 %	SAT3 %		
Lower Zambezi	25	88.0 (68.8–97.4)	84.0 (63.9–95.5)	8.0 (0.98–26)	100.0 (83.3–100)	84.0 (63.9–95.5)
Lundazi	25	88.0 (68.8–97.4)	100.0 (83.3–100)	12.0 (2.5–31.2)	100.0 (83.3–100)	100.0 (83.3–100)
Mosi-oa-tunya	25	32.0 (14.9–53.5)	76.0 (59.3–92.7)	44.0 (24.4–65.1)	92.0 (74.0–99.9)	60.0 (38.7–78.9)
Sichifulo	20	45.0 (23.1–68.3)	35.0 (15.4–59.2)	50.0 (27.2–72.8)	95.0 (75.1–99.9)	35.0 (15.4–59.2)
Sioma	4	0	0	0	0	0

TABLE 2: Prevalence of LPBE results, mixed infection, and PrioCHECK FMDV-NS test results in relation to age.

Age category	n	Prevalence (95% CI)—LPBE	Mixed infection	Prevalence (95% CI)—PrioCHECK FMDV-NS
Less than 1 year	4	0	0	0
1-2 years	37	100 (100-100)	64.9 (57.6–72.2)	100 (100-100)
3-4 years	49	93.9 (87.2–100)	87.7 (78.1–97.4)	85.7 (75.9–95.5)
5-6 years	9	100 (100-100)	88.9 (87.1–90.7)	100 (100-100)
p value		0.413	0.497	0.451

TABLE 3: Prevalence of LPBE results, mixed infection, and PrioCHECK FMDV-NS results in buffalo according to sex category.

| Sex | n | Prevalence (95% CI)—LPBE | | | Mixed infection | Prevalence (95% CI)—PrioCHECK FMDV-NS |
		SAT1	SAT2	SAT3		
Female	61	59 (46.7–71.0)	75 (64.1–85.9)	24.5 (13.7–35.2)	76.5 (64.5–88.5)	86.9 (78.4–95.4)
Male	38	63.2 (47.9–78.5)	71.1 (56.7–65.5)	28.9 (14.5–43.3)	62.4 (54.9–69.9)	81.6 (69.3–93.9)
p value		0.861	0.278	0.778	0.533	0.567

for FMDV antibodies on PrioCHECK FMDV-NS test. There was a significant difference in prevalence among the different sampling sites ($p < 0.05$) and this was statistically significant (p value = 0.001). Of the 84 buffaloes that tested positive for FMDV NPS antibodies, 69 were strong positives (>70) and 15 were weak positives (>50 and <70). The prevalence according to age categories was also not statistically different (p value = 0.413) (Table 2). The overall prevalence of females ($n = 61$) and males ($n = 38$) on PrioCHECK FMDV-NS test was 86.9% (95% CI 78.4–95.4) and 81.6% (95% CI 69.3–93.9), respectively. Further, there was no significant difference in the prevalence of antibodies against SAT serotypes tested in LBPE and against nonstructural proteins (PrioCHECK FMDV-NS test) in relation to age and sex (Table 3).

The cross-tabulation of combined test results for the LPBE SAT serotype ELISA and the PrioCHECK FMDV-NS ELISA among the buffaloes sampled in GMA and NP is shown in Table 4. The results showed a fair agreement between results obtained on PrioCHECK FMDV-NS and LPBE SAT serotypes (kappa = 0.296 at 0.001; McNemar = 0.057).

3.1.3. *Virus Isolation and Serotyping by Antigen ELISA in Probang Samples.* A total of 49 probang samples (Lundazi, $n = 24$, and Lower Zambezi, $n = 25$) were collected, treated,

TABLE 4: LPBE test and PrioCHECK FMDV-NS test cross-tabulation.

| | PrioCHECK FMDV-NS test | | |
	Negative	Positive	Total
LPBE test			
Negative	4	3	7
Positive	11	81	92
Total	15	84	99

and passaged. Overall cytopathic effects (CPE) suggestive of FMDV replication in primary RM cell cultures were observed in three samples from Lundazi ($n = 2$) and Lower Zambezi ($n = 1$). The CPE was characterised by the fast destruction of the cell monolayer from which infected cells were round and seen singly. Complete destruction of the cell sheet was mostly seen within 48 hours of inoculation of the 1st passage or 2nd passage. Samples with CPE were analysed using the antigen ELISA to identify the serotypes. The antigen ELISA analysis showed that two samples from Lundazi were of SAT2 serotypes, and one sample from Lower Zambezi was of the SAT1 serotype.

4. Discussion

The aim of this study was to determine the seroprevalence of the FMD in buffaloes and identify circulating FMDV serotypes in buffalo populations in Zambia. A high prevalence of antibodies against FMDV in buffaloes was observed in all the study areas except in Sioma where only few animals (all calves) were tested. Further, major FMDV SAT types observed to be circulating in buffaloes in Zambia based on the results from LPBE were SAT1, SAT2, and SAT3, while only SAT1 and SAT2 were isolated from probang samples. Our study reveals that FMD could be a problem in study areas. These results corroborate the findings of previous studies which demonstrated high FMDV seroprevalence in buffalo populations in Southern Africa [25, 26]. In our study SAT2 was the most predominant serotype, followed by SAT1 and then SAT3. Overall, all the Game Parks/Game Management Areas had high prevalence of mixed infections, which supports the earlier observation that individual buffaloes may be persistently infected with more than one type of FMDV in the pharyngeal region [27–29]. The LPBE was chosen as it has been used successfully for numerous animal species before, including the African buffalo. While the test shows an almost perfect sensitivity, the specificity in cattle usually is about 95% and similar values were assumed for the African buffalo. However, in cattle up to 18% [30, 31] false positive reactions have been reported. LPBE detects immunoglobulins directed against the capsid or structural proteins of the virus and therefore cannot distinguish antibodies induced by vaccinations using inactivated vaccines from those elicited by infection with live virus [32]. PrioCHECK FMDV-NS detects antibodies against the nonstructural 3ABC protein of FMDV but cannot distinguish between serotypes. However, antibodies to the 3ABC protein are considered to be the most reliable indicators of infection/exposure to FMDV [33, 34]. The specificity of the PrioCHECK FMDV-NS for bovine sera was given as 98.1 percent by [35] while the sensitivity in nonvaccinated, experimentally infected bovines also approached 100 percent. Bronsvoort et al. [36] published sensitivity and specificity estimates of 87.7 percent and 87.3 percent, respectively, for the African buffalo using Bayesian statistics, but their data would be consistent with values closer to those recorded for cattle, in particular if factors like antibody kinetics and sample quality are taken into account.

The study has also revealed that buffaloes within the age of one to two years are most likely to be infected by FMDV as all the buffaloes were positive to FMDV infection at this age. This is in agreement with the findings of previous studies which indicated that, after maternal antibodies wane, the young buffaloes were prone to FMDV infection from the carrier buffaloes [37]. Buffaloes in the age category of 5-6 years were positive for antibodies against FMDV and had mixed infection slightly higher compared to the other categories; this could have been due to the risk that the older the buffaloes are, the more the time they are likely to get infected by different FMDV serotypes is. African buffaloes are efficient maintenance hosts of the SAT type viruses, with an individual animal maintaining the virus up to five years and

isolated herds for up to 24 years, although persistence in an individual buffalo is probably not lifelong [37].

Probang samples were collected with the view of isolating FMDV and identifying serotypes in circulation [29, 37, 38]. However, only a small proportion of samples yielded positive results as two, SAT2, and one, SAT1, virus isolates were obtained. This is in line with the report that the excretion of virus by carriers is intermittent [1] and the findings by [10] that reported that the quantity of virus present in the pharynx of carrier animals can vary considerably over time. As part of future studies, it is recommended to obtain more probang samples for virus isolation and also generate nucleotide sequences of these isolates so that the FMDV circulating in these buffaloes can be differentiated to topotypes level to understand their diversity. In addition, the availability of more local FMDV isolates enables the calculation of r^1 values required to check and possibly adapt preventive and control measures in endemic or epidemic regions where strategic or general vaccination is required with vaccine containing the FMDV subtypes that are active in the area [29].

In this study, based on LPBE, very few SAT3 seropositive buffalo samples were only seropositive for SAT3 ($n = 5$), while slight proportions were SAT1 seropositive only ($n = 9$) or SAT2 seropositive only ($n = 10$). The majority of samples were positive to more than one serotype, and this raises the issue of to what extent the SAT results are cross-reactions [27]. Virus neutralisation assays using local FMDV isolates would be required to further dissect possible cross-reactivities. In addition, the isolation of a SAT3 FMDV from concurrent probang samples would confirm the presence of this serotype in Zambian buffaloes.

The study showed fair agreement between LPBE test and PrioCHECK FMDV-NS test cross-tabulation results. Lack of substantial or perfect agreement could be attributed to the fact that the kinetics and duration of the antibody response to structural and nonstructural viral proteins differ as does the rate of seroconversion [39].

Antibodies to all the three Southern African Territories (SAT) serotypes were detected in buffaloes in the four study areas (Mosi-oa-tunya, Sichifulo, Lower Zambezi, and Lundazi) where age and sex of the buffalo had no effect in FMDV infection/exposure status. This is in agreement with earlier observations in studies conducted in buffaloes in Sub-Saharan Africa [37]. The exception was Sioma where all the four samples collected from buffaloes in age range of six months to eight months were negative for antibodies against FMDV. Therefore no equivocal statement can be made regarding these results as the apparent absence could be attributed to the small sample size and may be that the young buffaloes had not yet been exposed to FMDV.

There is little published on non-SAT serotypes in buffalo in Zambia. From reported outbreaks in Saharan Africa [37], it appears that the majority of outbreaks in the southern regions are due to SAT serotypes with only sporadic introductions of O and A. Zambia being surrounded by other countries which have reported other serotypes cannot be excluded from harbouring other serotypes apart from SAT serotypes due to the reported outbreaks in Kenya (1994 to 2000), Tanzania

(1999 to 2000), and Uganda (1995 to 1999) of SAT1, SAT2, and O (as well as A and C in Kenya) [37]. This needs to be looked at in more detail as recent work on sera has shown consistency in results of antibody screening repeatedly over long storage period. The other interesting studies could be comparison of the prevalence of FMDV in buffalo to that in livestock held in Kazungula/Livingstone during the time period of the buffalo sampling as it could possibly shed light on the role that buffaloes have in transmission of the disease to domestic livestock. This is immanent from the fact that the Department of Veterinary Services in the Ministry of Agriculture and Livestock (MAL) had reported FMDV SAT1 outbreaks which belonged to topotype III (WZ) but were not closely related to other SAT1 viruses [17].

It is known that buffaloes play an important role in maintaining FMD infections and are able to infect other susceptible species in Sub-Saharan Africa [26, 40] and that buffaloes have been shown to be the source of infection for impala and domestic animals in proximity of the Kruger National Park (KNP) and other game parks in Southern Africa [40]. References [41–43] demonstrated natural and experimental transmission from carrier buffalo to cattle. However, it should be noted that even though transmission has been demonstrated, the transmission conditions from carrier buffalo are not well understood and difficult to replicate because many attempts at carrying out transmission from carrier buffalo to naive buffalo or cattle have failed, even under conditions of immunosuppression or coinfection with rinderpest and bovine herpes-1 virus [28, 44–47].

5. Conclusion

In conclusion, our study has demonstrated high FMDV seroprevalence in buffaloes in Zambia and characterised the SAT serotypes circulating in the country. These findings will play a role in the control of FMD in Zambia because knowledge of circulating FMDV is critical in vaccine matching, which is necessary to ensure vaccine efficacy. Most parts of Zambia are endemic to FMD; therefore strategic or general vaccination is required with vaccine containing the FMDV subtypes that are active in the area [29].

There is still need for molecular characterisation of the positive virus samples on antigen ELISA at the same time antigen titrations should also be performed and r^1 values should be determined to enable matching with the FMD.

Conflict of Interests

The authors declare that none of them have financial or personal relationships with individuals or organisations that may have inappropriately influenced them in writing this paper and, therefore, declare that there is no conflict of interests.

Acknowledgments

The authors would like to thank the GRZ, SACIDS (through a grant from the Wellcome Trust (Grant WTO 87546MA)) and SADC TADs program for funding this study. They thank the late Director of Veterinary Services Dr. Joseph Mubanga for his assistance with this work. Many thanks are due to Dr. Paul Fandamu, Ms. Mwauseya, Mr. M. Mukubwali, and Mr. M. Simweemba for the technical support. They thank Ms. L. Seoke of BVI for the assistance with laboratory work. They are grateful to the Quality Control Staff of BVI for the good supply of RM monolayer cells.

References

[1] S. Alexandersen, Z. Zhang, and A. I. Donaldson, "Aspects of the persistence of foot-and-mouth disease virus in animals—the carrier problem," *Microbes and Infection*, vol. 4, no. 10, pp. 1099–1110, 2002.

[2] F. Brown, "The history of research in foot-and-mouth disease," *Virus Research*, vol. 91, no. 1, pp. 3–7, 2003.

[3] N. J. Knowles and A. R. Samuel, "Molecular epidemiology of foot-and-mouth disease virus," *Virus Research*, vol. 91, no. 1, pp. 65–80, 2003.

[4] J. B. Brooksby, "Portraits of viruses: foot-and-mouth disease virus," *Intervirology*, vol. 18, no. 1-2, pp. 1–23, 1982.

[5] P. Chilonda, J. D. Woodford, B. Ahmadu, K. L. Samui, M. Syakalima, and J. E. D. Mlangwa, "Foot and mouth disease in Zambia: a review of the aetiology and epidemiology and recommendations for possible control," *Revue Scientifique et Technique*, vol. 18, no. 3, pp. 585–592, 1999.

[6] E. Overby and G. C. N. Zyambo, "Foot and mouth disease outbreaks in Zambia," *Revue Scientifique et Technique*, vol. 2, no. 1, pp. 189–197, 1999.

[7] M. Munyeme, J. B. Muma, H. M. Munangándu, C. Kankya, E. Skjerve, and M. Tryland, "Cattle owners' awareness of bovine tuberculosis in high and low prevalence settings of the wildlife-livestock interface areas in Zambia," *BMC Veterinary Research*, vol. 6, article 21, 2010.

[8] B. W. J. Mahy, "Foot and mouth disease virus," in *Current Topics in Microbiology and Immunology*, vol. 288, 2005.

[9] M. G. Mateu, "Antibody recognition of picornaviruses and escape from neutralization: a structural view," *Virus Research*, vol. 38, no. 1, pp. 1–24, 1995.

[10] R. P. Kitching, "Clinical variation in foot and mouth disease: cattle," *Revue Scientifique et Technique*, vol. 21, no. 3, pp. 499–504, 2002.

[11] Annonymous, *Annual Reports of the Department of Veterinary and Livestock Development*, Ministry of Agriculture, Livestock and Fisheries, 2005.

[12] *Annual Reports of the Department of Veterinary and Livestock Development*, Ministry of Agriculture, Livestock and Fisheries, 2008.

[13] Annonymous, *Annual Reports of the Department of Veterinary and Livestock Development*, Ministry of Agriculture, Livestock and Fisheries, 2006.

[14] *Annual Reports of the Department of Veterinary and Livestock Development*, Ministry of Agriculture, Livestock and Fisheries, 2007.

[15] *Annual Reports of the Department of Veterinary and Livestock Development*, Ministry of Agriculture, Livestock and Fisheries, 2009.

[16] *Annual Reports of the Department of Veterinary and Livestock Development*, Ministry of Agriculture, Livestock and Fisheries, 2010.

[17] Tech. Rep., OIE/FAO FMD Reference Laboratory Network, 2012.

[18] F. Banda, C. J. Kasanga, R. Sallu et al., "Investigation of foot-and-mouth disease outbreaks in the Mbala and Kazungula districts of Zambia," *Onderstepoort Journal of Veterinary Research*, vol. 81, no. 2, article 721, 2014.

[19] Y. Sinkala, M. Simuunza, D. U. Pfeiffer et al., "Challenges and economic implications in the control of foot and mouth disease in sub-Saharan Africa: Lessons from the Zambian experience," *Veterinary Medicine International*, vol. 2014, Article ID 373921, 12 pages, 2014.

[20] J. S. S. Dillman, "Foot and mouth disease investigations in game animals (lechwe and buffaloes)," Final Report vol.1, Germany Agency for Technical Cooperation, Government Publishers, Lusaka, Zambia, 1976.

[21] H. K. Mwima, "Wildlife research and management in Zambia with special reference to some protected areas where wild and domestic animals co-exist," in *The Effects of Enlargement of Domestic Animal Pasture on the Wildlife in Zambia, Lusaka, Zambia*, pp. 305–308, 1995.

[22] OIE, *Manual of Diagnostic Tests and vaccines for Terrestrial Animals*, Office International des Epizooties, Paris, France, 6th edition, 2010.

[23] C. Hamblin, I. T. R. Barnett, and R. S. Hedger, "A new enzyme-linked immunosorbent assay (ELISA) for the detection of antibodies against foot-and-mouth disease virus I. Development and method of ELISA," *Journal of Immunological Methods*, vol. 93, no. 1, pp. 115–121, 1986.

[24] M. de Diego, E. Brocchi, D. Mackay, and F. de Simone, "The non-structural polyprotein 3ABC of foot-and-mouth disease virus as a diagnostic antigen in ELISA to differentiate infected from vaccinated cattle," *Archives of Virology*, vol. 142, no. 10, pp. 2021–2033, 1997.

[25] J. J. Esterhuysen, G. R. Thomson, J. R. Flammand, and R. G. Bengis, "Buffalo in the northern Natal game parks show no serological evidence of infection with foot-and-mouth disease virus," *Onderstepoort Journal of Veterinary Research*, vol. 52, no. 2, pp. 63–66, 1985.

[26] G. R. Thomson, W. Vosloo, and A. D. S. Bastos, "Foot and mouth disease in wildlife," *Virus Research*, vol. 91, no. 1, pp. 145–161, 2003.

[27] R. S. Hedger, I. T. R. Barnett, D. V. Gradwell, and P. T. Dias, "Serological tests for foot-and-mouth disease in bovine serum samples, problems of interpretation," *Revue Scientifique et Technique*, vol. 1, pp. 387–393, 1992.

[28] E. C. Anderson, W. J. Doughty, J. Anderson, and R. Paling, "The pathogenesis of foot-and-mouth disease in the African buffalo (*Syncerus caffer*) and the role of this species in the epidemiology of the disease in Kenya," *Journal of Comparative Pathology*, vol. 89, no. 4, pp. 541–549, 1979.

[29] P. Sutmoller, S. S. Barteling, R. C. Olascoaga, and K. J. Sumption, "Control and eradication of foot-and-mouth disease," *Virus Research*, vol. 91, no. 1, pp. 101–144, 2003.

[30] A. Clavijo, P. Wright, and P. Kitching, "Developments in diagnostic techniques for differentiating infection from vaccination in foot and mouth disease," *Veterinary Journal*, vol. 167, no. 1, pp. 9–22, 2004.

[31] B. Haas, "Application of the liquid phase blocking sandwich ELISA. Problems encountered in import/export serology and possible solutions," in *Proceedings of the Session of the Research Group of the European Commission for the Control of Foot and Mouth Disease*, pp. 124–127, EuFMD, Vienna, Austria, 1994.

[32] R. M. Armstrong, S. J. Cox, N. Aggarwal et al., "Detection of antibody to the foot-and-mouth disease virus (FMDV) non-structural polyprotein 3ABC in sheep by ELISA," *Journal of Virological Methods*, vol. 125, no. 2, pp. 153–163, 2005.

[33] K. J. Sørensen, K. G. Madsen, E. S. Madsen, J. S. Salt, J. Nqindi, and D. K. J. Mackay, "Differentiation of infection from vaccination in foot-and-mouth disease by the detection of antibodies to the non-structural proteins 3D, 3AB and 3ABC in ELISA using antigens expressed in baculovirus," *Archives of Virology*, vol. 143, no. 8, pp. 1461–1476, 1998.

[34] T. Sun, P. Lu, and X. Wang, "Localization of infection-related epitopes on the non-structural protein 3ABC of foot-and-mouth disease virus and the application of tandem epitopes," *Journal of Virological Methods*, vol. 119, no. 2, pp. 79–86, 2004.

[35] E. Brocchi, I. E. Bergmann, A. Dekker et al., "Comparative evaluation of six ELISAs for the detection of antibodies to the non-structural proteins of foot-and-mouth disease virus," *Vaccine*, vol. 24, no. 47-48, pp. 6966–6979, 2006.

[36] B. M. D. C. Bronsvoort, S. Parida, I. Handel et al., "Serological survey for foot-and-mouth disease virus in wildlife in eastern Africa and estimation of test parameters of a nonstructural protein enzyme-linked immunosorbent assay for buffalo," *Clinical and Vaccine Immunology*, vol. 15, no. 6, pp. 1003–1011, 2008.

[37] W. Vosloo, A. D. S. Bastos, O. Sangare, S. K. Hargreaves, and G. R. Thomson, "Review of the status and control of foot and mouth disease in sub-Saharan Africa," *Scientific and Technical Review*, vol. 21, no. 3, pp. 437–449, 2002.

[38] M. Rémond, C. Kaiser, and F. Lebreton, "Diagnosis and screening of foot-and-mouth disease," *Comparative Immunology, Microbiology and Infectious Diseases*, vol. 25, no. 5-6, pp. 309–320, 2002.

[39] B. M. D. Bronsvoort, N. Toft, I. E. Bergmann et al., "Evaluation of three 3ABC ELISAs for foot-and-mouth disease non-structural antibodies using latent class analysis," *BMC Veterinary Research*, vol. 2, article 30, 2006.

[40] G. R. Thomson and A. D. S. Bastos, "Foot and mouth disease," in *Infectious Diseases of Livestock*, J. A. W. Coetzer and R. C. Tustin, Eds., pp. 1324–1365, Oxford University Press, Cape Town, South Africa, 2nd edition, 2004.

[41] P. S. Dawe, F. O. Flanagan, R. L. Madekurozwa et al., "Natural transmission of foot-and-mouth disease virus from African buffalo (*Syncerus caffer*) to cattle in a wildlife area of Zimbabwe," *Veterinary Record*, vol. 134, no. 10, pp. 230–232, 1994.

[42] P. S. Dawe, K. Sorensen, N. P. Ferris, I. T. Barnett, R. M. Armstrong, and N. J. Knowles, "Experimental transmission of foot-and-mouth disease virus from carrier African buffalo (*Syncerus caffer*) to cattle in Zimbabwe," *Veterinary Record*, vol. 134, no. 9, pp. 211–215, 1994.

[43] A. D. S. Bastos, D. T. Haydon, O. Sangaré, C. I. Boshoff, J. L. Edrich, and G. R. Thomson, "The implications of virus diversity within the SAT2 serotype for control of foot-and-mouth disease in sub-Saharan Africa," *Journal of General Virology*, vol. 84, no. 6, pp. 1595–1606, 2003.

[44] R. G. Bengis, G. R. Thomson, R. S. Hedger, V. De Vos, and A. Pini, "Foot-and-mouth disease and the African buffalo (*Syncerus caffer*). 1. Carriers as a source of infection for cattle," *The Onderstepoort Journal of Veterinary Research*, vol. 53, no. 2, pp. 69–73, 1986.

[45] J. B. Condy and R. S. Hedger, "The survival of foot and mouth disease virus in African buffalo with non transference of infection to domestic cattle," *Research in Veterinary Science*, vol. 16, no. 2, pp. 182–185, 1974.

[46] M. D. Gainaru, G. R. Thomson, R. G. Bengis, J. J. Esterhuysen, W. Bruce, and A. Pini, "Foot-and-mouth disease and the African buffalo (*Syncerus caffer*). II. Virus excretion and transmission during acute infection.," *The Onderstepoort Journal of Veterinary Research*, vol. 53, no. 2, pp. 75–85, 1986.

[47] G. R. Thomson, "The role of carrier animals in the transmission of foot and mouth diseases," OIE Comprehensive Reports on Technical Items Presented to the International Committee or to Regional Commissions, 1996.

12

Light and Electron Microscopic Studies on Prenatal Differentiation of Exocrine Pancreas in Buffalo

Divya Gupta, Varinder Uppal, Neelam Bansal, and Anuradha Gupta

Department of Veterinary Anatomy, College of Veterinary Sciences, Guru Angad Dev Veterinary and Animal Sciences University, Ludhiana, Punjab 141004, India

Correspondence should be addressed to Varinder Uppal; v.uppal@yahoo.com

Academic Editor: Remo Lobetti

The study was conducted on pancreas of 24 buffalo fetuses collected from abattoir and Veterinary clinics, GADVASU, Ludhiana. The buffalo fetuses were divided into three groups after measuring their CVRL, namely, group I (CVRL between 0 and 20 cm), group II (CVRL above 20 cm and up to 40 cm), and group III (CVRL above 40 cm) and their approximate age was calculated. The tissues were processed for light and ultrastructural studies. In group I, at 1.2 cm CVRL (34 days), the pancreas comprised tubules and solid nest of undifferentiated epithelial cells. At 7.5 cm CVRL (63 days) acinar cells with zymogen granules were observed. These acinar cells varied in shape from columnar to pyramidal. At 12.8 cm CVRL (86 days), parenchyma began to organize into lobes and lobules. The centroacinar cells were observed at 12.8 cm CVRL (86 days). In group II, at 28.3 cm CVRL (137 days), there was extensive branching of tubules that resulted in highly branched ductal tree connecting exocrine secretary units to the duct system. The interlobular and intralobular ducts were well observed at this age yet the intercalated ducts were not completely developed. In group III, exocrine pancreas showed a massive growth at 48 cm CVRL (182 days) with distinct pancreatic lobes and lobules. At 54 cm CVRL (195 days), well developed pancreatic architecture was seen with the presence of extensive development of exocrine part organized in lobes and lobules with interlobular and intralobular ducts whereas the intercalated ducts were observed in 80 cm CVRL (254 days).

1. Introduction

Pancreas is a bifunctional organ consisting of an exocrine part organized in acini and a duct system that secretes enzymes for digestion and an endocrine part that secretes hormones like insulin, glucagon, and so forth that helps in glucose homeostasis. Knowledge of development of pancreas is essential to understand congenital pancreatic abnormalities like anomalous pancreatobiliary junction, annular pancreas, and pancreas divisum arising from abnormal histogenesis and morphogenesis occurring during critical period of organization of the organ during prenatal life [1]. Nowadays, the biology of the pancreas has been studied intensely, largely driven by the hope of finding better treatments for devastating pancreatic diseases, such as diabetes mellitus, pancreatitis, and pancreatic adenocarcinoma. In particular, advancements in stem cell technology have recently sparked optimism that diabetes could be cured by harvesting stem cells for therapeutic use. This has led to heightened interest in understanding embryonic development of the pancreas [2].

In literature, prenatal development of exocrine pancreas has been reported in rat [3], pig [4], sheep [5], rabbit [6], and human [7, 8], but very scanty literature is available in buffaloes [9, 10]. So the present research work was conducted. Most of the work on development of exocrine pancreas has been reported in human. Since mammals, birds, reptiles, and amphibians have a pancreas with similar histology and mode of development, the findings of the present research have been discussed with the available literature in human. The recognition of normal development of the pancreas in mammals and other species can help understand congenital anomalies in humans and other species [11]. So, the present research may provide a basic data which can be used to evaluate any abnormality occurring in the development of the pancreas at a critical period of organization.

2. Materials and Methods

The present study was conducted on pancreas of 24 buffalo fetuses collected from slaughter house and Veterinary clinics, GADVASU, Ludhiana. The length of the fetuses was measured with the help of inelastic thread as a curved line along the vertebral column between the most anterior part of frontal bone and the rump at ischiatic tuberosity and designated as crown vertebral rump length (CVRL). After measuring the CVRL in centimeters, the approximate age of the fetuses was estimated by using the formula given by Soliman [12] in buffalo. Based on the CVR length, the samples were divided into three groups: group I, CVR length up to 20 cm, group II, CVR length above 20 cm and up to 40 cm, and group III, CVR length above 40 cm. The pancreas was dissected out from the abdominal cavity and the tissues were fixed in 10% neutral buffered formalin and Bouin's fixative immediately after collection. After the fixation, the tissues were processed for paraffin blocks preparation by acetone benzene schedule [13]. The blocks were prepared and the sections of 5-6 μm were cut with rotary microtome. The paraffin sections were stained with hematoxylin and eosin, Masson's trichrome, and Holme's stains.

For electron microscopic studies, fresh tissues were washed and fixed in Karnovsky's fixative. The secondary fixation was done for 2 hours in 2% osmium tetraoxide. The tissues were dehydrated, cleared, infiltrated, embedded, and polymerized. The ultrathin sections (70–90 nm) were cut and stained with uranyl acetate (15 min) followed by lead citrate (10 min) [14]. Finally, the grids with sections were examined under transmission electron microscope.

3. Results

In group I, at 1.2 cm CVRL (34 days), the pancreatic parenchyma comprised tubules/ductules and solid nest of undifferentiated epithelial cells in mesenchymal tissue between the developing stomach, duodenum, and mesonephric kidney. The cells of these tubules/ductules were cuboidal in shape having slightly eosinophilic cytoplasm and intensely basophilic nuclei. These tubules/ductules also comprised some cells which were more eosinophilic and these cells represented the differentiating acinar cells (Figure 1) but at this stage no granules were observed in these cells. At 2.6 cm CVRL (40 days), these eosinophilic cells started to assemble in groups but no well defined acini were found (Figure 2). A large number of mitotic figures were observed in these developing cells. The pancreatic duct observed at this stage was lined by simple columnar epithelium. With further branching of pancreatic primitive tubules, the pancreas grew more in size and the luminization of many epithelial buds was observed at 4.2 cm CVRL (48 days). At 7.5 cm CVRL (63 days), there was extensive branching of tubules and these tubules consisted of different types of precursor cells (Figure 3). Newly formed microlumens were initially unconnected but eventually fused into a luminal plexus. Many differentiated acinar cells were grouped to form acini with a well developed lumen. These acinar cells varied in shape from columnar to pyramidal. The supranuclear part of

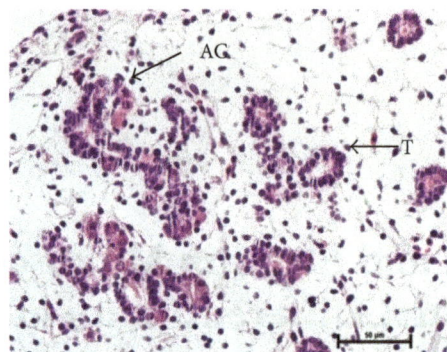

FIGURE 1: 1.2 cm CVRL (34 days) showing primitive tubules (T) and developing acinar cells (AC) in mesenchyme of pancreas. Hematoxylin and eosin ×400.

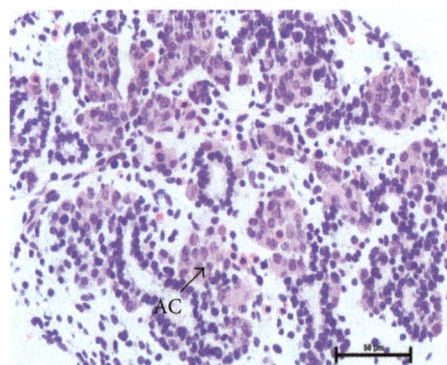

FIGURE 2: 2.6 cm CVRL (40 days) showing development of acinar cells (AC) from primitive tubules. Hematoxylin and eosin ×400.

the cell was filled with eosinophilic zymogen granules. The presence of these granules was confirmed by ultrastructural studies and it was found that these granules were of variable sizes and were not fully mature at this stage. Some granules were small, round, and membrane-bound and contained homogeneous electron dense material, whereas others were having moderately electron dense material (Figure 4). Some degranulated vesicles were also present at this stage. Nucleus was large and oval in shape. Endoplasmic reticulum and mitochondria were few in number. The Golgi apparatus was prominent at this stage.

At 9.6 cm CVRL (72 days), there was massive growth of the pancreatic tubules. During the study, the different types of branching patterns were observed. At 10.7 cm CVRL (77 days), the pancreatic duct was lined by simple columnar epithelium and at places glands were observed. At 12.8 cm CVRL (86 days), parenchyma had begun to organize into lobes and lobules with abundant connective tissue (Figure 5). Along with the formation of lobules, interlobular and intralobular ducts were also observed at this age. The intralobular duct was lined by simple cuboidal epithelium, whereas the interlobular duct was having either simple cuboidal or simple columnar epithelium (Figure 6). The cells were tall and pyramidal having a distinct basal lamina. Along with the acinar cells, the centroacinar cells were observed for

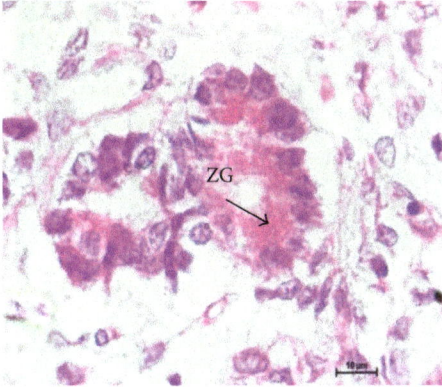

FIGURE 3: 7.5 cm CVRL (62 days) paraffin section showing acini and zymogen granules (ZG) in apical part of cell. Hematoxylin and eosin ×1000.

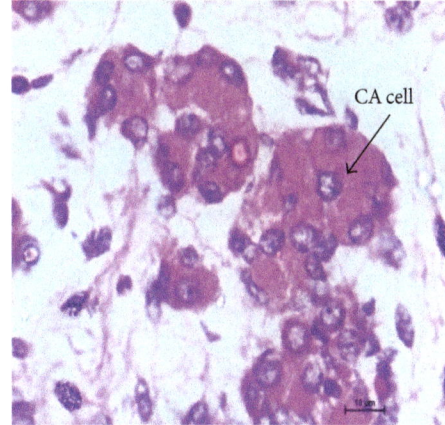

FIGURE 5: 12.8 cm CVRL (86 days) showing centroacinar (CA) cell. Hematoxylin and eosin ×1000.

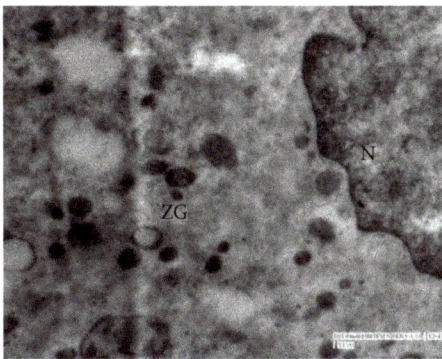

FIGURE 4: Electron micrograph 7.5 cm CVRL (62 days) showing nucleus (N), developing zymogen granules (ZG), and some of the empty vesicles (EV) in acinar cell ×1700.

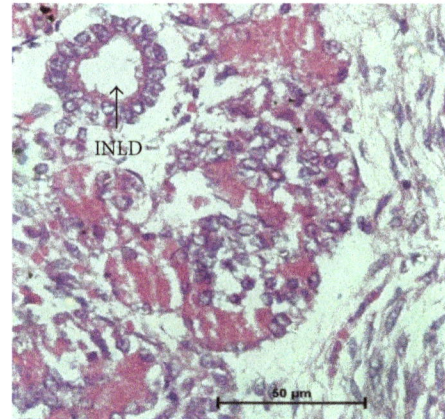

FIGURE 6: 19 cm CVRL (114 days) showing interlobular duct (ILD) and well formed acini (A). Hematoxylin and eosin ×400.

the first time at this stage. The nuclei of centroacinar cells were basophilic and vesicular. The collagen fibers were better developed.

In group II, at 28.3 cm CVRL (137 days), there was extensive branching of tubules that resulted in highly branched ductal tree connecting exocrine secretary units to the duct system. Although interlobular and intralobular ducts were well developed at this age, the intercalated ducts were not developed as still the acinar cells were budding off from these smaller ducts. At 32 cm CVRL (146 days), acini were more developed and arranged in groups separated by connective tissue (Figure 7). Ultrastructurally, zymogen granules were of different size and shape (Figure 8). These granules were round, oval, spherical, elongated, and spindle-shaped and were located between the Golgi cisternae and the apical membrane. Discharge of granules into the acinar lumen was not observed. The granules were membrane-bound. Some of granules were electron dense and others were moderately electron dense. They contained longitudinal fibrils. In some instances apparent fusion of these elongated granules was observed. Numerous mitochondria and endoplasmic reticulum were present. Moderate amount of glycogen was also observed in acinar cells at this stage especially around

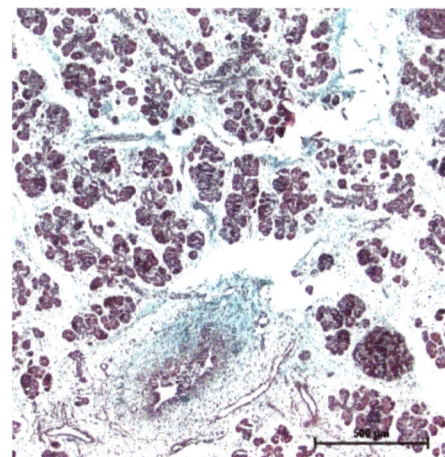

FIGURE 7: 32 cm CVRL (146 days) showing collagen fibers in connective tissue. Masson's trichrome ×40.

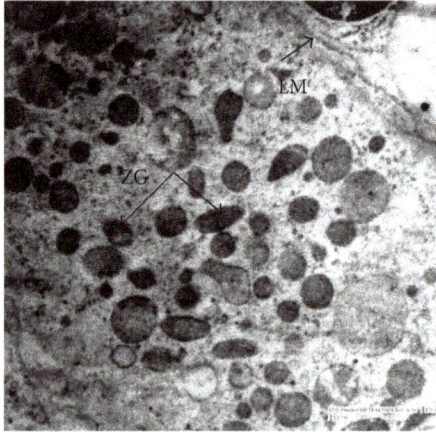

FIGURE 8: Electron micrograph at 32 cm CVRL (146 days) showing different shapes of zymogen granules (ZG) and lamellar membrane (LM) ×1700.

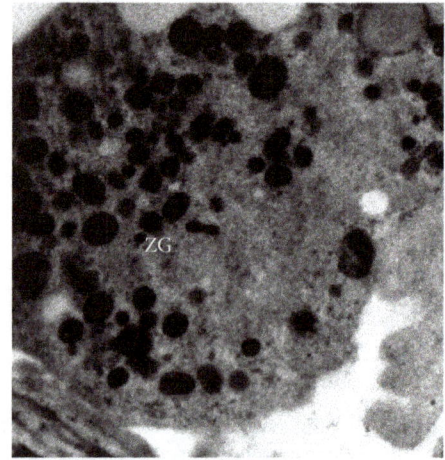

FIGURE 10: Electron micrograph of foetal pancreas at 48 cm CVRL (182 days) showing electron dense zymogen granules (ZG) in acinar cell ×1700.

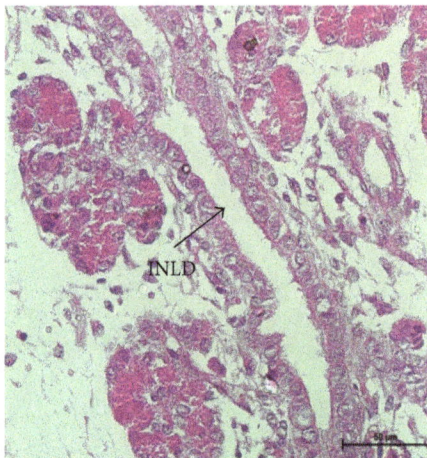

FIGURE 9: 48 cm CVRL (182 days) showing intralobular duct (INLD) and acini (A). Hematoxylin and eosin ×400.

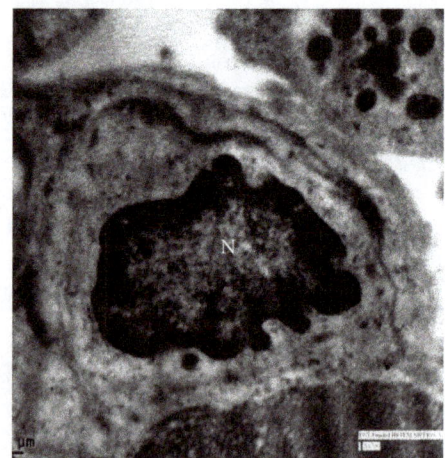

FIGURE 11: Electron micrograph of 48 cm CVRL (182 days) foetus showing irregular shape nucleus (N) and cell membrane (CM) of centroacinar cell ×1700.

the apically located zymogen granules. Nucleus was large and oval in shape. The basolateral membranes were simple with few interdigitations and junctional complexes with neighboring cells. At 35 cm CVRL (153 days), the interlobular duct was lined by simple columnar epithelium with few ciliated cells and goblet cells and intralobular duct was lined by simple cuboidal cells. Ganglia and nerve fibers were also observed in the vicinity of acinar cells.

In group III, exocrine pancreas showed a massive growth at 48 cm CVRL (182 days) (Figure 9). Pancreatic lobes and lobules were very distinct at this stage. Interlobular duct was lined by simple cuboidal epithelium. Their nuclei were large and spherical and with prominent nucleolus. The ducts were still showing the budding of new acinar cells. The nuclei of acinar cells were present near the basement membrane and were having a well developed nucleolus. The upper part of cell was filled with zymogen granules which were more developed than the previous two groups. Ultrastructurally, these granules were large and contained electron

dense material (Figure 10) and resembled mature zymogen granules. The granules were almost spherical but they varied in their size. There was a decrease in the number of free ribosomes and a concomitant increase in the amount of rough endoplasmic reticulum. Fewer mitochondria were found in the apex in these mature acinar cells than earlier stages. The junctional complexes were somewhat less prominent. The centroacinar cell had small number of organelles like Golgi apparatus, endoplasmic reticulum, and mitochondria as compared to the acinar cells. The nucleus was irregular in shape (Figure 11). More numbers of blood vessels started to accumulate around the acini and ducts. At 54 cm CVRL (195 days), well developed pancreatic architecture was seen with the presence of extensive development of exocrine part organized in lobes and lobules with interlobular and intralobular ducts (Figure 12). But intercalated ducts were still not observed at this age. The smaller ducts still had the precursors of different cells. A large number of goblet cells

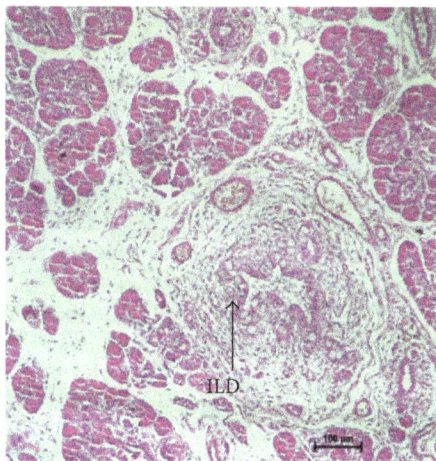

FIGURE 12: 54 cm CVRL (195 days) showing blood vessels (BV) and interlobular duct (ILD) in interlobular stroma. Hematoxylin and eosin ×100.

were observed in the interlobular ducts. At 70 cm CVRL (232 days), the blood vessels were more developed in the interlobular area with more collagen fibers around them and elastic fibers in the wall of blood vessels. The intercalated ducts were observed in 80 cm CVRL (254 days). These ducts were lined by low cuboidal epithelium. The duct system of the pancreas was well differentiated at this stage. The acinar cells were tall and pyramidal having spherical nucleus with prominent nucleolus present in the basal part of cell.

Micrometrical observations revealed the mean height of acinar cells as $13.4 \pm 0.38\,\mu m$ in group I, $14.03 \pm 0.67\,\mu m$ in group II, and $15.67 \pm 0.67\,\mu m$ in group III, while the mean diameter of acini was $33.5 \pm 2.03\,\mu m$ in group I, $36.4 \pm 3.75\,\mu m$ in group II, and $41.17 \pm 6.47\,\mu m$ in group III. Statistically, the height of acinar cells did not differ significantly between group I and group II and between group II and group III but it differed significantly between group I and group III ($p < 0.05$). So, there was substantial increase in height of acinar cells from group I to group III. The diameter of acini did not differ significantly between group I, group II, and group III ($p > 0.05$).

4. Discussion

The solid nest of undifferentiated epithelial cells in pancreatic parenchyma observed at 1.2 cm CVRL (34 days) in the present study has been referred to as cell buds by Conklin [15]. These cell cords are the common precursors of both acinar and islet cells. Such cell cords have been observed by Laitio et al. [16] at 9 weeks and Gupta et al. [17] at 12-13 weeks in human foetal pancreas. Once these cell buds are formed, the next step is the luminization of these epithelial buds. Cleaver and MacDonald [18] have reported that the entire pancreatic tree arose from an endodermally derived protodifferentiated epithelium and multipotent progenitor cells located at branched tips and gave rise to different pancreatic cells including acinar, endocrine, and ductal lineages. Villasenor et al. [19] have demonstrated that the process

of pancreatic branching involves the number of cellular events including transient epithelial stratification, dynamic cell polarity shift, asynchronous apical cell constriction, and rosette organization as well as microlumen formation and fusion. Pancreatic tubulogenesis begins with individual cells acquiring apicobasal polarity. Cells develop a defined apical membrane that faces a centre lumen and a basal surface attached to a layer of extracellular matrix. Then these newly formed polarized cells form rosettes wherein adjacent cells are linked by intercellular junctional complexes around a nascent central lumen. Newly formed microlumens are initially unconnected but eventually fuse into a luminal plexus. Remodelling of the luminal plexus produces a tubular network lined by polarized monolayered epithelia attached to basement membrane. It has also been speculated by above authors that mesenchymal tissue is a signaling tissue which helps localize expression of various factors that induce the branching pattern of the pancreatic primitive tubules. Laitio et al. [16] have reported the lumen formation at third foetal month in human pancreas. The presence of zymogen granules in the acinar cells has been reported by Conklin [15] at 110–150 mm CRL in human foetal pancreas and at 12 foetal weeks by Laitio et al. [16]. Tadokoro et al. [1] have reported in rats that the number and density of zymogen granules before birth depend on the serum glucocorticoid concentration. Many enzymes like lipase, trypsin, and amylase are stored in zymogen granules in foetal acinar cells and thus autodigestion of the cells does not occur [3]. It has been well documented that the rough endoplasmic reticulum and the Golgi apparatus are both involved in the early stage of zymogen granule synthesis in the adult [20]. The basolateral membrane junctional complexes have been reported at 20 weeks of gestation in human foetal pancreas [21].

The organization of pancreatic parenchyma into lobes and lobules has been reported by Lucini et al. [9] at 3rd month of gestation in buffalo foetal pancreas. In the present study, the formation of interlobular and intralobular ducts was observed at 12.8 cm CVRL (86 days), whereas in the earlier studies Conklin [15] has reported these ducts at 12.5–14.5 weeks and Gupta et al. [17] have reported them at 18 weeks of age in human foetal pancreas. The pancreatic duct has been observed at 43 days of gestation in human foetal pancreas [22]. With further advancement, the size and shape of zymogen granules were changed. Laitio et al. [16] have described different shapes of granules in human foetal pancreas at 12–16 weeks. Structurally the zymogen granules were fully formed so it may be suggested that these granules may secrete enzymes in the new born calves that may help in digestion of milk in new born animals. Presence of neuronal elements, that is, nerve fibres and ganglion, helps in pancreatic exocrine secretion through parasympathetic stimulation [23]. There was massive growth of exocrine pancreas at 48 cm CVRL (182 days) with well developed acini having better developed zymogen granules as reported earlier by Inagaki et al. [3] in foetal and neonatal rat pancreas and by Laitio et al. [16] in human foetal pancreas. In the present study well developed duct system was observed at 80 cm CVRL (254 days), whereas in an earlier report by Singh and Sethi [10] well established duct system has been reported at 75 cm CVRL (243 days) in buffalo foetal pancreas.

Micrometrical values of diameter of acini observed in present study in all the groups are higher than those reported by Prashar [24] who has reported mean diameter of acini as $22.37 \pm 0.74 \mu m$ in neonatal buffalo pancreas. So it may be inferred that diameter of acini is increased with advancement of gestation period but after the birth it decreases.

Conflict of Interests

The authors do not have any conflict of interests.

References

[1] H. Tadokoro, M. Takase, and B. Nobukawa, "Development and congenital anomalies of the pancreas," *Anatomy Research International*, vol. 2011, Article ID 351217, 7 pages, 2011.

[2] H. P. Shih, A. Wang, and M. Sander, "Pancreas organogenesis: from lineage determination to morphogenesis," *Annual Review of Cell and Developmental Biology*, vol. 29, pp. 81–105, 2013.

[3] T. Inagaki, T. Tajiri, G. Tate, T. Kunimura, and T. Morohoshi, "Dynamic morphologic change and differentiation from fetal to mature pancreatic acinar cells in rats," *Journal of Nippon Medical School*, vol. 79, no. 5, pp. 335–342, 2012.

[4] G. L. Carlsson, R. S. Heller, P. Serup, and P. Hyttel, "Immunohistochemistry of pancreatic development in cattle and pig," *Anatomia, Histologia, Embryologia*, vol. 39, no. 2, pp. 107–119, 2010.

[5] P. W. Aldoretta, T. D. Carver, and W. W. Hay Jr., "Maturation of glucose-stimulated insulin secretion in fetal sheep," *Biology of the Neonate*, vol. 73, no. 6, pp. 375–386, 1998.

[6] M. Titlbach and E. Maňáková, "Development of the rabbit pancreas with particular regard to the argyrophilic cells," *Acta Veterinaria Brno*, vol. 76, no. 4, pp. 509–517, 2007.

[7] K. Desdicioglu, M. A. Malas, and E. H. Evcil, "Foetal development of the pancreas," *Folia Morphologica*, vol. 69, no. 4, pp. 216–224, 2010.

[8] S. Manupati, R. Sugavasi, D. B. Indira, B. Sirisha, D. B. Subhadhra, and Y. Suneetha, "Morphometry and histogenesis of human foetal pancreas," *International Journal of Health Sciences and Research*, vol. 2, no. 9, pp. 18–24, 2012.

[9] C. Lucini, L. Castaldo, O. Lai, and G. De Vico, "Ontogeny, postnatal development and ageing of endocrine pancreas in *Bubalus bubalis*," *Journal of Anatomy*, vol. 192, no. 3, pp. 417–424, 1998.

[10] O. Singh and R. S. Sethi, "Histogenesis of pancreas of Indian buffalo (*Bubalus bubalis*) during prenatal development," *Indian Veterinary Journal*, vol. 89, no. 11, pp. 56–59, 2012.

[11] J. M. W. Slack, "Developmental biology of the pancreas," *Development*, vol. 121, no. 6, pp. 1569–1580, 1995.

[12] M. K. Soliman, "Studies on the physiological chemistry of the allantoic and amniotic fluid of buffaloes at various periods of pregnancy," *Indian Veterinary Journal*, vol. 52, pp. 111–117, 1975.

[13] L. G. Luna, *Manual of Histologic Staining: Methods of the Armed Forces Institute of Pathology*, McGraw Hill Book, New York, NY, USA, 3rd edition, 1968.

[14] J. J. Bozolla and L. D. Russell, *Electron Microscopy: Principles and Techniques for Biologists*, Jones and Bartlett Publishers, Boston, Mass, USA, 1999.

[15] J. L. Conklin, "Cytogenesis of the human fetal pancreas," *The American Journal of Anatomy*, vol. 111, pp. 181–193, 1962.

[16] M. Laitio, R. Lev, and D. Orlic, "The developing human fetal pancreas: an ultrastructural and histochemical study with special reference to exocrine cells," *Journal of Anatomy*, vol. 117, no. 3, pp. 619–634, 1974.

[17] V. Gupta, K. Garg, S. Rajeha, R. Choudhry, and A. Tuli, "The histogenesis of islets in the human fetal pancreas," *Journal of Anatomical Society of India*, vol. 51, no. 1, pp. 23–26, 2002.

[18] O. Cleaver and R. J. MacDonald, "Developmental molecular biology of the pancreas," in *Pancreatic Cancer*, pp. 71–117, Springer, New York, NY, USA, 2010.

[19] A. Villasenor, D. C. Chong, M. Henkemeyer, and O. Cleaver, "Epithelial dynamics of pancreatic branching morphogenesis," *Development*, vol. 137, no. 24, pp. 4295–4305, 2010.

[20] L. G. Caro and G. E. Palade, "Protein synthesis, storage, and discharge in the pancreatic exocrine cell: an autoradiographic study," *The Journal of Cell Biology*, vol. 20, pp. 473–495, 1964.

[21] W. G. Liang, P. Eugene, and M. D. Dimagno, *The Pancreas: Biology, Pathobiology, and Disease*, Raven Press, New York, NY, USA, 1993.

[22] M. Polak, L. Bouchareb-Banaei, R. Scharfmann, and P. Czernichow, "Early pattern of differentiation in the human pancreas," *Diabetes*, vol. 49, no. 2, pp. 225–232, 2000.

[23] W. J. Banks, *Applied Veterinary Histology*, Mosby, St. Louis, Mo, USA, 1993.

[24] A. Prashar, *Age related histomorphological and histochemical studies on the pancreas of Indian buffalo (Bubalis bubalis) [M.V.Sc. Thesis]*, Punjab Agricultural University, Ludhiana, India, 1995.

13

Hematological, Biochemical, and Serological Findings in Healthy Canine Blood Donors after the Administration of CaniLeish® Vaccine

Chiara Starita, Alessandra Gavazza, and George Lubas

Department of Veterinary Sciences, University of Pisa, Via Livornese Lato Monte, San Piero a Grado, 56122 Pisa, Italy

Correspondence should be addressed to Alessandra Gavazza; agavazza@vet.unipi.it

Academic Editor: Timm C. Harder

The aim of the study was to evaluate hematological, biochemical, and serological findings in healthy canine blood donors after the administration of CaniLeish® vaccine. Twenty-seven client-owned dogs were included in the study and arranged into 3 groups according to the vaccination stage. Complete blood count (CBC) with blood smear examination, serum biochemical profile (SBP), serum protein electrophoresis (SPE), and serological tests for *L. infantum* were performed at different times. Additionally, in a subgroup of dogs IgA, IgM, and IgG were quantified. No statistical significance for CBC and SBP was found. In 10.7% of cases slight hyperproteinemia occurred. In SPE absolute values β-1-globulins (Group 2 and Group 2-3) and β-2-globulins (Group 3) were found modified ($P < 0.05$). IgG values were statistically different ($P < 0.05$) 6–8 months after the third immunisation (Group 2) and IgM and IgG values were statistically different after 2 months (Group 3). IFAT positive samples were 20.8% (Group 1), 15.0% (Group 2), and 52.8% (Group 3). Speed Leish K™ tests were always negative. The modifications found were probably attributed to the development of immune or inflammatory response due to the vaccine. Administration of CaniLeish vaccine in canine blood donors could be a safe practice and did not affect their health status.

1. Introduction

Canine leishmaniosis is caused by an intracellular protozoan called *Leishmania infantum* transmitted by sand flies of the genus *Phlebotomus*. The progression from infection to clinical disease occurs if the canine cell-mediated immune response is inadequate and the parasite increases in number within macrophages in many organs and tissues [1].

The prevention of canine leishmaniosis requires a combined approach including measures focused both on dogs and on environment [2–4]. A canine vaccine that modulates cell-mediated immune response against the protozoan has been available in Italy since 2012 (CaniLeish, Virbac, France). It reduces the risk of developing, after the contact with the parasite, from an active infection to a symptomatic disease [5–7]. In addition, it may help those dogs that get infected despite vaccination, as suggested by a recent study using xenodiagnosis, since disease severity appears to be generally

associated with high parasite loads in the skin and their infectivity [8].

Hence, the control of leishmaniosis is particularly important in canine blood donors because the risk of transmission of infectious agents through transfused blood products from blood donors, that are carriers of infection, is demonstrated [9–11]. Overall, protozoan diseases have long incubation periods, subclinical persistence in infected animals, and likelihood of remaining viable in bloodstocks [10, 11].

The recently revised Italian guidelines about veterinary transfusion medicine established by the Ministry of Health [12] stated that blood donor dogs should be healthy animals and should undergo complete clinical examination and laboratory tests including hematobiochemical profile and serological assay, using IFAT, or PCR for *Leishmania infantum*, *Ehrlichia canis*, *Anaplasma phagocytophilum*, *Rickettsia rickettsii*, and *Babesia canis* [13].

In order to increase the prevention of leishmaniosis in blood donors, the vaccine against leishmaniosis could be used. To the author's knowledge no data has been published about the evaluation of hematological and biochemical findings after administration of CaniLeish. Therefore, the aim of this study was to evaluate hematological, biochemical, and serological findings in a group of healthy dogs participating in a voluntary blood donor program at the Transfusion Veterinary Centre, University of Pisa, receiving a full coverage of immunisation with CaniLeish.

2. Materials and Methods

2.1. Selection Criteria. The study took place between February 2013 and July 2014 in the area of northern Tuscany, Italy. Twenty-seven client-owned dogs participating in a voluntary blood donor program at the University of Pisa were included (written consent was previously collected from all the owners). The following selection criteria were used to include dogs as blood donors: Dog Erythrocyte Antigen (DEA) 1 negative, absence of any clinical signs or symptoms of disease, values of complete blood count (CBC) (ProCyte Dx®, Idexx, Italy) and blood smear examination, serum biochemical profile (SBP) (total protein, albumin, urea, alkaline phosphatase, and alanine aminotransferase) (Liasys®, Assel, Italy), and serum protein electrophoresis (SPE) in agarose gel (Pretty®, Interlab, Italy) within the reference ranges of the Veterinary Clinical Pathology University Laboratory: negative serology for *Leishmania infantum* using immunofluorescence antibody test (IFAT) [14] and Speed Leish K™ test, negative serology for *Ehrlichia canis* and *Anaplasma phagocytophilum* using IFAT [15]. Any serological positivity titre starting from 1 : 40 was an exclusion cause from the blood donors program. Moreover, all dogs received a regular protection against ectoparasites, both repellent and/or antifeeding drugs applied locally.

2.2. Vaccine Administration. Lyophilized CaniLeish vaccine (Virbac, France) stored at +4/+10°C was reconstituted with its solvent (approximately 1 mL) and administered subcutaneously in the withers region followed by a gentle massage of the site. Dogs were monitored for 30 minutes in order to observe the onset of possible anaphylactic reactions. The owners were advised to report to the authors any suspected reaction or adverse effect that might occur and in that case they would have undergone a control. The vaccine was administered according to the protocol indicated in the manufacturer's instructions: first cycle of 3 inoculations, each of them every 3 weeks, and annual boosters for further administration.

2.3. Study Design. Twenty-seven canine blood donors (17 females, 10 males; 14 Boxers, 8 mixed breeds, 3 Golden Retrievers, 1 Weimaraner, 1 Border Collie; 2–7 years old) were included in the study. Dogs were divided into three groups according to the vaccination stage. Group 1 included 6 dogs that underwent first and second annual boosters because they had already completed the first cycle of immunisation by

their referring veterinarian. Group 2 included 12 dogs, which underwent the first cycle of immunisation and first annual booster. Group 3 included 9 dogs, which underwent only the first cycle of immunisation. The times (T) in days of controls were $T0$ (first immunisation), $T21$ (second immunisation), $T42$ (third immunisation), $T100$ (two months after the third immunisation), $T250$ (6–8 months after the third immunisation), $T405$ (first annual booster), and $T770$ (second annual booster). About 10 mL of blood was withdrawn from the jugular or cephalic vein for laboratory analysis. For Group 1 only serological assays (IFAT *L. infantum* and Speed Leish K) were performed at $T0$, $T250$, $T405$, and $T770$. For Group 2, CBC with blood smear examination, serum biochemical profile (total protein, albumin, urea, alkaline phosphatase, and alanine aminotransferase), serum electrophoresis, IFAT for *L. infantum*, and Speed Leish K were provided at $T0$, $T21$, $T42$, $T250$, and $T405$. In Group 3, the same laboratory tests of Group 2 were performed at $T0$, $T21$, $T42$, and $T100$. Group 2 and Group 3 were evaluated together as Group 2-3 whenever possible, for comparison purposes. Moreover, for a subgroup of dogs (10/12 of Group 2 and 7/9 of Group 3) IgA (immunoglobulin), IgM, and IgG fractions were quantified, respectively, at $T0$–$T100$ and $T0$–$T250$ using the method described by Tvarijonaviciute [16]. Briefly, commercial kits (Olympus Europe GmbH) were run on an automatic analyzer (Olympus AU600, Olympus Europe GmbH, Hamburg, Germany) following the manufacturer's instruction.

2.4. Statistics. Data distribution was assessed through the D'Agostino-Pearson test. The Kruskal-Wallis test was performed for CBC, SBP, and SPE data, while for immunoglobulin the Wilcoxon test was provided. For all tests, significance was set as $P < 0.05$. Statistical analysis was performed using commercial software (MedCalc® Software v.14.8.1.0, Mariakerke, Belgium).

3. Results

3.1. Hematobiochemical Analysis. No statistical significance for data from CBC and SBP was found (data not shown). However, slight hyperproteinemia up to 8.4 g/dL (reference range 5.8–7.8 g/dL) occurred in 10.7% of cases. Results from SPE are shown in Table 1 as absolute values using median and 95% confidence interval. Our data show a statistical significance ($P < 0.05$) of β-1-globulins in Group 2 and Group 2-3 and of β-2-globulins in Group 3. Tables 2 and 3 report the results of the quantification of IgA, IgM, and IgG in Groups 2 and 3, respectively. The IgG values were statistically different ($P < 0.05$) at $T250$ for Group 2, while IgM and IgG values were statistically different ($P < 0.05$) at $T100$ in Group 3.

3.2. Serological Tests. The results of IFAT are reported in Table 4 (and Figures 1, 2, and 3). In Group 1, 20.8% of canine samples were positive at low titres (up to 1 : 80), in Group 2, 15.0% of samples were positive at rather low titres (mostly up to 1 : 80, one dog up to 1 : 320), and, in Group 3, 52.8% of samples were positive at rather low and high titres (mostly 1 : 80 and 1 : 160, one dog up to 1 : 320). In detail, in

TABLE 1: Major serum proteins and electrophoresis fractions reported as absolute values in Groups 2 and 3.

Analyte[§]	Time	Group 2 median (n = 12)	95% CI median	Group 3 median (n = 9)	95% CI median	Group 2-3 median (n = 21)	95% CI median
Total protein (5.8–7.8 g/dL)	T0	7.2	6.6–7.8	6.5	6.3–6.8	6.7	6.5–7.2
	T21	7.1	6.8–7.6	6.8	6.0–7.7	7.0	6.7–7.5
	T42	7.1	6.6–7.6	6.5	6.2–7.4	6.8	6.5–7.3
	T100	NT	NT	6.8	6.5–7.5	NT	NT
	T250	6.6	6.5–7.8	NT	NT	NT	NT
	T405	7.2	6.6–7.5	NT	NT	NT	NT
Albumin (2.6–4.1 g/dL)	T0	3.5	3.2–4.1	3.4	3.1–3.5	3.4	3.3–3.5
	T21	3.5	3.2–3.7	3.3	2.9–3.9	3.4	3.3–3.7
	T42	3.5	3.3–3.7	3.3	3.0–3.7	3.4	3.2–3.6
	T100	NT	NT	3.3	3.1–3.7	NT	NT
	T250	3.4	3.1–3.6	NT	NT	NT	NT
	T405	3.3	3.1–3.5	NT	NT	NT	NT
Globulins (2.5–4.5 g/dL)	T0	3.6	3.0–4.2	3.2	2.8–3.6	3.2	3.0–3.6
	T21	3.7	3.5–3.9	3.4	3.0–3.8	3.5	3.3–3.8
	T42	3.5	3.2–4.0	3.3	3.2–3.7	3.5	3.3–3.7
	T100	NT	NT	3.6	3.2–4.0	NT	NT
	T250	3.5	3.1–4.4	NT	NT	NT	NT
	T405	3.9	3.5–4.3	NT	NT	NT	NT
Alpha-1-globulins (0.1–0.3 g/dL)	T0	0.3	0.32–0.3	0.2	0.2–0.3	0.3	0.2–0.3
	T21	0.3	0.2–0.3	0.2	0.2–0.23	0.2	0.2–0.3
	T42	0.3	0.2–0.3	0.2	0.2–0.3	0.2	0.2–0.3
	T100	NT	NT	0.2	0.2–0.3	NT	NT
	T250	0.2	0.2–0.3	NT	NT	NT	NT
	T405	0.3	0.2–0.3	NT	NT	NT	NT
Alpha-2-globulins (0.6–1.4 g/dL)	T0	1.0	0.7–1.2	1.0	0.8–1.1	1.0	0.9–1.1
	T21	1.0	0.9–1.0	1.1	1.0–1.3	1.0	0.9–1.1
	T42	0.9	0.8–1.0	1.1	1.0–1.1	1.0	0.9–1.1
	T100	NT	NT	1.0	0.9–1.3	NT	NT
	T250	1.0	0.9–1.2	NT	NT	NT	NT
	T405	1.1	1.0–1.2	NT	NT	NT	NT
Beta-1-globulins (0.3–1.0 g/dL)	T0	0.6*	0.4–0.8	0.6	0.3–0.9	0.6*	0.5–0.8
	T21	0.5*	0.4–0.5	0.5	0.4–0.6	0.5*	0.4–0.5
	T42	0.5*	0.4–0.5	0.4	0.4–0.5	0.5*	0.4–0.5
	T100	NT	NT	0.4	0.3–0.7	NT	NT
	T250	0.9*	0.5–1.0	NT	NT	NT	NT
	T405	0.9*	0.4–1.1	NT	NT	NT	NT
Beta-2-globulins (0.4–1.1 g/dL)	T0	1.0	0.3–1.8	0.7*	0.7–0.9	0.7	0.7–1.0
	T21	1.1	1.0–1.2	1.0*	0.7–1.1	1.0	0.9–1.1
	T42	1.0	0.9–1.2	1.0*	0.9–1.1	1.0	1.0–1.1
	T100	NT	NT	1.2*	0.8–1.4	NT	NT
	T250	0.9	0.6–1.1	NT	NT	NT	NT
	T405	0.8	0.7–1.0	NT	NT	NT	NT
Gamma globulins (0.4–0.9 g/dL)	T0	0.9	0.6–1.1	0.6	0.4–0.7	0.7	0.5–0.7
	T21	0.9	0.8–0.9	0.7	0.5–0.9	0.8	0.7–0.9
	T42	0.9	0.6–1.0	0.6	0.5–0.7	0.7	0.6–0.9
	T100	NT	NT	0.7	0.5–0.9	NT	NT
	T250	0.7	0.5–1.0	NT	NT	NT	NT
	T405	0.8	0.6–0.9	NT	NT	NT	NT

[§]Values in brackets are reference ranges.
NT = not tested.
*Kruskal-Wallis test was $P > 0.05$ for all time comparison for each group except where the asterisk next to the median values is reported ($P < 0.05$).

TABLE 2: Immunoglobulin concentration in Group 2 (10 dogs).

Analyte[§]	Time	Median	95% CI median
IgA (0.1–1.8 mg/dL)	T0	11.3	0.1–18.3
	T250	8.8	1.3–18.0
IgM (61–99 mg/dL)	T0	184.5	113.8–211.6
	T250	180.5	119.0–212.9
IgG (323–659 mg/dL)	T0	411.5*	317.3–466.7
	T250	444.5*	352.8–467.5

[§]Values in brackets are reference ranges.
* = Wilcoxon test $P < 0.05$.

TABLE 3: Immunoglobulin concentration in Group 3 (7 dogs).

Analyte[§]	Time	Median	95% CI median
IgA (0.1–1.8 mg/dL)	T0	8.1	3.1–14.1
	T100	10.8	3.7–14.5
IgM (61–99 mg/dL)	T0	110.0*	91.5–136.6
	T100	140.0*	116.9–158.6
IgG (323–659 mg/dL)	T0	497.0*	448.9–566.5
	T100	575.0*	504.0–704.1

[§]Values in brackets are reference ranges.
* = Wilcoxon test $P < 0.05$.

TABLE 4: IFAT *L. infantum* for the three groups of dogs.

Time	Group 1 (n)	Group 2 (n)	Group 3 (n)
T0	Negative (6)	Negative (12)	Negative (9)
T21	Not tested	Negative (10) 1:80 (1) 1:320 (1)	Negative (2) 1:80 (2) 1:160 (5)
T42	Not tested	Negative (9) 1:40 (1) 1:80 (1) 1:320 (1)	Negative (1) 1:40 (1) 1:80 (3) 1:160 (3) 1:320 (1)
T100	Not tested	Not tested	Negative (5) 1:40 (3) 1:80 (1)
T250	Negative (5) 1:80 (1)	Negative (10) 1:40 (1) 1:80 (1)	Not tested
T405	Negative (4) 1:40 (2)	Negative (10) 1:40 (2)	Not tested
T770	Negative (4) 1:40 (2)	Not tested	Not tested

Group 2 two dogs at T21 and three dogs at T100 (during the initial immunisation) showed variable titres up to 1:320. At the following monitoring, only one dog was continuously positive for all the observations. In Group 3 most of the dogs were showing positive titre for IFAT after the initial immunisation (T21) and this trend was observed for the other two collection points as well. All Speed Leish K tests were negative throughout the study period.

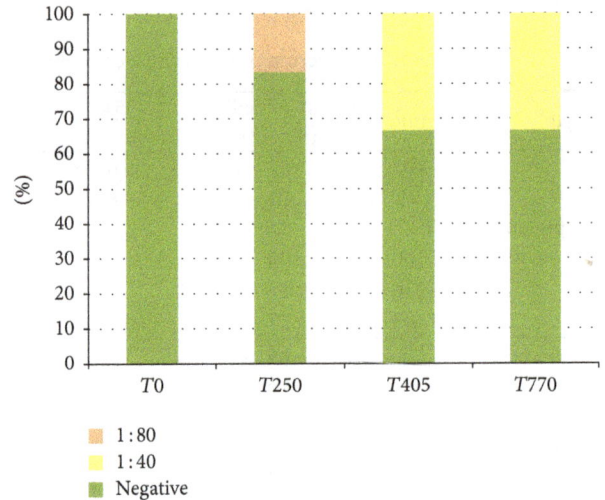

FIGURE 1: IFAT positivity (%), Group 1.

Legend:
- 1:80
- 1:40
- Negative

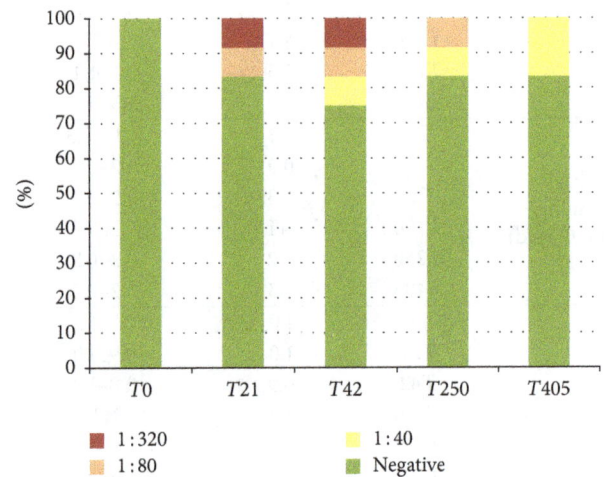

FIGURE 2: IFAT positivity (%), Group 2.

Legend:
- 1:320
- 1:80
- 1:40
- Negative

4. Discussion

In the present study the serological status of dogs after the administration of CaniLeish was monitored up to the second annual booster. No publications have so-far assessed long-term IFAT titres modifications in vaccinated dogs. The positivity was generally low and the trend is various for all dogs. The prevalence recorded was 20.8% in Group 1, 15.0% in Group 2, and 52.8% in Group 3. Many previous studies reported an increase of IFAT titres after vaccination. Sagols et al. demonstrated the seroconversion of dogs vaccinated from 2 weeks to 4 months after the third shot and the gradual decrease of titres in the following monitoring [17]. Moreno et al. indicated the increase of IFAT titres in all 20 vaccinated dogs at weeks 8 and 12 (maximum titre 1:500) after the first injection and one dog still had a titre of 1:200 at week 30 [6]. All dogs became negative at IFAT (titre <1:200) at week 42. Furthermore, in another study Sagols et al. tested 31 vaccinated dogs after 3-4 weeks from the first annual booster evidencing the increase of IFAT titres [18].

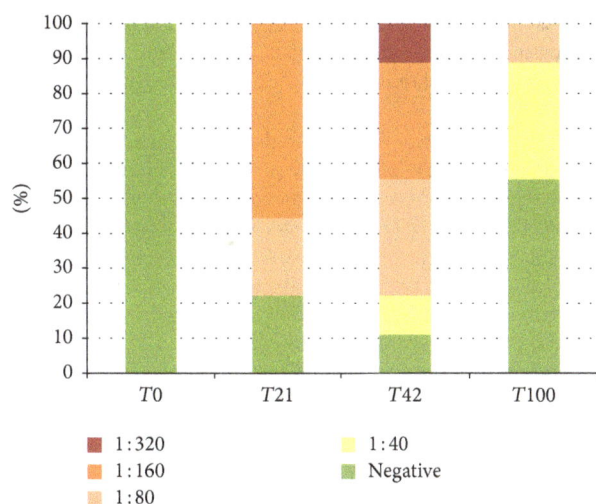

FIGURE 3: IFAT positivity (%), Group 3.

Recently, Sagols et al. investigated the follow-up of the humoral immune response after the first annual booster recording an evolution of IFAT titres similar to the transient profile obtained after the primary vaccination [19]. However, IFAT results should be interpreted with caution in vaccinated dogs, because they are obtained from a nonspecific test that detects all IgG antibodies against the whole parasite, both due to the contact with the parasite and due to the development of immunological response. According to previous studies by Sagols et al. all Speed Leish K assays remained negative, so the antibodies detected by IFAT technique were not identified by this test (immunochromatographic anti-kinesin antibody test) [17–19]. Therefore, Sagols et al. demonstrated that this rapid test is reliable for detecting antibodies due to the contact with the parasite. On the other hand, Solano-Gallego et al. have indicated that the sensitivity of rapid serological tests used for dog screening prior to vaccination with CaniLeish is rather low [20]. Thus, it is likely that some dogs will be already Leishmania-infected at the time of vaccination, and this will be a complicating factor for assessing vaccine efficacy in the field. Moreover, the EFSA AHAW panel shows that antibodies elicited on vaccinated dogs cannot be discriminated with current serological methods [21]. Until the advent of vaccination in Europe, standard guidelines suggested that IFAT titres of at least 4 times the laboratory cut-off level were indicative of the disease and that levels between the threshold and 4 times the threshold raised a suspicion of the disease [22]. Nowadays, the literature agrees that the most useful diagnostic approaches for investigation of infection in sick and clinically healthy infected dogs include both the detection of specific serum anti-Leishmania antibodies by quantitative serological techniques and the demonstration of the parasite DNA in tissues by applying specific molecular techniques [1, 4, 21, 22].

To the author's knowledge, no previous data about the follow-up and monitoring of dogs vaccinated through hematobiochemical and SPE analysis were published. Our results for SPE showed the increase of few globulins fractions (β-globulins) that could be attributed to the immune response induced by the vaccine. Proteins that migrate in each fraction should be investigated individually, but this was not the goal of this study. Additionally, modifications observed in Ig quantification could be attributed to the immune stimulation induced by the vaccine. The significant increase of total IgG anti-Leishmania antibodies after vaccination with CaniLeish is also demonstrated in other studies [5, 7].

In our study the limits were the low number of dogs included, their different vaccination stages, the lack of PCR analysis of blood to rule out the possibility of transmission of L. infantum through bloodstocks, and the lack of ELISA testing for dosing the level of IgG1 and IgG2 to assess the type of immune response. The study is still continuing and further data will be published.

5. Conclusions

In conclusion, the adoption of the vaccine CaniLeish in a group of blood donors, typically healthy dogs as they are frequently monitored all year long, could be a safe practice. After vaccination there are only minimal modifications in total protein contents, some globulins fractions, IgM and IgG, and mild increase of IFAT titres.

Disclosure

This paper was partially presented in abstract form at the 16th ESVCP Annual Congress, 1st–4th October 2014, Milan, Italy.

Competing Interests

The authors declare that they have no competing interests.

Acknowledgments

The present study was supported by the Canine Leishmaniosis Working Group and Hill's Pet Nutrition.

References

[1] S. Paltrinieri, L. Solano-Gallego, A. Fondati et al., "Guidelines for diagnosis and clinical classification of leishmaniasis in dogs," Journal of the American Veterinary Medical Association, vol. 236, no. 11, pp. 1184–1191, 2010.

[2] M. Maroli, L. Gradoni, G. Oliva et al., "Guidelines for prevention of leishmaniasis in dogs," Journal of the American Veterinary Medical Association, vol. 236, no. 11, pp. 1200–1206, 2010.

[3] D. Otranto and F. Dantas-Torres, "The prevention of canine leishmaniasis and its impact on public health," Trends in Parasitology, vol. 29, no. 7, pp. 339–345, 2013.

[4] L. Solano-Gallego, G. Miró, A. Koutinas et al., "LeishVet guidelines for the practical management of canine leishmaniosis," Parasites & Vectors, vol. 4, no. 1, article 86, pp. 1–16, 2011.

[5] V. Martin, I. Vouldoukis, J. Moreno, D. McGahie, S. Gueguen, and A.-M. Cuisinier, "The protective immune response produced in dogs after primary vaccination with the LiESP/QA-21

vaccine (CaniLeish®) remains effective against an experimental challenge one year later," *Veterinary Research*, vol. 45, no. 1, article 69, 2014.

[6] J. Moreno, I. Vouldoukis, P. Schreiber et al., "Primary vaccination with the LiESP/QA-21 vaccine (CaniLeish®) produces a cell-mediated immune response which is still present 1 year later," *Veterinary Immunology and Immunopathology*, vol. 158, no. 3-4, pp. 199–207, 2014.

[7] G. Oliva, J. Nieto, V. Foglia Manzillo et al., "A randomized, double-blind, controlled efficacy trial of the LiESP/QA-21 vaccine in naïve dogs exposed to two Leishmania infantum transmission seasons," *PLoS Neglected Tropical Diseases*, vol. 8, no. 10, p. 13, 2014.

[8] G. Bongiorno, R. Paparcone, V. Foglia Manzillo, G. Oliva, A.-M. Cuisinier, and L. Gradoni, "Vaccination with LiESP/QA-21 (CaniLeish®) reduces the intensity of infection in *Phlebotomus perniciosus* fed on *Leishmania infantum* infected dogs-A preliminary xenodiagnosis study," *Veterinary Parasitology*, vol. 197, no. 3-4, pp. 691–695, 2013.

[9] S. D. Owens, D. A. Oakley, K. Marryott et al., "Transmission of visceral leishmaniasis through blood transfusions from infected English Foxhounds to anemic dogs," *Journal of the American Veterinary Medical Association*, vol. 219, no. 8, pp. 1076–1083, 2001.

[10] E. De Freitas, M. N. Melo, A. P. Da Costa-Val, and M. S. M. Michalick, "Transmission of Leishmania infantum via blood transfusion in dogs: potential for infection and importance of clinical factors," *Veterinary Parasitology*, vol. 137, no. 1-2, pp. 159–167, 2006.

[11] M. D. Tabar, X. Roura, O. Francinoy, L. Altety, and R. R. De Gopegui, "Detection of *Leishmania infantum* by real-time PCR in a canine blood bank," *Journal of Small Animal Practice*, vol. 49, no. 7, pp. 325–328, 2008.

[12] Ministero della Salute (Italian Ministry of Health), "Linea guida per l'esercizio delle attività sanitarie riguardanti la medicina trasfusionale in campo veterinario (Guidelines concerning the practice of health procedures about veterinary transfusion medicine)," *Official Journal*, vol. 25, pp. 5–18, 2016.

[13] G. Lubas, G. Oliva, M. T. Antognoni et al., "Selection of canine blood donors considering epidemiological issues in Italy: a working group consensus on infectious diseases screening," in *Proceedings of the 25th ECVIM-CA Congress*, Lisbon, Portugal, September 2015.

[14] F. Mancianti and N. Meciani, "Specific serodiagnosis of canine leishmaniasis by indirect immunofluorescence, indirect hemagglutination, and counterimmunoelectrophoresis," *American Journal of Veterinary Research*, vol. 49, no. 8, pp. 1409–1411, 1988.

[15] V. V. Ebani, F. Bertelloni, B. Torracca, and D. Cerri, "Serological survey of Borrelia burgdorferi sensu lato, Anaplasma phagocytophilum, and Ehrlichia canis infections in rural and urban dogs in Central Italy," *Annals of Agricultural and Environmental Medicine*, vol. 21, no. 4, pp. 671–675, 2014.

[16] A. Tvarijonaviciute, S. Martínez-Subiela, M. Caldin, F. Tecles, and J. J. Ceron, "Evaluation of automated assays for immunoglobulin G, M, and A measurements in dog and cat serum," *Veterinary Clinical Pathology*, vol. 42, no. 3, pp. 270–280, 2013.

[17] E. Sagols, V. Martin, E. Claret et al., "Evaluation of the humoral immune response after vaccination with LiESP/QA-21 (CaniLeish®): interest of *Leishmania* specific anti-kinesin antibodies detection," in *Proceedings of the WSAVA/FECAVA/BSAVA Congress*, Birmingham, UK, April 2012.

[18] E. Sagols, F. Ferraz, E. Claret et al., "Evaluation of the humoral immune response after the first annual CaniLeish® booster vaccination," in *Proceedings of the SCIVAC Congress*, Pisa, Italy, March 2013.

[19] E. Sagols, F. Ferraz, E. Claret et al., "Follow up of the humoral immune response after the first annual CaniLeish® booster vaccination," in *Proceedings of the Southern European Veterinary Conference (SEVC '13)*, Barcelona, Spain, October 2013.

[20] L. Solano-Gallego, S. Villanueva-Saz, M. Carbonell et al., "Serological diagnosis of canine leishamniosis: comparison of three commercial ELISA tests (Leiscan®, ID screen® and *Leishmania* 96®), a rapid test (Speed Leish K™) and an in-house IFAT," *Parasites & Vectors*, vol. 7, no. 111, p. 10, 2014.

[21] EFSA AHAW Panel (EFSA Panel on Animal Health and Welfare), "Scientific opinion on canine leishmaniosis," *EFSA Journal*, vol. 13, no. 4, p. 77, 2015.

[22] L. Solano-Gallego, A. Koutinas, G. Miró et al., "Directions for the diagnosis, clinical staging, treatment and prevention of canine leishmaniosis," *Veterinary Parasitology*, vol. 165, no. 1-2, pp. 1–18, 2009.

14

Preliminary Study of Pet Owner Adherence in Behaviour, Cardiology, Urology, and Oncology Fields

Zita Talamonti, Chiara Cassis, Paola G. Brambilla, Paola Scarpa, Damiano Stefanello, Simona Cannas, Michela Minero, and Clara Palestrini

Università degli Studi di Milano, Dipartimento di Scienze Veterinarie e Sanità Pubblica (DIVET), Via Celoria 10, 20133 Milan, Italy

Correspondence should be addressed to Zita Talamonti; zita.talamonti@gmail.com

Academic Editor: Remo Lobetti

Successful veterinary treatment of animals requires owner adherence with a prescribed treatment plan. The aim of our study was to evaluate and compare the level of adherence of the owners of patients presented for behavioural, cardiological, urological, and oncological problems. At the end of the first examination, each owner completed a questionnaire. Then, the owners were called four times to fill out another questionnaire over the phone. With regard to the first questionnaire, statistically significant data concern behavioral medicine and cardiology. In the first area the owner's worry decreases during the follow-up and the number of owners who would give away the animal increases. In cardiology, owners who think that the pathology harms their animal's quality of life decreased significantly over time. With regard to the 9 additional follow-up questions, in behavioural medicine and urology the owner's discomfort resulting from the animal's pathology significantly decreases over time. Assessment of adherence appears to be an optimal instrument in identifying the positive factors and the difficulties encountered by owners during the application of a treatment protocol.

1. Introduction

Owner compliance or adherence to treatment recommendations can determine the success of veterinary treatment [1]. The term compliance describes the observance of a medical recommendation, but it also includes how well laws, regulations, and guidelines are applied when administering prescribed treatments. The concept of compliance in veterinary medicine involves the consistency and accuracy with which a client follows the regime recommended by the veterinarian or other veterinary health care team members [2]. The term "compliance" (or "observance") suggests that a patient adapts to, submits to, or obeys the instructions of a doctor and implies a submissive role with a professional in a position of authority. The negative connotation of the term has caused the medical world to increasingly distance itself from the term compliance, replacing it with "adherence"; in other words, the tendency to adhere to the doctor's instructions, carrying them out quickly, respectfully, and accurately [3]. The World

Health Organization defines adherence as "the extent to which a person's behaviour, taking medication, following a diet, and/or executing lifestyle changes, corresponds with agreed recommendations given by a health care provider" [4]. For these reasons, the term adherence is preferred to compliance and will be used throughout the text in this paper.

In veterinary medicine, adherence is the centrepiece for fulfilling the veterinary profession's obligation to advocate on behalf of the pet's best interest. Adherence is based on effective communication of recommendations, resulting in informed client acceptance and efficient follow-through for patient care [2]. The successful outcome of a prescribed treatment depends on several factors, including a correct diagnosis, the prescription of the right treatment, and the adherence shown by the patient. The veterinarian plays a fundamental role in owner adherence to treatment of and the management of the patient, so it appears to be the result of cooperation between both persons. Since the application of any diagnostic and therapeutic option requires the owner's consent, it is of prime importance for the attending doctor to achieve their adherence to treatment, so as to achieve a successful therapeutic outcome and client satisfaction [1]. A high level of adherence in the veterinary field is dependent on two basic factors: the owner's view of his/her animal (and the resulting importance of the said animal to the owner) and the owner's understanding of the medical situation [5, 6]. The goal is to provide what the client wants, which happens to be congruent with the health care team's delivering the care the patient needs and deserves; by increasing the client's understanding of veterinary recommendations and through the health care team's reinforcement of clarifications, adherence ratios increase [2]. Adherence to treatment also appears to be influenced by the duration and frequency of the treatment, by the consultation time offered by the clinician and by the quality of interaction between the veterinarian, the pet, and the owner. With regard to the duration of the treatment, several studies have shown a negative correlation between the level of adherence and a long treatment period. In fact, if a long-term treatment is prescribed, nonadherence of the owner may occur over time which, in the case of prolonged administration of drugs, leads to reduced intake by the patient. However, with regard to the relationship between adherence and the frequency with which the treatment must be administered, it seems that a higher frequency of drug administration leads to reduced adherence to treatment; adherence is therefore inversely proportional to the increase of daily doses [7]. There is also a relationship between adherence and the time devoted by the veterinarian to the consultation: the level of adherence is generally higher in owners who believe that the veterinarian has devoted more time to the consultation [8]. In the same way, the therapist's ability to adequately explain the reasons underlying a given behaviour/symptom manifested by the animal may have a positive influence on the owner's adherence to the treatment [9]. One of the reasons that causes an owner not to adhere to the treatment is his/her belief that the treatment is not necessary, thus emphasising the need to provide a better explanation of the benefits that can be obtained through the treatment and its correct application [10]. In this way, the owners see themselves as an active part of the healing process or the maintenance of the animal's state of well-being, which has a clear positive effect on adherence to protocols that are often demanding in terms of time and economy. In line with the aim of enhancing adherence levels, the veterinarian should provide maximum clarity concerning the pathology and the necessary therapeutic protocols, so that the owner can really understand the problem and the importance of applying the correct treatments. The veterinarian should then try to empathise with the owner, through an understanding of the difficulties that the owner may encounter in the application of specific therapeutic protocols [10]. Studies performed on human psychotherapy have shown how a reliable, empathic, and flexible attitude from the therapist has a positive impact on the cooperation of the patient, while a professional with an attitude perceived as rigid, aloof, tense, distracted, and insecure has a negative influence on the adherence shown by the patient [11]. Excessive lifestyle changes can have a negative influence on adherence to treatment: asking a patient to change their lifestyle in order to improve a treatment (e.g., combining proper physical exercise and diet) is more difficult than following the pharmacological treatment alone [1]. Good adherence to treatment can also be obtained by inviting the owner to regular, scheduled follow-up visits to ensure that the treatment is being implemented correctly by the owner, modifying certain aspects based on the animal's response and encouraging the owner to express any doubts about the correct application of the treatment [12]. Only a few studies on compliance in veterinary medicine have been published and, to the authors' knowledge, no study to date has compared the pet owners' adherence in different veterinary areas. This study assessed and compared the adherence levels of the owners of patients with behavioural, cardiological, urological, and oncological problems. We investigated how the owners perceive the disease of their animal and what they think about the feasibility of the treatment proposed. Finally, we have assessed the perception of the owner related to the usefulness of the treatment and the difficulties they have encountered in implementing it.

2. Materials and Methods

The study was conducted on dogs that attended the clinical visit at the Behavioural, Cardiology, Urology, and Oncology Services of the Veterinary Sciences and Public Health Department of the University of Milan from November 2012 to October 2013.

The observational prospective study was comprised of an initial enrolment phase and a second follow-up monitoring phase.

Phase 1. Cases were chosen among dog patients presented at the veterinary clinic for specialist consultation in the different fields considered in this study. We used a convenience sampling technique as subjects were selected because of their convenient accessibility and proximity to the researcher. Enrolment coincided with the first examination and implied a written consent of the owners. The consultations were conducted by veterinarians, specialists in the field, and were of variable duration from 45 to 120 minutes. The clinical visit was composed of medical history-taking, clinical examination, classification of the pathology, explanation of the prescribed treatment and scheduled follow-up (with health checks on varying dates depending on the pathology and the observed need), and definition of clinical outcome and prognosis.

At the end of the first examination, the veterinarian carried out an initial questionnaire with the owner, composed of 6 multiple-choice questions. Each question was worded as a statement to which the respondent assigned a score expressed by means of a Likert scale, where 1 = strongly disagree; 2 = disagree; 3 = neither; 4 = agree; 5 = strongly agree.

Phase 2. Then, the owners were called by phone 15 days, 1 month, 3 months, and 6 months after the examination. During the telephone calls, a questionnaire was carried out which included, in addition to the initial 6 questions, further 9 follow-up questions (Table 1).

TABLE 1: Questionnaire: 1 = strongly disagree; 2 = disagree; 3 = neither; 4 = agree; and 5 = strongly agree.

| | Questionnaire | Follow-up | | | | |
		1	2	3	4	5
First visit	(1) I am concerned about the disorder of my animal					
	(2) I could abandon my animal because of the disorder					
	(3) I could euthanize my animal because of the disorder					
	(4) My daily routine have changed because of the disorder of my animal					
	(5) It is challenging to apply the new management rules					
	(6) My animal quality of life is compromised by its disorder					
	(7) The disorder of my animal has been explained in detail					
	(8) The disorder of my animal bothers me					
	(9) The disorder of my animal bothers my neighbors or roommates					
	(10) The pharmacological treatment has been explained in detail					
	(11) It is simple to follow pharmacological recommendation					
	(12) I am consistent in administering drugs					
	(13) It is useful to administer prescribed drugs					
	(14) My animal refuses to take drugs					
	(15) The new management rules has been explained in detail					

3. Data Analysis

The answers to the questionnaire were classified with scores from 1 to 5 and entered into a database for later statistical analysis. The data analysis was performed by means of IBM SPSS Statistics 22 software [13]. The data was subject to a descriptive analysis and then a Chi Square test to compare the observed and expected frequencies in each response category.

4. Results

This study analysed a total of 48 cases (26 spayed females, 2 intact females, 3 neutered males, and 17 intact males, with different ages ranging from 8 months to 14 years old), including 20 in the behavioural medicine area, 14 in cardiology, 8 in urology, and 6 in oncology. Some owners decided to terminate their involvement in the study (8.6%), some animals died (8.5%), and others were given away (3%) or euthanized (0.8%) (Table 2).

Phase 1. The analysis of the questionnaires gathered during the first examination showed how most owners (60.6%) proved to be concerned by their animal's disease (agree 33.5% and strongly agree 27.1%). Nevertheless, 42.2% of owners believe that the disease does not harm the animal's quality of life (strongly disagree 32.8%, disagree 9.4%) and are not thinking of giving it away or euthanizing it as a result of the pathology (70.3% strongly disagree). Of those interviewed, 40.4% believe that their day-to-day habits have not changed (strongly disagree 37.7%, disagree 7.6%) as a result of the animal's pathology and 53.5% find it easy to apply the new management rules recommended by the veterinarian (50.8% strongly disagree, 2.7% disagree).

These percentages vary depending on the area analysed. Table 3, in which the "strongly agree" responses are aggregated with the "agree" responses and "disagree" is aggregated with "strongly disagree," details the results obtained in the four areas. Owners of urological patients were the most worried about the disorder of their dogs; furthermore they did not consider abandonment or euthanasia as an option or a solution for their animals' problems.

Daily routine was more affected in owners in cardiological and behavioral areas. In addition, owners in the latter category found it more difficult than others to apply the new management rules and many of them were convinced that the disease could compromise the quality of life of their animal (Table 3).

Phase 2. The changes in the responses given by owners over time showed that, in relation to the behavioural medicine area, the concern caused by the animal's pathology significantly falls during the follow-up visits ($p < 0.05$) (Figure 1). On the contrary, the percentage of owners who consider giving their dog away as a result of the pathology increases significantly over time ($p < 0.05$). The responses to any changes in day-to-day habits and the commitment to the new management rules remain constant throughout the entire duration of the study, as is also the case with owner's responses in the cardiology and urology areas. In cardiology, the number of owners who think that the pathology harms their animal's quality of life falls significantly over time ($p < 0.05$) (Figure 2). In the oncology area, although there are a higher number of owners who, during the follow-up visits, consider the possibility of euthanizing the animal, this variation is not significant.

With regard to the 9 additional questions in the follow-up questionnaires, the only significant data relates to the behavioural medicine and urology areas, in which the owner's discomfort resulting from the animal's pathology significantly decreases over time ($p < 0.05$). In the behavioural medicine area, the discomfort caused to cohabitants and neighbours also significantly decreases ($p < 0.05$).

TABLE 2: Number of owners who abandoned the study and number of patients abandoned, euthanized, and dead (BM = behavioural medicine; C = cardiology; U = urology; and O = oncology).

	First visit				15 days				1 month				3 months				6 months				Total			
	BM	C	U	O	BM	C	U	O	BM	C	U	O	BM	C	U	O	BM	C	U	O	BM	C	U	O
Owners who abandoned the study	0	0	0	0	2	1	0	0	0	0	0	0	2	0	0	0	0	0	0	0	**4**	**1**	**0**	**0**
Patients abandoned	0	0	0	0	0	0	0	0	0	0	0	0	3	0	0	0	1	0	0	0	**4**	**0**	**0**	**0**
Patients euthanized	0	0	0	0	0	0	0	0	0	0	0	0	1	0	0	0	0	0	0	0	**1**	**0**	**0**	**0**
Patients dead	0	0	0	0	1	0	0	1	0	1	0	0	0	1	1	0	0	3	0	3	**1**	**5**	**1**	**4**

TABLE 3: Results obtained by the four fields during the first visit.

	Behavioural medicine		Cardiology		Urology		Oncology	
	Agree	Disagree	Agree	Disagree	Agree	Disagree	Agree	Disagree
I am concerned about the disorder of my animal	49%	26%	71,2%	9,1%	77,5%	15,5%	53,3%	21%
I could abandon my animal because of the disorder	9%	61%	4,5%	75,8%	2,5%	90%	0%	76,7%
I could euthanize my animal because of the disorder	1%	74%	6%	71,2%	2,5%	82,5%	23,3%	50%
My daily routine have changed because of the disorder of my animal	37%	36%	37,9%	42,4%	22,5%	67,5%	20%	53,3%
It is challenging to apply the new management rules	32,9%	36,7%	15,4%	62,5%	9,4%	75%	4,2%	62,5%
My animal quality of life is compromised by its disorder	41,4%	29,3%	36,5%	42,4%	17,5%	70%	16,6%	43,6%

5. Discussion

The aim of our study was to assess the adherence levels of owners of patients in the behavioural, cardiological, urological, and oncological sectors of veterinary medicine. Given the lack of published research on pet owners' adherence in different veterinary areas, this pilot study was planned as a first step to determine if and how it is possible to assess and compare adherence in each of the considered sectors of veterinary medicine. The main limitation of this study is the relatively small sample of animals included, and this means that caution should therefore be exercised so as not to generalize these results and more patients should be involved in order to transfer the results to the entire population.

Overall, the owners who participated in the study appeared to be concerned by their animal's disorder; this information could be very important in improving the owner's adherence, because the concern for the pathology could represent a concrete reason for the person to adhere to the prescribed treatment [1]. However, the owner's concern does not appear to go hand in hand with the harm to the animal's quality of life. In fact, most interviewees believe that the pathology does not affect the animal's quality of life. This could be linked to poor knowledge and an erroneous interpretation of the animal's body language by the owner, which can make it difficult to recognise signs of the animal's discomfort or pain. In fact, owners often have an anthropomorphic view of their animal's behaviour and, consequently, they expect human behaviours and reactions from their animals, often creating misunderstandings in the communication and relationship with the dog [14]. Giving the animal away and putting it down are possibilities that are rarely considered by the owner. The man-animal bond of companionship changes considerably over the years and the new way of experiencing the relationship with the pet often translates into greater attention to its health and greater emotional involvement in living with its disease and its loss [15]. This greater involvement of the owner not only causes him/her not to feel the influence of the pathology on their own day-to-day habits or to encounter difficulties in adapting to the needs pertaining to their animal's pathology, but also represents an effective instrument that can be used to obtain greater adherence.

When comparing the four clinical areas investigated, the owners of patients with behavioural problems stated that they were less worried about the problem manifested by their animal and this concern tends to fall over time. This could be linked to the fact that, to date, behavioural medicine and behavioural problems are not well-known by owners and this may lead them to underestimate or not recognize the seriousness of their dog or cat's disorder or the necessary commitment to their treatment, thus reducing their adherence level. It would therefore be necessary for owners to receive more in depth information from the attending veterinarians related to the possibility of onset of behavioural pathologies [9]. Owners who, in the first visit, appeared to be most concerned were those of the urology area. In our study, patients in this

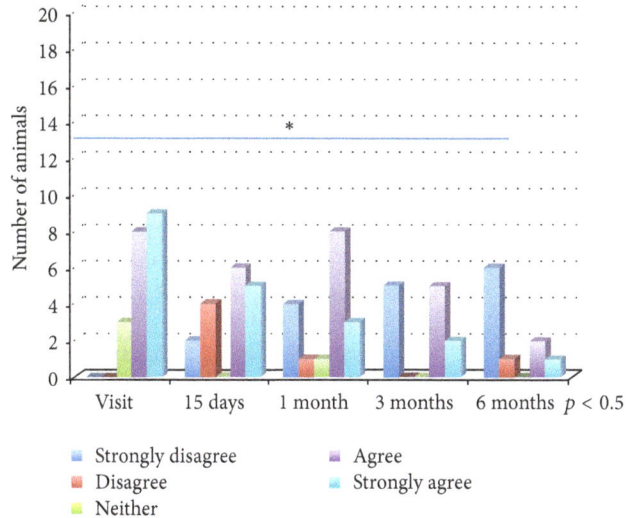

FIGURE 1: Behavioural medicine: "I am concerned about the disorder of my animal."

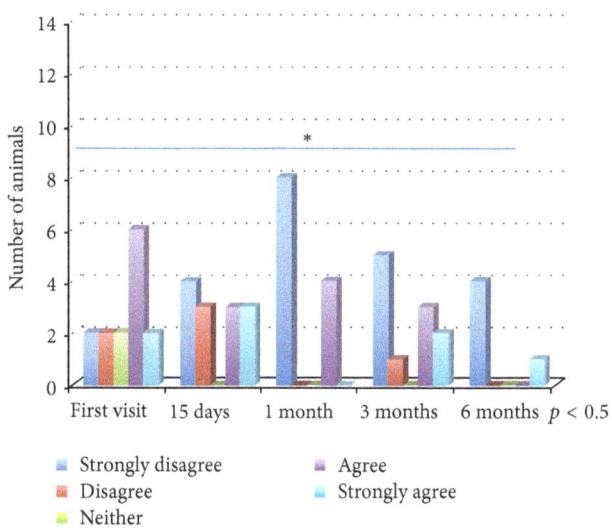

FIGURE 2: Cardiology: "My animal's quality of life is compromised by its disorder."

area were mainly cats and currently, as a result of veterinary information, the owners of these animals have a certain level of awareness of the possibility of elderly cats developing renal pathologies; their concern could therefore be based on knowledge of such serious pathologies. A simple explanation of the pathology may encourage the owner to follow the therapeutic protocol with a greater level of participation and attention. In fact, it seems that one of the reasons that causes an owner not to adhere to the treatment is his/her belief that the treatment is not necessary or useless, thus underlining the importance of providing a clear explanation of the benefits that can be obtained through the treatment and its correct application [10]. In this way, the owners see themselves as an active part of the healing process or the maintenance of the animal's state of well-being, which has a clear positive effect

on adherence to protocols that are often demanding in terms of time and money. In order to increase the adherence level, it seems important to ask owners to express their concerns about the health condition of the animal. This makes it possible to establish a dialogue with the owner, to make them feel free to express any concerns about the health of the animal and therefore add any important elements to the diagnostic process and the resulting treatment [16].

Among the four areas investigated, the owners who, upon the first visit, least consider the idea of putting down or giving the animal away as a result of the pathology are those in the urology area, followed by those of cardiology, oncology, and behavioural medicine. During the follow-up visits, the situation remains unchanged for the first three areas (in which no subject was given away or euthanized), while, in the behavioural area, four animals were given away and one was put down. For this purpose, it is important to consider the social aspect of behavioural pathology; behavioural problems often have a strong impact on the animal itself, the owner, and their cohabitants and neighbours, and this is why an owner could be more willing to give away or put down their animal [17]. Furthermore, owners often do not have sufficient information to manage the behavioural problem, they are not referred to specific, specialised professionals, and they attend specialist consultations when the problem has already been apparent for some time (thus compromising the prognosis [17, 18]). In addition to this, this factor could be influenced by the effect of time on the owner-dog relationship. In fact, in most cases, heart, urological, and oncological pathologies occur at an advanced age, that is to say, after years of close cohabitation between the person and the animal, with the resulting creation of a strong and deep-rooted bond; conversely, behavioural pathologies often arise in young animals or those recently adopted and, sometimes, this brief period is not sufficient to create a close and deep relationship. The increase in owners of patients in behavioural medicine who have given their animal away by the third follow-up can be traced back to the fact that, at this point in the treatment, the owner expects results that do not materialise because, in most cases, behavioural treatment requires time and commitment and results may not be visible after only one month from the start [18]. In this regard, it seems that the veterinarian can help to increase adherence levels by also inviting the owner to regular, scheduled follow-up visits: this would enable the veterinarian to ensure that the treatment is being implemented correctly by the owner and possibly change any aspects depending on the animal's response [1, 19].

When comparing the four areas investigated, the management rules laid down by the behavioural veterinary doctor as well as the day-to-day habits appear to be the most demanding. This may be derived from the fact that behavioural treatment, unlike that which is generally prescribed by specialists in the other three areas, is comprised of changes to the rules of management and interaction with the animal, in addition to administration of a pharmacological treatment where necessary [19]. Since the ease of applying the treatment has a positive effect on adherence levels, it is advisable to limit the amount of information provided, use clear and plain language, and speak slowly to enable the owner to absorb each indication given [2, 9, 20, 21]. Clear and simple explanations often give rise not only to greater adherence to the treatment, but also to an increase in the value attributed by the owner to the veterinary recommendations [10]. In fact, adherence to treatment appears to be significantly influenced by the importance and value given by the owner to the veterinary recommendations [10].

When comparing the four areas investigated, there are a greater number of owners in the behavioural medicine and cardiology groups who believe that the pathology harms the animal's quality of life. In the case of cardiology, there is a significant reduction of this value over time and this points to the effectiveness of the treatment enabling the owner to take into account the clinical improvements of their animal. This consideration is also reinforced by the fact that, in the same area, there is a significant decrease in the discomfort caused to the owner during the follow-up visits. The same information has also been obtained in the behavioural medicine area, in which there is also a reduction in the discomfort caused to the owner by the pathology [18].

6. Conclusions

In the veterinary field, the management of the patient is the result of cooperation between the veterinarian and the owner. The role of the veterinarian is therefore fundamental in enabling an increase in the levels of adherence to the therapeutic protocols by the owners of animals.

To achieve good adherence levels, constant contact between the doctor and owner is necessary. It is therefore essential that the owner be allowed to clarify any doubts with the veterinarian that may arise during treatment and to receive constant support in the administration of the treatment and coping with the animal's pathology. Assessment of adherence appears to be an optimal instrument in identifying the positive factors and the difficulties encountered by owners during the application of a treatment requiring the administration of specific drugs and the implementation of precise management rules. The results set out here should be considered as preliminary to research that we are conducting on a wider sample of animals for a longer follow-up period.

Conflict of Interests

The authors declare that there is no conflict of interests regarding the publication of this paper.

Acknowledgment

The authors acknowledge the assistance of Kirk T. Ford for the revision of the English paper.

References

[1] American Animal Hospital Association, *The Path to High-Quality Care. Practical Tips for improving Compliance*, American Animal Hospital Association, Lakewood, Colo, USA, 2003.

[2] C. J. Wayner and M. L. Heinke, "Compliance: crafting quality care," *Veterinary Clinics of North America: Small Animal Practice*, vol. 36, no. 2, pp. 419–436, 2006.

[3] T. Klauer and U. K. Zettl, "Compliance, adherence, and the treatment of multiple sclerosis," *Journal of Neurology*, vol. 255, no. 6, supplement, pp. 87–92, 2008.

[4] World Health Organization, *Adherence to Long-Term Therapies*, World Health Organization, Geneva, Switzerland, 2003.

[5] R. A. S. White, "The approach to the tumor patient," in *Manual of Small Animal Oncology*, R. A. S. White, Ed., pp. 13–16, British Small Animal Veterinary Association (BSAVA), 1991.

[6] P. A. Ciekot, "Consulenza al cliente per il cancro: considerazioni per una presentazione professionale ed intelligente delle opzioni, dei rischi e degli scopi terapeutici," in *Oncologia Chirurgica*, S. D. Gilson, Ed., vol. 9, no. 2, pp. 215–227, Medicina-Scienze, 1998.

[7] V. J. Adams, J. R. Campbell, C. L. Waldner, P. M. Dowling, and C. L. Shmon, "Evaluation of client compliance with short-term administration of antimicrobials to dogs," *Journal of the American Veterinary Medical Association*, vol. 226, no. 4, pp. 567–574, 2005.

[8] K. Grave and H. Tanem, "Compliance with short-term oral antibacterial drug treatment in dogs," *Journal of Small Animal Practice*, vol. 40, no. 4, pp. 158–162, 1999.

[9] B. A. Berger, "Assessing and interviewing patients for meaningful behavioral change: part 1," *The Case Manager*, vol. 15, no. 5, pp. 46–50, 2004.

[10] T. W. Lue, D. P. Pantenburg, and P. M. Crawford, "Impact of the owner-pet and client-veterinarian bond on the care that pets receive," *Journal of the American Veterinary Medical Association*, vol. 232, no. 4, pp. 531–540, 2008.

[11] S. J. Ackerman and M. J. Hilsenroth, "A review of therapist characteristics and techniques negatively impacting the therapeutic alliance," *Psychotherapy*, vol. 38, no. 2, pp. 171–185, 2001.

[12] L. Pagliaro, "Medicina basata sule evidenze," *Recenti Progressi in Medicina*, vol. 89, no. 3, 1998.

[13] IBM, *IBM SPSS Statistics 22 Command Syntax Reference*, IBM, Chicago, Ill, USA, 2013.

[14] J. W. S. Bradshaw and R. A. Casey, "Anthropomorphism and anthropocentrism as influences in the quality of life of companion animals," *Animal Welfare*, vol. 16, pp. 149–154, 2007.

[15] L. Lagoni, C. Butler, and S. J. Withrow, "Companion animal death and pet owner grief," in *Small Animal Clinical Oncology*, S. J. Withrow and E. G. MacEwen, Eds., pp. 547–559, WB Saunders, 2nd edition, 1996.

[16] J. R. Shaw, B. N. Bonnett, C. L. Adams, and D. L. Roter, "Veterinarian-client-patient communication patterns used during clinical appointments in companion animal practice," *Journal of the American Veterinary Medical Association*, vol. 228, no. 5, pp. 714–721, 2006.

[17] L. Notari and B. Gallicchio, "Owners' perceptions of behavior problems and behavior therapists in Italy: a preliminary study," *Journal of Veterinary Behavior: Clinical Applications and Research*, vol. 3, no. 2, pp. 52–58, 2008.

[18] K. L. Overall, *La clinica comportamentale del cane e del gatto*, C.G. Edizioni Medico Scientifiche, 2001.

[19] Y. Takeuchi, K. A. Houpt, and J. M. Scarlett, "Evaluation of treatments for separation anxiety in dogs," *Journal of the American Veterinary Medical Association*, vol. 217, no. 3, pp. 342–345, 2000.

[20] R. P. C. Kessels, "Patients' memory for medical information," *Journal of the Royal Society of Medicine*, vol. 96, no. 5, pp. 219–222, 2003.

[21] C. Bower, "Il ruolo della medicina comportamentale nella pratica veterinaria," in *Terapia comportamentale del cane e del gatto*, D. F. Horwitz, D. S. Mills, and S. Heath, Eds., UTET, 2004.

15

Serological and Molecular Evidence of Q Fever in Domestic Ruminants in Bangladesh

Md. Arifur Rahman,[1] **Md. Mahbub Alam,**[1] **Md. Aminul Islam,**[1]
A. K. Fazlul Haque Bhuiyan,[2] **and A. K. M. Anisur Rahman**[1]

[1]*Department of Medicine, Faculty of Veterinary Science, Bangladesh Agricultural University (BAU), Mymensingh 2202, Bangladesh*
[2]*Department of Animal Breeding and Genetics, Faculty of Animal Husbandry, BAU, Mymensingh 2202, Bangladesh*

Correspondence should be addressed to A. K. M. Anisur Rahman; arahman_med@bau.edu.bd

Academic Editor: Giuliano Bettini

The objective of this study was to know the herd and animal level prevalence of Q fever in domestic ruminants in some selected districts in Bangladesh. Randomly collected 111 bulk milk and 94 sera samples of cattle, sheep, and goats were tested by indirect ELISA (iELISA). DNA extracted from 23 aborted fetal membranes was analyzed by real time (rt) PCR. The positive cut-off value of iELISA in bulk milk and individual animal sera was $\geq 30\%$ and $\geq 40\%$, respectively. The overall herd level prevalence of Q fever in dairy cattle was 15.6%. The prevalence of Q fever in dairy cattle was significantly higher in Sirajganj in comparison to Satkhira District ($P < 0.01$). The overall seroprevalence of Q fever in domestic ruminants was 5.06%. Although statistically insignificant, the seroprevalence of Q fever was relatively higher in sheep (9.52%) in comparison to goats (3.33%) and cattle (3.57%). Out of 23 aborted fetal membranes, only one sheep placenta was positive in rt PCR. Q fever is present in all of the three important species of domestic ruminants in Bangladesh. It may have some role in sheep abortion as the seroprevalence is relatively higher and also one sheep placenta is rt PCR positive.

1. Introduction

Q (for Query) fever is a ubiquitous zoonosis caused by an obligate intracellular bacterium *Coxiella* (*C.*) *burnetii*. It has been reported from all over the world except Antarctica and possibly New Zealand [1, 2]. The primary reservoirs of *C. burnetii* are cattle, sheep, and goats. However, the infection has been reported in other mammals (humans, cats, dogs, rodents, rabbits, horses, swine, camels, water buffalo, and marine mammals), ticks and other arthropods, birds, fish, and reptiles [3, 4]. The common manifestations of Q fever in ruminants are abortion, stillbirth, premature delivery, and delivery of weak offspring [2]. Indeed these clinical manifestations are usually observed in sheep and goats and Q fever is mostly asymptomatic in cattle. Clinically infected cows may develop infertility, metritis, and mastitis [5].

In humans, Q fever is mostly asymptomatic but may be responsible for acute or chronic disease conditions such as influenza-like illness, pneumonia, hepatitis, meningoencephalitis, myocarditis, endocarditis, and chronic fatigue syndrome in persistently infected patients and may contribute to abortion and stillbirth in pregnant women [2, 6].

Diagnosis of Q fever in animals is based on detection of bacteria, bacterial DNA, or antibodies [7]. Although these bacteria can grow in axenic (host cell-free) media, isolation is time consuming and hazardous for the laboratory workers [8]. In addition, Q fever isolation techniques require a Biosafety Level 3 Laboratory (BSL-3). Mostly, *C. burnetii* exposure in animals can be screened indirectly by serological tests. The CFT (OIE recommended test) and ELISA (EU recommended test) are the two most commonly used serological tests in this purpose. However, CFT protocol is complex and fails to detect antibodies in sheep or goats [9]. The ELISA is reported to be highly sensitive and specific for the diagnosis of Q fever [10]. Moreover, ELISA can be used to detect antibodies in bulk milk and individual animal serum. The bacterial DNA can be detected by using PCR [11].

Although Q fever is present worldwide, its status in animals, humans, arthropods, birds, wild animals, and other reservoirs in Bangladesh is not known except one report on serological evidence in cattle and goats [12]. Nevertheless, the reproductive diseases in dairy cattle [13–15] are endemic in Bangladesh. So the objectives of this paper are to determine the herd level prevalence of Q fever in dairy cattle and goats, to estimate the animal level prevalence of Q fever in cattle, sheep, and goats originated from herds having previous history of abortion, and to detect *C. burnetii* DNA from aborted fetal membranes of cattle, goat, and sheep.

2. Materials and Methods

2.1. Milk Samples. This study used milk samples from two previous studies, which were undertaken in the Department of Medicine, BAU, Mymensingh 2202. In one study, 399 randomly collected bulk milk samples were examined for somatic cell count from where 94 samples were used in this study. The history of reproductive failure in the selected dairy herds was not known. In another study, 17 milk ring test positive samples were sent to Belgium for isolation of *Brucella* spp., which were also used for this study. The districts of Bangladesh included in this study are shown in Figure 1.

2.2. Serum Sample Collection. Serum samples were collected from a serum bank in the Department of Medicine, BAU, Mymensingh. Those samples were randomly collected to study brucellosis in cattle, sheep, and goats in different districts of Bangladesh in 2007 and 2008 [16]. Ninety-four (94) serum samples were collected from 40 herds of the Mymensingh and Sherpur Districts out of 58 having some abortion (known from the owners) in the last year.

2.3. DNA Samples of Placentas. Twenty-three DNA samples (5 from cattle, 10 from goats, and 8 from sheep) extracted from aborted fetal membranes for the detection of *Brucella* spp. were also used in this study. DNA was extracted using the DNeasy spin column kit (QIAGEN) according to the manufacturer's protocol.

2.4. Herd and Animal Level Data Collection. Animal level data on age, breed, sex, and pregnancy status and herd level data on herd size, herd composition, and location of the herd were collected from available database of serum samples.

For milk samples, the location of the farm and number of lactating cows in herd were collected from the bovine mastitis database.

2.5. Indirect ELISA Test

2.5.1. Preparation of Milk and Sera Samples. The milk and sera samples were prepared according to the instructions of commercial kit. In brief, 10 milliliters of milk from each selected herd was collected for testing antibody against *C. burnetii* exposure. The samples were centrifuged and the nonfat

fraction was stored at −20°C until tested for antibodies against *C. burnetii*. Before testing, herd milk samples were prepared at 1 : 5 dilution using diluted (1 : 10) wash solution. Sera of the selected animals were removed from the serum bank and prepared at 1 : 400 dilution by using diluted wash solution.

2.5.2. Test Procedure. All reagents were taken into 18–26°C before use. The reagents were mixed by shaking gently. All samples were tested in duplicate and the optical densities (OD) of the samples were averaged and corrected by subtracting the OD of the negative control. Both milk and serum based tests were performed using the commercial CHEKIT Q Fever Antibody ELISA Test Kit (IDEXX, Liebefeld-Bern, Switzerland) based on *C. burnetii* inactivated phase 1 and phase 2 antigens [10]. The positive cut-off value (S/P ratio) of iELISA in bulk milk and individual animal sera was ≥30% and ≥40%, respectively.

2.6. Real Time PCR. The real time (rt) PCR assay was performed using a 7500 rt PCR System (Applied Biosystems). Samples were considered positive with a cycle threshold (Ct) < 40 [17]. It was performed in Veterinary Agrochemical Research Centre (CODA-CERVA) in Brussels, Belgium.

2.7. Statistical Analysis. The association of herd and animal level factors with Q fever prevalence was analyzed by χ^2 test using R 3.1.0 (The R Foundation for Statistical Computing 2014).

3. Results

3.1. Descriptive Statistics. The serum samples were collected from 40 herds where there was history of abortion in any of the three domestic ruminant species in the last year. The herd size varied from 1 to 20 with a median of 3 animals. Thirteen herds consisted of only cattle, 13 of only goats, 8 of both cattle and goats, and 6 of only sheep. In 55.0% (22/40) herd's aborted materials were disposed by burial but in the rest of the herds the materials were thrown away in the field or in nearby water bodies. About 35% (14/40) farmers were found to keep sheep (7.5%) or goats (27.5%) inside their house at night.

The age of cattle varied from 4 months to 12 years with a median of 6 years. The range and median age of goats and sheep, respectively, were 2.5 months to 4 years and 2 years, 1 month to 4 years and 8 months. Among cattle 82.0% were female and indigenous and all of the sheep were indigenous and 74.2% of them were female but 80.0% and 94.0% goats were female and Black Bengal breed type, respectively. The range of positive S/P value in cattle herds was 41.4 to 123.0.

3.2. Herd Level Prevalence of Q Fever in Dairy Cattle. A summary of ELISA test results on the presence of *C. burnetii* antibodies in herd milk is presented in Table 1. An overall herd level prevalence of Q fever in dairy cattle was 15.6% (95% Confidence Interval (CI): 9.4–23.8) (Table 1). The distribution of Q fever in dairy herds is shown in Table 2. The prevalence of Q fever was significantly higher in Sirajganj

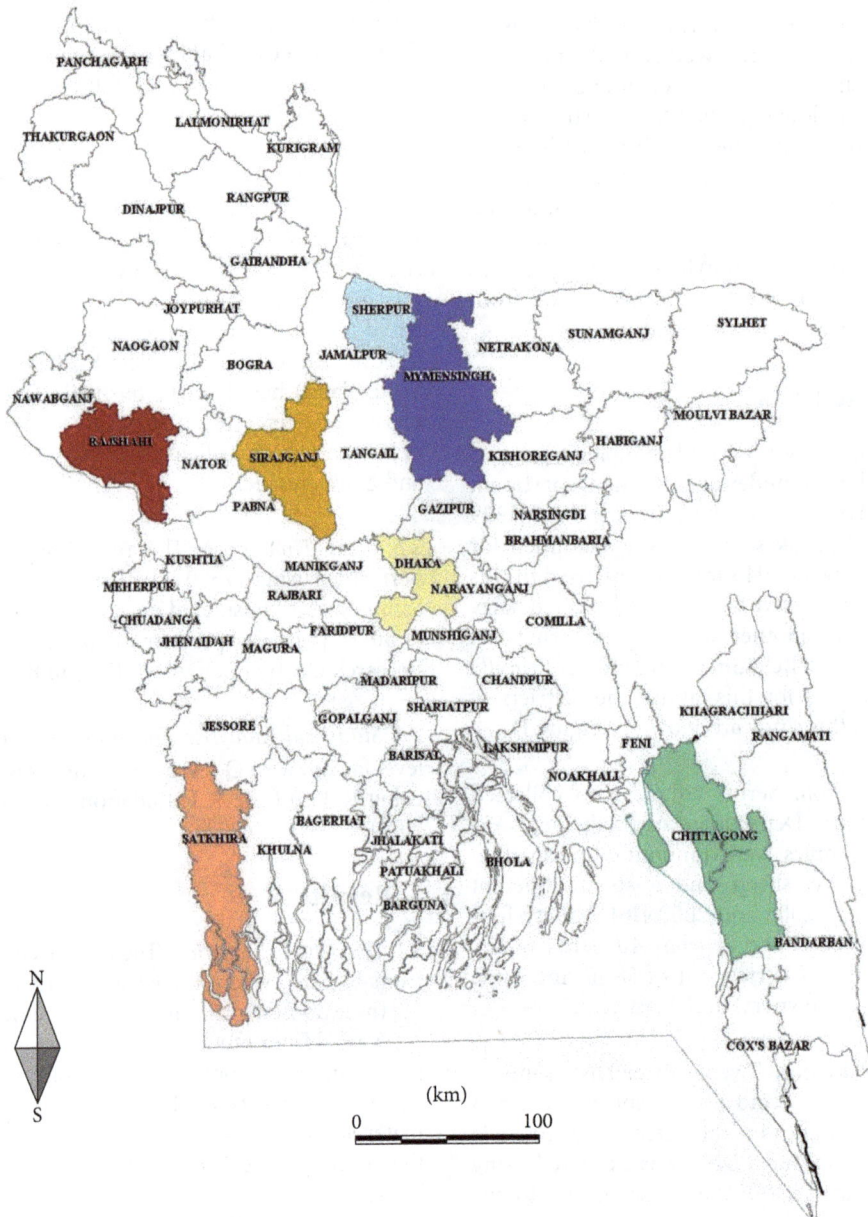

Q fever study areas

☐ Seroprevalence 11.1% in goats

■ Seroprevalence 8.3% and 9.5% in cattle and sheep, respectively

■ Herd level prevalence 7.1%

■ Herd level prevalence 10.1%

☐ Government goat farm positive and a sheep placenta of BLRI sheep farm PCR positive

■ Herd level prevalence 34.6%

■ Bulk milk of government goat farm positive

FIGURE 1

TABLE 1: Summary of iELISA tests results on the presence of *Coxiella burnetii* antibodies (S/P values) in milk samples.

Test result	Number of herds/flocks	Apparent prevalence	95% CI	Range of S/P values (%)	Mean S/P values (%)
Positive (S/P ≥ 30%)	17 (cattle)	15.6%	9.4–23.8	41.4–123.0	81.3
Negative (S/P < 30%)	92	84.4%	76.2–90.6	0–25.9	5.6
Positive (S/P ≥ 30%)	2 (goats)*			421.6 and 424.2	

*Both goat flocks were positive; CI: Confidence Interval.

TABLE 2: Distribution of herd level prevalence of Q fever based on iELISA using bulk milk.

Variable	Tested	Positive (>40%)	Prevalence	95% CI	χ^2 test P value
District					<0.01
Satkhira	28	2	7.1	0.9–23.5	
Chittagong	55	6	10.9	4.1–22.2	
Sirajganj	26	9	34.6	17.2–55.6	
Number of lactating cows					1
>5	22	3	13.6	2.9–34.9	
1 to 5	87	14	16.1	9.1–15.5	
Breed composition					0.29
Sahiwal cross	18	2	11.1	1.4–34.7	
Friesian cross	73	10	13.7	6.8–23.8	
Both	18	5	27.8	9.7–53.5	

The other two bulk milk samples were collected from two government goat farms in Savar, Dhaka, and Rajshahi Districts; CI: Confidence Interval.

(34.6%) in comparison to Satkhira District ($P < 0.01$). Although statistically insignificant, the prevalence of Q fever was relatively higher in herds having only Friesian cross (13.7%) and both Sahiwal and Friesian breed together (27.8%) in comparison to Sahiwal cross.

3.3. Seroprevalence of Q Fever in Cattle, Goats, and Sheep. The summary of ELISA test results on the presence of *C. burnetii* antibodies in serum samples is provided in Table 3. Out of 94 sera samples tested, the ages of 15 (10 sheep and 5 goats) animals were below six months (two seropositive sheep), which were excluded from the result in estimating seroprevalence (maternal immunity). The overall seroprevalence of Q fever in domestic ruminants was 5.06% (95% CI: 1.63–13.14). Three point seven nine percent (3.79%) sera samples were Q fever suspect and 91.13% were Q fever negative. The range of positive S/P value was 42.70 to 49.80%. The distribution of Q fever seroprevalence in domestic ruminants is shown in Table 4. The seroprevalence of Q fever was found to be higher in sheep (9.52%, 95% CI: 1.67–31.83) in comparison to goat (3.33%, 95% CI: 0.17–19.05) and cattle (3.57%, 95% CI: 0.18–20.24) but it was statistically insignificant. The seroprevalence of Q fever varied according to sex, pregnancy status, and study areas but none was significant statistically.

The demographic characteristics of the four Q fever seropositive domestic ruminants are shown in Table 5. Both seropositive sheep were from the same location (Unions/Sub-Upazila of Mymensingh Sadar Upazila/subdistrict).

3.4. Real Time PCR Result. *Coxiella burnetii* DNA was detected from only one sheep placenta. The remaining 22 samples were negative.

4. Discussion

In this study the herd level prevalence of Q fever in cattle based on bulk milk and animal level seroprevalence of Q fever in cattle, goats, and sheep were estimated by using indirect ELISA test. The overall prevalence of Q fever in bulk cow milk was 15.6% indicating that Q fever is an existing disease in dairy cattle population in Bangladesh. The herds under study were originated from major milk pockets of Bangladesh like Sirajganj, Chittagong, and Satkhira Districts (Figure 1). The sample size was very small and the sample does not represent the dairy herds of Bangladesh. It was also a limitation of this study. Due to the lack of fund it was not possible to include more samples in this study. So the herd level prevalence of Q fever we obtained may not represent the true status of this disease in dairy herds of the study areas. A widely variable and much higher herd level prevalence of Q fever (57.8 to 78.6%) was reported from different corners of the world [18–21]. Dairy cattle are usually chronically infected with Q fever and shed *C. burnetii* in the milk [22]. It is also stated that chronically infected dairy cattle are the most important source of human infection [1]. Another important source of human infection is the manipulation of fetus and its fluids and placentas from aborted small ruminants without safety

TABLE 3: Summary of iELISA tests results on the presence of *Coxiella burnetii* antibodies (S/P values) in serum samples.

Test result	Number	Prevalence (%)	95% Confidence Interval	Range of S/P values (%)	Mean S/P values (%)
Positive (S/P ≥ 40%)	4	5.06	1.63–13.14	42.70–49.80	45.35
Suspect (30% ≤ S/P < 40%)	3	3.79	0.98–11.45	30.10–34.50	32.40
Negative (S/P < 30%)	72	91.13	82.04–96.06	0–29.80	5.13

TABLE 4: The distribution of seroprevalence of Q fever in domestic ruminants.

Variable	Tested	Positive	Prevalence (95% CI)	χ^2 test P value
Species				0.55
Cattle	28	1	3.57 (0.18–20.24)	
Sheep	21	2	9.52 (1.67–31.83)	
Goats	30	1	3.33 (0.17–19.05)	
Sex				1.00
Male	15	1	6.67 (0.34–33.96)	
Female	64	3	4.69 (1.22–13.96)	
Pregnancy				0.63
No	38	1	2.63 (0.14–15.43)	
Yes	26	2	7.69 (1.34–26.59)	
Male	15	1	6.67 (0.34–33.96)	
District				1.00
Sherpur	25	1	4.0 (0.21–22.32)	
Cattle	16	0	0 (0–24.07*)	
Sheep	0	0		
Goats	9	1	11.11 (0.58–49.33)	
Mymensingh	54	3	5.56 (1.44–16.34)	
Cattle	12	1	8.33 (0.44–40.25)	
Sheep	21	2	9.52 (1.67–31.83)	
Goats	21	0	0 (0–19.24*)	

CI: Confidence Interval; *97.5% Confidence Interval.

protection measures. As Q fever is a zoonosis and it exists in animals of Bangladesh it is also supposed to be present in humans. Due to lack of reporting, awareness, and nonspecific influenza-like symptoms of this disease in humans, it may be overlooked and remained undiagnosed in human diagnostic laboratories. Due to lack of reporting from animals, the physicians are also unaware about this disease in humans. As a result, physicians usually do not refer flu-like cases for Q fever diagnosis. Both in humans and in animals, inhalation of bacteria present in the environment is the main route of infection. So dairy workers, animal caretakers, and pyrexia of unknown origin cases should be regularly tested for Q fever. Moreover, consumption of contaminated raw milk may produce infection in humans [1]. Indeed, the Bangladeshi population seldom ingests the raw milk.

We have tested only bulk milk, which does not allow identification of individual cows infected with Q fever. However, it is very useful for screening herds under disease surveillance system. A large epidemiologic study including representative dairy herds of Bangladesh will help to reveal the herd level status of this disease in Bangladesh. Out of three study areas, significantly higher prevalence of Q fever was found in dairy herds of Sirajganj than Satkhira District. The cattle management system in Sirajganj area slightly varies from that of other parts of Bangladesh. In the dry season, the cattle graze freely and remain in the pasture ("Bathan") for almost six months (December to May). As a result, a lot of intermingling among cattle of different owners occurs during that period. Intermixing of cattle from different owners may facilitate the transmission of infection in dairy cattle herds of this area. In some herd, presence of sheep is also noticed in that period. Environment conditions in dry season could play a role in the survival of the bacteria and facilitate the transmission between animals as well. Similarly, higher prevalence of Q fever in loose housing system was also reported by Paul et al. [10]. Capuano et al. [23] also reported relatively higher seroprevalence of Q fever in herds housed in winter but turned out in spring than those housed permanently. Like other infectious diseases, Q fever was reported to be significantly associated with increased herd size [23, 24]. In this study, the prevalence of Q fever in contrast was a bit higher in smaller herds. However, the difference was not significant statistically. The prevalence of Q fever was relatively higher in herds having Friesian cross and in herd containing both Sahiwal and Friesian breed together although the difference was not significant statistically. Other authors had also reported significantly higher level of Q fever prevalence in Holstein breed [10, 23].

We have observed relatively higher seroprevalence of Q fever in sheep than cattle and goats. Similar observations were also reported by other authors [25, 26]. The prevalence of Q fever was reported to be significantly higher with the age of the animals [27–29]. We have also observed that the age of the seropositive animals is ≥10 months.

In our study, serum samples of the animals were originated from herds where there was history of abortion in previous year. Out of four seropositive cases two were in sheep indicating that Q fever might have some role in sheep abortion. Our rt PCR result also supports this hypothesis. An rt PCR Q fever positive result in the placenta means a contact with the bacteria. To confirm an abortion caused by *Coxiella burnetii* is necessary to detect histopathology lesions in the aborted fetus and placenta. Significantly higher seroprevalence of Q fever in sheep had also been reported by Berri et al. [30]. The immunosuppressive effects of pregnancy may be responsible for the increased multiplication of the organism in the placenta and thereby the higher seroprevalence [31].

It is revealed from this study that Q fever is present in all of the three important domestic ruminant species in Bangladesh. It may have some role in sheep abortion as

TABLE 5: Characteristics of the four Q fever seropositive domestic ruminants.

Farmer ID	Area	Species	Age	Breed	Sex	Body weight	S/P value (%)
Fa 50	Sirta, Mymensingh Sadar	Cattle	6 years	Indigenous	Female	200	42.7
Fa 268	Noyabil, Sherpur	Goat	1 year	Black Bengal	Female	6	49.8
Fa 543	Buror Chor, Mymensingh Sadar	Sheep	10 months	Indigenous	Male entire	12	43.4
Fa 548	Buror Chor, Mymensingh Sadar	Sheep	1.5 years	Indigenous	Female	18	45.5

the seroprevalence is relatively higher and one sheep placenta is rt PCR positive.

Competing Interests

The authors declare that they have no competing interests.

Acknowledgments

This research work was funded by the Seed Bull Production Project (SPGR fund) in the Department of Animal Breeding and Genetics, BAU, and the NST Authority. The authors are grateful to Professor Dr. Md. Taohidul Islam, Department of Medicine, BAU, Mymensingh, for providing bulk milk samples and to Dr. David Fretin of Veterinary Agrochemical Research Centre, Brussels, Belgium, for the support on real time PCR.

References

[1] M. Maurin and D. Raoult, "Q fever," *Clinical Microbiology Reviews*, vol. 12, no. 4, pp. 518–553, 1999.

[2] E. Angelakis and D. Raoult, "Q fever," *Veterinary Microbiology*, vol. 140, no. 3-4, pp. 297–309, 2010.

[3] B. Babudieri, "Q fever: a zoonosis," *Advances in Veterinary Science*, vol. 5, pp. 81–182, 1959.

[4] S. R. Porter, G. Czaplicki, J. Mainil, R. Guattéo, and C. Saegerman, "Q fever: current state of knowledge and perspectives of research of a neglected zoonosis," *International Journal of Microbiology*, vol. 2011, Article ID 248418, 22 pages, 2011.

[5] H. To, K. K. Htwe, N. Kako et al., "Prevalence of *Coxiella burnetii* infection in dairy cattle with reproductive disorders," *Journal of Veterinary Medical Science*, vol. 60, no. 7, pp. 859–861, 1998.

[6] M. J. Wildman, E. G. Smith, J. Groves, J. M. Beattie, E. O. Caul, and J. G. Ayres, "Chronic fatigue following infection by *Coxiella burnetii* (Q fever): ten-year follow-up of the 1989 UK outbreak cohort," *Quarterly Journal of Medicine*, vol. 95, no. 8, pp. 527–538, 2002.

[7] A. Rodolakis, "Q fever, state of art: epidemiology, diagnosis and prophylaxis," *Small Ruminant Research*, vol. 62, no. 1-2, pp. 121–124, 2006.

[8] A. Omsland, T. Hackstadt, and R. A. Heinzen, "Bringing culture to the uncultured: *Coxiella burnetii* and lessons for obligate intracellular bacterial pathogens," *PLoS Pathogens*, vol. 9, no. 9, Article ID e1003540, 2013.

[9] E. Kováčová, J. Kazár, and A. Šimková, "Clinical and serological analysis of a Q fever outbreak in western Slovakia with four-year follow-up," *European Journal of Clinical Microbiology and Infectious Diseases*, vol. 17, no. 12, pp. 867–869, 1998.

[10] S. Paul, J. F. Agger, B. Markussen, A.-B. Christoffersen, and J. S. Agerholm, "Factors associated with *Coxiella burnetii* antibody positivity in Danish dairy cows," *Preventive Veterinary Medicine*, vol. 107, no. 1-2, pp. 57–64, 2012.

[11] E. Rousset, V. Duquesne, P. Russo, and M. F. Aubert, "Q fever," in *Manual of Diagnostic Tests and Vaccines for Terrestrial Animals*, World Organisation for Animal Health (OIE), Paris, France, 2010.

[12] N. Haider, M. S. Rahman, S. U. Khan et al., "Serological evidence of *Coxiella burnetii* infection in cattle and goats in Bangladesh," *EcoHealth*, vol. 12, no. 2, pp. 354–358, 2015.

[13] M. A. S. Talukder, M. A. M. Y. Khandoker, M. G. M. Rahman, M. R. Islam, and M. A. A. Khan, "Reproductive problems of cow at Bangladesh Agricultural University Dairy Farm and possible remedies," *Pakistan Journal of Biological Sciences*, vol. 8, pp. 1561–1567, 2005.

[14] A. Khair, M. M. Alam, A. K. M. A. Rahman, M. T. Islam, A. Azim, and E. H. Chowdhury, "Incidence of reproductive and production diseases of cross-bred dairy cattle in Bangladesh," *Bangladesh Journal of Veterinary Medicine*, vol. 11, no. 1, pp. 31–36, 2014.

[15] M. A. S. Sarker, M. Aktaruzzaman, A. K. M. A. Rahman, and M. S. Rahman, "Retrospective study of clinical diseases and disorders of cattle in Sirajganj district in Bangladesh," *Bangladesh Journal of Veterinary Medicine*, vol. 11, no. 2, pp. 137–144, 2014.

[16] A. K. M. A. Rahman, C. Saegerman, D. Berkvens et al., "Bayesian estimation of true prevalence, sensitivity and specificity of indirect ELISA, Rose Bengal Test and Slow Agglutination Test for the diagnosis of brucellosis in sheep and goats in Bangladesh," *Preventive Veterinary Medicine*, vol. 110, no. 2, pp. 242–252, 2013.

[17] S. Boarbi, M. Mori, E. Rousset, K. Sidi-Boumedine, M. Van Esbroeck, and D. Fretin, "Prevalence and molecular typing of *Coxiella burnetii* in bulk tank milk in Belgian dairy goats, 2009–2013," *Veterinary Microbiology*, vol. 170, no. 1-2, pp. 117–124, 2014.

[18] J. F. Agger, A.-B. Christoffersen, E. Rattenborg, J. Nielsen, and J. S. Agerholm, "Prevalence of *Coxiella burnetii* antibodies in Danish dairy herds," *Acta Veterinaria Scandinavica*, vol. 52, article 5, 2010.

[19] J. Muskens, E. Van Engelen, C. Van Maanen, C. Bartels, and T. J. G. M. Lam, "Prevalence of *Coxiella burnetii* infection in Dutch dairy herds based on testing bulk tank milk and individual samples by PCR and ELISA," *Veterinary Record*, vol. 168, no. 3, p. 79, 2011.

[20] G. Czaplicki, J.-Y. Houtain, C. Mullender et al., "Apparent prevalence of antibodies to *Coxiella burnetii* (Q fever) in bulk tank milk from dairy herds in southern Belgium," *The Veterinary Journal*, vol. 192, no. 3, pp. 529–531, 2012.

[21] I. Astobiza, F. Ruiz-Fons, A. Piñero, J. F. Barandika, A. Hurtado, and A. L. García-Pérez, "Estimation of *Coxiella burnetii* prevalence in dairy cattle in intensive systems by serological and molecular analyses of bulk-tank milk samples," *Journal of Dairy Science*, vol. 95, no. 4, pp. 1632–1638, 2012.

[22] G. H. Lang, "Q fever: an emerging public health concern in Canada," *Canadian Journal of Veterinary Research*, vol. 53, no. 1, pp. 1–6, 1989.

[23] F. Capuano, M. C. Landolfi, and D. M. Monetti, "Influence of three types of farm management on the seroprevalence of Q fever as assessed by an indirect immunofluorescence assay," *Veterinary Record*, vol. 149, no. 22, pp. 669–671, 2001.

[24] E. D. Ryan, M. Kirby, D. M. Collins, R. Sayers, J. F. Mee, and T. Clegg, "Prevalence of *Coxiella burnetii* (Q fever) antibodies in bovine serum and bulk-milk samples," *Epidemiology and Infection*, vol. 139, no. 9, pp. 1413–1417, 2011.

[25] M. Khalili and E. Sakhaee, "An update on a serologic survey of Q fever in domestic animals in Iran," *The American Journal of Tropical Medicine and Hygiene*, vol. 80, no. 6, pp. 1031–1032, 2009.

[26] F. Ruiz-Fons, I. Astobiza, J. F. Barandika et al., "Seroepidemiological study of Q fever in domestic ruminants in semi-extensive grazing systems," *BMC Veterinary Research*, vol. 6, article 3, 2010.

[27] A. L. García-Pérez, I. Astobiza, J. F. Barandika, R. Atxaerandio, A. Hurtado, and R. A. Juste, "Short communication: investigation of *Coxiella burnetii* occurrence in dairy sheep flocks by bulk-tank milk analysis and antibody level determination," *Journal of Dairy Science*, vol. 92, no. 4, pp. 1581–1584, 2009.

[28] E. Kennerman, E. Rousset, E. Gölcü, and P. Dufour, "Seroprevalence of Q fever (coxiellosis) in sheep from the Southern Marmara region, Turkey," *Comparative Immunology, Microbiology and Infectious Diseases*, vol. 33, no. 1, pp. 37–45, 2010.

[29] S. Esmaeili, F. B. Amiri, and E. Mostafavi, "Seroprevalence survey of Q fever among sheep in northwestern Iran," *Vector-Borne and Zoonotic Diseases*, vol. 14, no. 3, pp. 189–192, 2014.

[30] M. Berri, A. Souriau, M. Crosby, and A. Rodolakis, "Shedding of *Coxiella burnetii* in ewes in two pregnancies following an episode of *Coxiella* abortion in a sheep flock," *Veterinary Microbiology*, vol. 85, no. 1, pp. 55–60, 2002.

[31] K. Polydorou, "Q fever in Cyprus: a short review," *The British Veterinary Journal*, vol. 137, no. 5, pp. 470–477, 1981.

16

Determining Proportion of Exfoliative Vaginal Cell during Various Stages of Estrus Cycle Using Vaginal Cytology Techniques in Aceh Cattle

Tongku N. Siregar, Juli Melia, Rohaya, Cut Nila Thasmi, Dian Masyitha, Sri Wahyuni, Juliana Rosa, Nurhafni, Budianto Panjaitan, and Herrialfian

Faculty of Veterinary Medicine, Syiah Kuala University, Banda Aceh 23111, Indonesia

Correspondence should be addressed to Budianto Panjaitan; antopjt@gmail.com

Academic Editor: Francesca Mancianti

The aim of this study was to investigate the period of estrus cycle in aceh cattle, Indonesia, based on vaginal cytology techniques. Four healthy females of aceh cattle with average weight of 250–300 kg, age of 5–7 years, and body condition score of 3-4 were used. All cattle were subjected to ultrasonography analysis for the occurrence of corpus luteum before being synchronized using intramuscular injections of PGF2 alpha 25 mg. A vaginal swab was collected from aceh cattle, stained with Giemsa 10%, and observed microscopically. Period of estrus cycle was predicted from day 1 to day 24 after estrus synchronization was confirmed using ultrasonography analysis at the same day. The result showed that parabasal, intermediary, and superficial epithelium were found in the vaginal swabs collected from proestrus, metestrus, and diestrus aceh cattle. Proportions of these cells in the particular period of estrus cycle were 36.22, 32.62, and 31.16 (proestrus); 21.33, 32.58, and 46.09 (estrus); 40.75, 37.58, and 21.67 (metestrus); and 41.07, 37.38, and 21.67 (diestrus), respectively. In conclusion, dominant proportion of superficial cell that occurred in estrus period might be used as the base for determining optimal time for insemination.

1. Introduction

The changes during normal estrus cycle relate to the basic concept of the ovulation process, regression of the corpus luteum, pregnancy, and birth. The ovulation process is related to estrus and mating. A good estrus detection will be able to determine the optimum time for insemination [1]. However, the accuracy to detect estrus to determine the optimum time for insemination is below 50% [2].

There are many methods to identify the estrus cycle and the optimal determination mating time; they are estrus observation [3], measurement of steroid level, vaginal cytology [4], ultrasound, and rectal palpation. In aceh cattle, the estrus observation for optimal mating time determination is limited by the low performance of estrus [5] especially in the event of environmental heat stress [6] whereas the steroid examination is relatively noneconomical and has a longer execution time. The vaginal cytology is a simple technique and alternative that can be used by practitioners to characterize the reproduction cycle of the estrus [7]. The research on female collared peccary showed that vaginal cytology can be used as an estrus cycle predictor [8].

The research in the vaginal cytology method using animals has been done for many times, for example, in a dog [9], cow [10, 11], goat [12], and deer [13]. The examination of the vaginal cytology during estrus cycle has been conducted for clinically appearing estrus symptoms [14] and steroid concentration [4, 12]. However, there are many chances of making a mistake in determining the estrus cycle based on the observation of the clinical symptoms compared to determining the estrus cycle based on the ultrasound observation (USG), whereas the steroid examination is relatively noneconomical and has more execution time. In aceh cattle, the determination of the estrus cycle based on vaginal cytology imaging has not been reported.

2. Material and Methods

This research uses four adult females of aceh cattle; they were not in a pregnant condition, clinically healthy, and aging from 5 to 7 years with a weight of 250–300 kg. The cattle had a good body condition score with good criteria between 3 and 4 on a score scale of 5. Additionally, all cattle have normal reproductive organs marked by showing at least twice regular estrous cycle, ever pregnant and having birth, and also free from endometritis and pyometra.

2.1. Estrus Synchronization. In order to get a day 0 estrus cycle (estrus period, standing heat), all cattle had estrus synchronization using luteolytic dosage PGF2α injections (25 mg, Lutalyse™, Pharmacia & Upjohn Company, Pfizer Inc.). The injections were done twice with interval of 11 days. Twenty-four hours after the last PGF2α injections, examination using USG was performed every day during the estrus cycle.

2.2. The Vaginal Cytology Preparation. The vaginal cytology preparation was done according to the instructions of Ola et al. [15]. Observations were done using light microscope with objective lens magnification of 40×100. The observed vaginal epithelial cells (superficial, intermediate, and parabasal) were counted according to each group to the determined phases of the estrus cycle based on the USG observation results.

2.3. USG Examinations. The cattle were placed in a pinned cage and the USG device (MINDRAY DP3300VET, Shenzhen Mindray Bio-Medical Electronic Co., Ltd., China) was placed on a safe place away from the cattle and easy to be operated by the operator. Feces were released from the cattle's rectum; then, a manual exploration was done from the topography of the cattle's reproduction tracts before the USG examination. Ovaries were located on the underside of the left and right uterine cornua. Diameter CL and follicles in the ovaries were measured using internal caliper on ultrasound, that is, the distance between the two points of the longest axis by axis with units cm. Furthermore, imaging of vagina, cervix, and uterus body was captured in long axis of craniocaudal view of pubic region. When the transducer was moved to the lateral, the cornua uterus would be seen in a cross section state.

2.4. Measurement of Serum Progesterone and Estradiol. Collection of blood (10 mL) for examination of progesterone and estradiol concentrations conducted during the estrus cycle begins on day 0 (time of estrus) and ends at the next estrus. Serum was recovered by centrifugation (15 minutes at 2,500 rpm) and stored at $-20°C$ until being assayed for serum progesterone and estradiol concentrations using commercial progesterone and estradiol ELISA kit (DRG Instruments GmbH, Germany).

2.5. Data Analysis. Vaginal cells percentages among the stages of estrus cycle were compared by Chi-square test. The mean progesterone and estradiol concentrations between groups were analyzed by one-way ANOVA.

3. Results and Discussion

Several types of cells were observed in the mucosal surface of vagina during estrous phases. Those cells were parabasal, intermediate, and superficial cells. This observation was according to the reports of Najamudin et al. [13]. The vaginal epithelial cell consists of three types and they were the parabasal, intermediate, and superficial cell. The parabasal cell was the small epithelial cell found in the vagina, having a round shape, and nucleus was bigger than the cytoplasm. The intermediate cell has variation of shapes and has size 2-3 times compared to the parabasal cell. The superficial cell was the large sized cells and had a polygonal and flat shape but did not always have the pyknotic nucleus. The proportion of each epithelial cell during the estrus cycle is shown in Table 1.

Based on the standard and characteristic of epithelial cell in proestrus and estrus phase, the proportion of parabasal, intermediate, and superficial cell was found with measurement of 36.22, 32.62, and 31.16 and 21.33, 32.58, and 46.09, respectively. The collected proportion from this research was according to Widiyono et al. [12], in which the largest epithelial cell proportion in the estrus phase is the superficial cells or superficial and intermediate cells in proestrus and estrus phase. The results showed that the proportion of the superficial cells was higher during proestrus (31.16) and increased during estrus (46.09) and showed significant differences with metestrus and diestrus phase ($P < 0.05$). The proportion of superficial cells during metestrus and diestrus was, respectively, 21.67 and 21.54 ($P > 0.05$).

Even though the population of the superficial cells is dominant in this phase, it is still relatively low in contrast to the superficial cell in estrus of dogs that reached 90% [9].

In estrus phase, estrogen hormone will increase activeness in uterus wall; it causes hypersecretion in epithelial cells of the uterus and vagina, so that the superficial cells followed the vaginal peel. In this research, the estradiol concentrations in proestrus, estrus, metestrus, and diestrus phase were 171.99 + 11.30, 223.13 + 9.50, 10.05 + 98.03, and 67.37 + 8.75 pg mL^{-1}, respectively. Increasing concentrations of estradiol in proestrus and estrus phase may be related to the high proportion of superficial cells. In bligon goat, the percentage of superficial cell was found to be 32.25% when estradiol was on level 247.77 pg dL^{-1}, 25.50% when the uterus and estradiol level was 246.17 pg dL^{-1}, and lowered to level of 12.22% when the lowest estradiol level was at 211.25 pg dL^{-1}. The average concentration of progesterone was different on the stage of aceh cattle cycle. At the time of proestrus (2-3 days), progesterone level was 0.97 + 0.21 ng mL^{-1}. The concentration reached its lowest level during estrus (1-2 days), that is, 0.12 + 0.02 ng mL^{-1}. Metestrus and diestrus phase length were 13–16 days with average concentration of progesterone being 0.10 $\pm$ 1.67 ng mL^{-1}. When progesterone becomes dominant in metestrus and diestrus phase, the number of larger cells was sharply reduced [16], so that the epithelial cells were dominated by parabasal cells. In this study, the proportion of parabasal cells in metestrus and diestrus phase was, respectively, 40.75 and 41.07 and significantly ($P < 0.05$) higher in comparison with proestrus and diestrus phase. From the USG confirmation results, it could be seen that the estrus phase

TABLE 1: Characteristic and proportion of the Indonesian aceh cattle vaginal epithelial cell during the estrus cycle.

Phase	Duration period Estrus (days)	Vaginal epithelial cell proportion (%)			USG imaging	Steroid concentration	
		Parabasal	Intermediate	Superficial		Estrogen	Progesterone (ng/mL)
Proestrus	2-3	36.22[a,A]	32.62[a,A]	31.16[a,A]	Dominant follicle with a diameter of 10.60 ± 1.63 mm; CL starts to be lysis, and uterus is not yet enlarged		0.97 ± 0.21[a]
Estrus	1-2	21.33[b,A]	32.58[a,B]	46.09[b,C]	Dominant follicle (3rd DF) sized 13.75 + 1.71 mm; CL starts to be lysis; enlargement of the corpus uterus, a decrease in endometrial thickness		0.12 ± 0.02[a]
Metestrus	3-4	40.75[c,A]	37.58[a,A]	21.67[c,B]	Dominant follicle (1st DF) sized 10.00 ± 1.83 mm; CL present; a decrease in diameter of the uterus		1.40 ± 0.0[b]
Diestrus	10-12	41.07[c,A]	37.38[a,A]	21.54[c,B]	Diameter of the dominant follicle (2nd DF) with a size up to 8.75 ± 0.50 mm; CL present in the fixed/functional phase; stabilized uterus		1.94 + 0.1[b]

[a,b,c]The different superscript in the same column indicates significant differences ($P < 0.05$).

[A,B,C]The different superscript in the same line indicates significant differences ($P < 0.05$).

was marked by outbreak of the dominant follicle or ovulation. This indicated that the determination of the cycle phase in this research was correctly located in the estrus phase. The estrus phase in aceh cattle was 1-2 days. Different from the obtained results by Mingoas and Ngayam [11] with zebu cattle, the estrus phase in this research did not account for the cells undergoing cornification. The superficial epithelial cell which is not nucleus often undergoes cornification or keratinization which serves to protect the vaginal mucosa from irritation at the time of copulation. The loss of the epithelial cell nucleus in the estrus phase can be caused by the keratinization process. The keratinized cells were found individually separated from the other cells. Degeneration of those cells is caused by keratin substance blocking nutrient diffusion from the capillaries in the bondage tissue. In this phase, desquamation of superficial epithelial cells was also detected.

In the diestrus phase, population of superficial cells decreased and happened vice versa on the increase of intermediate and parabasal cells. Towards the end of diestrus, degeneration was caused by shaping vacuole on cytoplasm and nucleus was cornered to the side. In metestrus and diestrus phase, the proportions of parabasal, intermediate, and superficial cells each were 40.75, 37.58, and 21.67 and 41.07, 37.38, and 21.6, respectively. These proportions were according to Solis et al. [17] that parabasal cells were very dominant in phase before estrus in sheep, followed by intermediate and superficial cells. Parabasal cells (epithelial cells with huge nucleus) were the smallest of the epithelial cell type in vaginal peel. Parabasal cells are usually found on the estrus and anestrus phase. The observation results showed that the intermediate cells dominated during the estrus cycle. The same phenomenon was also reported by Widiyono et al. [12] in bligon goats. The results showed that the proportion of intermediate cells dominates the cell vaginal swabs during the estrus cycle. The same phenomenon was also reported by Widiyono et al. [12] in bligon goats. The proportions of intermediate cells were similar ($P > 0.05$) during proestrus (32.62), estrus (32.58), metestrus (37.58), and diestrus (37.38) obtained in this research.

4. Conclusion

The Indonesia aceh cattle vaginal epithelial cells during the estrus cycle consist of parabasal, intermediate, and superficial cell. In estrus phase, the superficial epithelial cell is the most dominant in comparison to the metestrus, diestrus, or even proestrus phase.

Conflict of Interests

The authors declare that there is no conflict of interests regarding the publication of this paper.

Acknowledgments

The authors acknowledged the Hibah Antar Lembaga 2011 for financial aid for the grant and the head of BPT-HMT Indrapuri Aceh Besar for facilitating this research.

References

[1] Z. O. Keister, S. K. DeNise, D. V. Armstrong, R. L. Ax, and M. D. Brown, "Pregnancy outcomes in two commercial dairy herds following hormonal scheduling programs," *Theriogenology*, vol. 51, no. 8, pp. 1587–1596, 1999.

[2] G. S. Lewis and M. C. Wulster-Radcliffe, "Lutalyse can upregulate the uterine immune system in the presence of progesterone," *Journal of Animal Science*, vol. 79, article 116, 2001.

[3] M. Sönmez, E. Demirci, G. Türk, and S. Gür, "Effect of season on some fertility parameters of dairy and beef cows in Elazig Province," *Turkish Journal of Veterinary and Animal Sciences*, vol. 29, no. 3, pp. 821–828, 2005.

[4] K. C. S. Reddy, K. G. S. Raju, K. S. Rao, and K. B. R. Rao, "Vaginal cytology, vaginoscopy and progesterone profile: Breeding tools in bitches," *Iraqi Journal of Veterinary Sciences*, vol. 25, no. 2, pp. 51–54, 2011.

[5] U. Hafizuddin, T. N. Siregar, M. Akmal, J. Melia, R. Husnurrizal, and T. Armansyah, "Perbandingan intensitas berahi sapi aceh yang disinkronisasi dengan prostaglandin F2 alfa dan berahi alami," *Jurnal Kedokteran Hewan*, vol. 6, no. 2, pp. 81–83, 2012.

[6] N. Meutia, T. N. Siregar, Sugito, and J. Melia, "Pengaruh stress panas terhadap intensitas berahi sapi aceh," in *Prosiding Konferensi Ilmiah Veteriner Nasional Perhimpunan Dokter Hewan Indonesia (KIVNAS ke-13 PDHI)*, pp. 57–58, Palembang, Indonesia, November 2014.

[7] S. D. Johnston, M. V. Root Kustritz, and P. N. S. Olson, *Canine and Feline Theriogenology*, W.B. Saunders Company, New York, NY, USA, 2001.

[8] P. Mayor, H. Galvez, D. A. Guimaraes, F. Lopez-Gatius, and M. Lopez-Bejar, "Serum estradiol-17β, vaginal cytology and vulval appearance as predictors of estrus cyclicity in the female collared peccary (*Tayassu tajacu*) from the eastern Amazon region," *Animal Reproduction Science*, vol. 97, no. 1-2, pp. 165–174, 2007.

[9] V. R. Beimborn, H. L. Tarpley, P. L. Bain, and K. S. Latimer, "The Canine Estrous Cycle: Staging Using Vaginal Cytological Examination. Class of 2003. Veterinary Clinical Pathology Clerkship Program," Ross University, School of Veterinary Medicine, St. Kitts, West Indies (Beimborn) and Department of Pathology, College of Veterinary Medicine, The University of Georgia, Athens, GA, USA, (Tarpley, Bain, Latimer), 2003, http://vet.uga.edu/vpp/clerkbeimborn.

[10] N. B. Blazquez, E. H. Batten, S. E. Long, G. C. Perry, and O. J. Whelehan, "A quantitative morphological study of the bovine vaginal epithelium during the oestrous cycle," *Journal of Comparative Pathology*, vol. 100, no. 2, pp. 187–193, 1989.

[11] J. L. K. Mingoas and L. L. Ngayam, "Preliminary findings on vaginal epithelial cells and body temperature changes during oestrous cycle in Bororo zebu cow," *International Journal of Biological and Chemical Sciences*, vol. 3, no. 1, 2009.

[12] I. Widiyono, P. P. Putro, Sarmin, P. Astuti, and C. M. Airin, "Kadar estradiol dan progesteron serum, tampilan vulva dan sitologi apus vagina kambing bligon selama siklus birahi," *Jurnal Veteriner*, vol. 2, no. 4, pp. 263–268, 2011.

[13] R. Najamudin, A. Sriyanto, S. Agungpriyono, and T. L. Yusuf, "Penentuan siklus estrus pada kancil (*Tragulus javanicus*) berdasarkan perubahan sitologi vagina," *Veterinary Journal*, vol. 11, no. 2, pp. 81–86, 2010.

[14] H. Y. Hamid and M. Z. A. B. Zakaria, "Reproductive characteristics of the female laboratory rat," *African Journal of Biotechnology*, vol. 12, no. 19, pp. 2510–2514, 2013.

[15] S. I. Ola, W. A. Sanni, and G. Egbunike, "Exfoliative vaginal cytology during the oestrous cycle of West African dwarf goats," *Reproduction Nutrition Development*, vol. 46, no. 1, pp. 87–95, 2006.

[16] B. F. Zohara, A. Azizunnesa, M. F. Islam, M. G. Alam, and F. Y. Bari, "Exfoliative vaginal cytology and serum progesterone during the estrous cycle of indigenous ewes in Bangladesh," *Journal of Embryo Transfer*, vol. 29, no. 2, pp. 183–188, 2014.

[17] G. Solis, J. I. Aguilera, R. M. Rincon, R. Banuelos, and C. F. Arechiga, "Characterizing cytology (ECV) in ewes from 60 d of age through parturition," *Journal of Animal Science*, vol. 82, supplement 1, 2008.

17

Efficacy of a Feed Dispenser for Horses in Decreasing Cribbing Behaviour

Silvia Mazzola,[1] **Clara Palestrini,**[1] **Simona Cannas,**[1] **Eleonora Fè,**[1]
Gaia Lisa Bagnato,[1] **Daniele Vigo,**[1] **Diane Frank,**[2] **and Michela Minero**[1]

[1]*Dipartimento di Medicina Veterinaria, Università degli Studi di Milano, Via Celoria 10, 20133 Milan, Italy*
[2]*Faculté de Médecine Vétérinaire, Département de Sciences Cliniques, Université de Montréal, No. 3200, rue Sicotte,
Saint-Hyacinthe, QC, Canada J2S 2M2*

Correspondence should be addressed to Silvia Mazzola; silvia.mazzola@unimi.it

Academic Editor: William Ravis

Cribbing is an oral stereotypy, tends to develop in captive animals as a means to cope with stress, and may be indicative of reduced welfare. Highly energetic diets ingested in a short time are one of the most relevant risk factors for the development of cribbing. The aim of this study was to verify whether feeding cribbing horses through a dispenser that delivers small quantities of concentrate when activated by the animal decreases cribbing behaviour, modifies feeding behaviour, or induces frustration. Ten horses (mean age 14 y), balanced for sex, breed, and size (mean height 162 cm), were divided into two groups of 5 horses each: *Cribbing* and *Control*. Animals were trained to use the dispenser and videorecorded continuously for 15 consecutive days from 1 h prior to feeding to 2 h after feeding in order to measure their behaviours. The feed dispenser, Quaryka®, induced an increase in time necessary to finish the ration in both groups of horses ($P < 0.05$). With Quaryka, cribbers showed a significant reduction of time spent cribbing ($P < 0.05$). After removal of the feed dispenser (Post-Quaryka), cribbing behaviour significantly increased. The use of Quaryka may be particularly beneficial in horses fed high-energy diets and ingesting the food too quickly.

1. Introduction

Stereotypies are defined as invariant and repetitive behaviour patterns that seem to have no function [1]. They are reported in more than 15% of domesticated horses [2] and are known as the disease of domestication [3], since they have never been observed in free-ranging feral horses. They may be indicative of reduced welfare [4, 5] but it is not self-evident whether stereotypies are representative of the current situation or of a previous suboptimal condition. This is based on the findings that once a stereotypic behaviour is established, it will become a habit, and it is difficult to stop or rectify it [6–8]. Cribbing horses may be stressed more easily than unaffected horses [9, 10]. It has been shown that attempts to inhibit this behaviour through the use of anticribbing collars or other physical devices may significantly impact equine welfare, by reducing the horse's ability to cope with stress without addressing the underlying cause [11].

Epidemiological and experimental studies provide quite an accurate understanding of the prevalence, underlying mechanisms, and owner perceptions of cribbing behaviour. These studies have shown that many factors can be associated with an increased risk of cribbing, including management conditions that prevent foraging opportunities and social contact, provision of high concentrate diets, and abrupt weaning [12]. Since cribbers perform the behaviour most frequently following delivery of concentrated feed, it has been suggested that diet may be implicated [13]. As a consequence of high-energy carbohydrate feed administration, cribbing horses ingest food quickly and have a lower production of saliva, a higher gastric fermentability [14], and acid fermentation in the cecum and large intestine [13]. The latter phenomenon may be related to a higher transit time of feed in the large intestine, indicating that the orocecal digestion in cribbing horses is less efficient compared to healthy subjects. The action of cribbing could therefore be an attempt to stimulate the receptors of the oral tissues to increase the flow of saliva and thus buffer the acidity of the gastrointestinal tract [15]. Equine behaviour and welfare scientists agree that management of cribbing horses should focus on improvement of life conditions and feeding management rather than on attempts at physical prevention of the behaviour.

The aim of this study was to verify whether feeding cribbing horses through a dispenser that delivers small quantities of concentrate when activated by the animal decreases or eliminates cribbing behaviour, modifies feeding behaviour, or induces frustration. This study describes the effect of a feed dispenser, Quaryka, on feeding time budget of cribbing horses.

2. Research Methods

Ten horses, balanced for breed and sex, aged between six and 20 years (mean age: 14 years), were recruited. All subjects were deemed healthy following a physical examination and were exempt of medical treatment, except for vaccination and deworming.

Horses were divided into two groups: five *Cribbing horses* and five *Control horses* (Table 2). Cribbing horses had been stereotyping for at least one month and had never been treated for the condition whereas Control horses had never exhibited the stereotypy. All subjects were kept under the same housing and management conditions. They were housed in standard single horse boxes (3×3 m) in visual contact with other conspecifics. They were fed twice a day, morning and afternoon, with hay and concentrate. Water was provided ad libitum by automatic drinkers. During the observation period, all horses were managed avoiding any changes in terms of workload, housing, rations, and daily routine. The owners were asked to fill out a questionnaire including information on the horse's characteristics and history as well as on the physical and social environment of the horse. Questions touched on home environment, management and feeding, and horse's use and exercise. Other specific questions regarded the medical history and development and presence of cribbing or other behaviour problems.

The design was a cross-over case-control study. In a preliminary phase, the horses were trained to use the dispenser Quaryka (Figure 1) that delivered small quantities of concentrate when a wheel was activated by the horse's mouth.

The training included four main steps lasting approximately two hours overall.

(1) *Approach to the Dispenser.* The horse's attention was directed to the wheel by placing some concentrate feed on its spokes.

(2) *Habituation to the Wheel Rotation.* When the horse approached the wheel with the muzzle, the wheel was manually rotated, so that the concentrate fell into the manger (this process allowed the animal to associate the movement of the wheel with the availability of food).

(3) *Reward-Dependent Approach to the Wheel.* As soon as the horse touched the spokes with the lips, the experimenter turned the wheel.

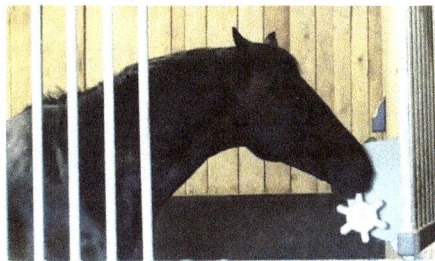

FIGURE 1: A horse approaches the dispenser wheel.

(4) *Autonomous Use of the Dispenser.* The horse approached the dispenser independently and the experimenter intervened only if the animal was distracted or did not apply enough force in turning the wheel. Each step was repeated several times, until the horse exhibited consistent learned behaviour.

After the preliminary phase, the observation period lasted 15 days divided into phases of five days each, for both groups of horses. During the first five days of testing (Pre-Quaryka), each subject was videorecorded in the box while fed concentrate in the usual location. During the next five days, the concentrate feed was distributed only through Quaryka (During-Quaryka) and, during the last five days, the dispenser was removed from the box and the horse was fed concentrate in the usual feeder (Post-Quaryka). During the study, the horses were continuously videotaped for one hour prior to and two hours after afternoon administration of the concentrate feed. Behaviour was recorded by a remotely operated video camera (Panasonic, HDC-SD99, Panasonic, Japan), mounted on a wall over the box and linked to a sequential switcher and time-lapse video recorder.

2.1. Data Analysis. The video recording analysis was carried out using dedicated software, the Solomon Coder (beta 12.09.04, copyright 2006–2008 by András Péter), customized with a specific behaviour configuration. An observer trained in animal behaviour and use of the software analysed all the videotapes. Behavioural categories are listed and described in Table 1. Owners' answers to the questionnaire were scored and reported.

2.2. Statistical Analysis. All statistical analyses were conducted using SPSS 21 (SPSS Inc., Chicago, USA). Differences were considered to be statistically significant if $P \leq 0.05$. For each behaviour, mean duration and standard deviation were calculated. ANOVA (analysis of variance) was used to investigate potential differences in horse behaviour between groups or time periods.

3. Results and Discussion

Results from the questionnaire are summarized in Table 2. The majority of the horses (70%) were stabled on sawdust litter, while only 30% of them, of both groups, were stabled on wheat wood shavings. All boxes had an open window (overlooking indoor or outdoor) and the large majority of

TABLE 1: Behavioural categories and definitions.

Behavioural category	Definition	State/event
Time to finish the ration	Time taken by horse to finish the food ration	State
Time at the dispenser	Elapsed time at the dispenser, every time the horse shows interest in Quaryka (sniffs, spins the wheel, etc.)	State
Time to learn how to use Quaryka	Time spent learning to use the dispenser, until the horse understood the relationship between turning the wheel and the presence of concentrate in the manger	State
Latency to use Quaryka	Time needed by the horse to approach Quaryka the first time	State
Latency to use Quaryka after filling	Elapsed time between filling Quaryka and the horse turning the wheel to obtain the food for the first time	State
Time spent cribbing	Bout of cribbing	State
Standing alert	Rigid stance with the neck elevated and the head oriented toward the source of interest The ears are held stiffly upright and forward, and the nostrils may be slightly dilated	State
Fear	Fearful head posture and facial expression (increasing head distance from Quaryka, ears flattened and held back, and sclera visible)	State
Cribbing	Single crib-bite	Event
Lip playing	Part of tongue is shown and moved along the upper lip	Event

the subjects (80%) had daily access to grass paddocks, with shade and water available. Horses were fed with hay (a mean of 9 kg/day each) and concentrate (a mean of 3 kg/day each) to meet their specific energy requirements. All owners described their horse as "easy to manage" and "getting along with other horses." All owners of *Cribbing horses* reported that the stereotypy was present at the time of purchase.

Most of the horses approached Quaryka with curiosity (60%), while the others (40%) showed signs of diffidence (no tactile exploration, standing alert) during the first 20 minutes.

The video analysis revealed that, during the entire observation period, none of the horses showed any of the behaviours related to frustration or fear described in Table 1 and none of the *Control horses* showed any displacement or stereotypic behaviour.

Figure 2 reports time to finish the ration recorded in horses during Pre-Quaryka.

Compared to *Control horses*, *Cribbing horses* tended to need a longer time to finish their concentrate, in agreement with findings of Clegg et al. [13] who found that cribbers and weavers took longer time than Control horses to fully consume their ration. This result can be explained considering that cribbers stereotype most frequently during and following the consumption of meals [16–20]. Only cribbers displayed lip playing during the observation time.

Quaryka induced an increase in time needed to finish the ration in both groups of horses (Figure 3, $P < 0.05$). Also cribbers needed significantly more time to finish the ration than Control horses ($P < 0.05$). After Quaryka removal, horses in both groups showed a feeding behaviour similar to that expressed before the introduction of the dispenser (Figure 3).

Interestingly, cribbers showed a significant reduction of time spent cribbing ($P < 0.05$), indicating that horses' interaction with Quaryka induced lengthening of the time taken

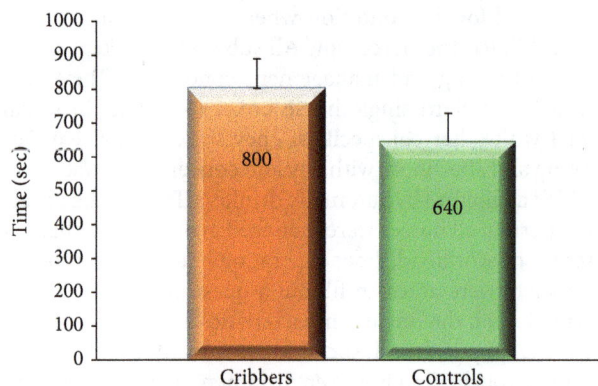

FIGURE 2: Time needed to finish the concentrate ration observed in Cribbing and Control horses during Pre-Quaryka phase of the study.

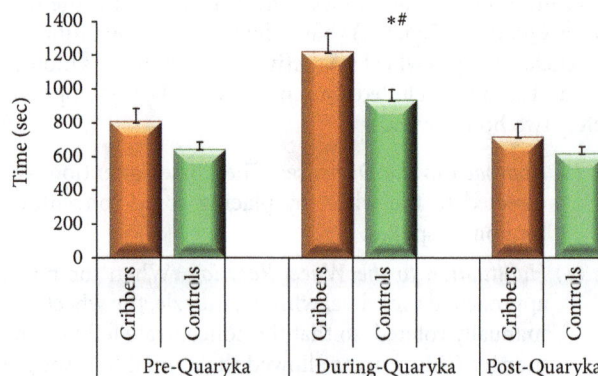

FIGURE 3: Time needed to finish the concentrate ration in Cribbing and Controls horses during the three phases of the study. $^*P > 0.05$ Cribbers versus Controls in During-Quaryka observation period. $^\#P > 0.05$ Cribbers and Control horses in During-Quaryka versus Pre-Quaryka observations.

TABLE 2: Results of the questionnaire, filled out by the owners of the horses.

Horse #	#1	#2	#3	#4	#5	#6	#7	#8	#9	#10
Group	Control	Control	Control	Control	Control	Cribbing	Cribbing	Cribbing	Cribbing	Cribbing
Age (years)	6	13	17	17	17	18	10	11	6	20
Sex	Mare	Gelding	Stallion	Gelding	Mare	Gelding	Mare	Mare	Gelding	Gelding
Breed	English thoroughbred	Friesian	Sella Italiano	Selle Française	Hannover	Irish Horse	Sella Italiano	Dutch Warmblood	Selle Française	English thoroughbred
Height (meters)	1,62	1,60	1,52	1,65	1,65	1,62	1,58	1,67	1,63	1,61
Attitude (original)	Gallop	Equitation	Jumping	Jumping	Dressage	Dressage	Jumping	Jumping	Equitation	Jumping
Attitude (actual)	Equitation	Equitation	Jumping	Equitation	Dressage	Equitation	Equitation	Jumping	Equitation	Companion
Box size (square meters)	9	9	10,5	12	12	9	9	12	9	9
Bedding type	Wood shavings	Wood shavings	Wood shavings	Straw	Wood shavings	Straw	Straw	Wood shavings	Wood shavings	Wood shavings
Access to paddock	Daylight hours	Daylight hours	4 hours	4 hours	No routine access	Daylight hours	Daylight hours	No routine access	Daylight hours	Daylight hours
Cribbing since						Cribbing at purchase	Cribbing at purchase	Cribbing at purchase	Cribbing at purchase	Cribbing at purchase
Severity of cribbing behaviour						Mild	Severe	Mild	Mild	Severe
Initial reaction to Quaryka	Curiosity	Curiosity	Diffidence	Curiosity	Diffidence	Curiosity	Curiosity	Diffidence	Curiosity	Diffidence

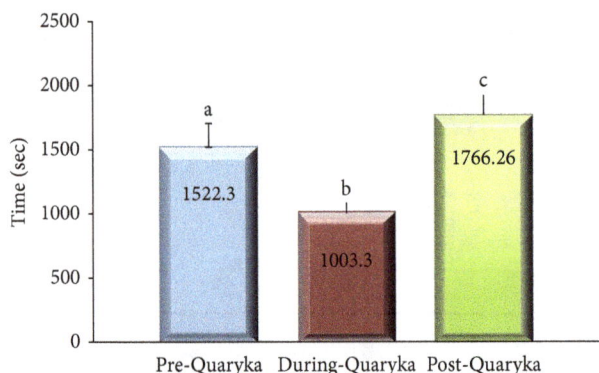

FIGURE 4: Cribbing group: cribbing behaviour observed during the three phases of the study. Bars with different superscripts differ significantly ($P < 0.05$).

to finish the ration, in the absence of stereotyped behaviours associated with food consumption. After removal of the feed dispenser (Post-Quaryka), cribbing behaviour significantly increased compared to the previous phases (Figure 4). This result is compatible with a posttreatment rebound caused by a rise in the motivation to cribbing. Posttreatment rebound was observed in horses prevented from cribbing by the use of inhibitory systems [19]. This hypothesis should be considered with caution as in this study cribbing was never prevented. A possible alternative explanation may be related to the short exposure of the subjects to the dispenser not allowing a lasting effect on the stereotypic behaviour.

The effectiveness of Quaryka in reducing cribbing behaviour cannot be generalised due to the limited animal sample. It should be noted that, in all the horses included in this study, the use of Quaryka was associated with an increase of time needed to finish the ration. This may be particularly beneficial in horses fed high-energy diets and ingesting their food too quickly.

Competing Interests

The authors declare that they have no competing interests.

Acknowledgments

This project has received funding support from the Grant Line 2-Action A, awarded by University of Milan. Quaryka was kindly furnished by the manufacturer. The authors would like to thank the horse owners for their kind collaboration.

References

[1] A. Sarrafchi, *Equine stereotypic behavior as related to horse welfare: a review [M.S. thesis]*, 2012.

[2] U. A. Luescher, D. B. McKeown, and J. Halip, "Reviewing the causes of obsessive-compulsive disorders in horses," *Veterinary Medicine*, vol. 86, pp. 527–531, 1991.

[3] D. Marsden, "A new perspective on stereotypic behaviour problems in horses," *In Practice*, vol. 24, no. 10, pp. 558–569, 2002.

[4] A. J. Waters, C. J. Nicol, and N. P. French, "Factors influencing the development of stereotypic and redirected behaviours in young horses: findings of a four year prospective epidemiological study," *Equine Veterinary Journal*, vol. 34, no. 6, pp. 572–579, 2002.

[5] G. J. Mason and N. R. Latham, "Can't stop, won't stop: is stereotypy a reliable animal welfare indicator?" *Animal Welfare*, vol. 13, pp. S57–S69, 2004.

[6] J. J. Cooper and M. J. Albentosa, "Behavioural adaptation in the domestic horse: potential role of apparently abnormal responses including stereotypic behaviour," *Livestock Production Science*, vol. 92, no. 2, pp. 177–182, 2005.

[7] A. J. Z. Henderson, "Don't fence me in: managing psychological well being for elite performance horses," *Journal of Applied Animal Welfare Science*, vol. 10, no. 4, pp. 309–329, 2007.

[8] P. D. McGreevy, N. P. French, and C. J. Nicol, "The prevalence of abnormal behaviours in dressage, eventing and endurance horses in relation to stabling," *The Veterinary Record*, vol. 137, no. 2, pp. 36–37, 1995.

[9] A. Sarrafchi and H. J. Blokhuis, "Equine stereotypic behaviors: causation, occurrence, and prevention," *Journal of Veterinary Behavior: Clinical Applications and Research*, vol. 8, no. 5, pp. 386–394, 2013.

[10] I. Bachmann, P. Bernasconi, R. Herrmann, M. A. Weishaupt, and M. Stauffacher, "Behavioural and physiological responses to an acute stressor in crib-biting and control horses," *Applied Animal Behaviour Science*, vol. 82, no. 4, pp. 297–311, 2003.

[11] K. Nagy, G. Bodo, G. Bardos, A. Harnos, and P. Kabai, "The effect of a feeding stress-test on the behavior and heart rate variability of control and crib-biting horses (with or without inhibition)," *Applied Animal Behaviour Science*, vol. 121, pp. 140–147, 2010.

[12] C. L. Wickens and C. R. Heleski, "Crib-biting behavior in horses: a review," *Applied Animal Behaviour Science*, vol. 128, no. 1–4, pp. 1–9, 2010.

[13] H. A. Clegg, P. Buckley, M. A. Friend, and P. D. McGreevy, "The ethological and physiological characteristics of cribbing and weaving horses," *Applied Animal Behaviour Science*, vol. 109, no. 1, pp. 68–76, 2008.

[14] B. Hothersall and C. Nicol, "Role of diet and feeding in normal and stereotypic behaviors in horses," *Veterinary Clinics of North America: Equine Practice*, vol. 25, no. 1, pp. 167–181, 2009.

[15] B. A. Moeller, C. A. McCall, S. J. Silverman, and W. H. McElhenney, "Estimation of saliva production in crib-biting and normal horses," *Journal of Equine Veterinary Science*, vol. 28, no. 2, pp. 85–90, 2008.

[16] M. J. Kennedy, A. E. Schwabe, and D. M. Broom, "Crib-biting and wind-sucking stereotypies in the horse," *Equine Veterinary Education*, vol. 5, no. 3, pp. 142–147, 1993.

[17] S. B. Gillham, N. H. Dodman, L. Shuster, R. Kream, and W. Rand, "The effect of diet on cribbing behavior and plasma β-endorphin in horses," *Applied Animal Behaviour Science*, vol. 41, no. 3-4, pp. 147–153, 1994.

[18] P. D. McGreevy, N. P. French, and C. J. Nicol, "The identification of abnormal behaviour and behavioural problems in stabled horses and their relationship to horse welfare: a comparative review," *The Veterinary Record*, vol. 137, no. 2, pp. 36–37, 1995.

[19] P. McGreevy and C. Nicol, "Physiological and behavioral consequences associated with short-term prevention of crib-biting in horses," *Physiology & Behavior*, vol. 65, no. 1, pp. 15–23, 1998.

[20] J. J. Cooper, N. Mcall, S. Johnson, and H. P. B. Davidson, "The short-term effects of increasing meal frequency on stereotypic behaviour of stabled horses," *Applied Animal Behaviour Science*, vol. 90, no. 3-4, pp. 351–364, 2005.

18

Altered Biomechanical Properties of Gastrocnemius Tendons of Turkeys Infected with Turkey Arthritis Reovirus

Tamer A. Sharafeldin,[1,2] Qingshan Chen,[3] Sunil K. Mor,[1] Sagar M. Goyal,[1] and Robert E. Porter[1]

[1]Department of Veterinary Population Medicine and Minnesota Veterinary Diagnostic Laboratory, Saint Paul, MN 55108, USA
[2]Department of Pathology, Faculty of Veterinary Medicine, Zagazig University, Zagazig 44519, Egypt
[3]Excelen, Center for Bone & Joint Research and Education, Minneapolis, MN 55415, USA

Correspondence should be addressed to Tamer A. Sharafeldin; shara022@umn.edu

Academic Editor: Cinzia Benazzi

Turkey arthritis reovirus (TARV) causes lameness and tenosynovitis in commercial turkeys and is often associated with gastrocnemius tendon rupture by the marketing age. This study was undertaken to characterize the biomechanical properties of tendons from reovirus-infected turkeys. One-week-old turkey poults were orally inoculated with O'Neil strain of TARV and observed for up to 16 weeks of age. Lameness was first observed at 8 weeks of age, which continued at 12 and 16 weeks. At 4, 8, 12, and 16 weeks of age, samples were collected from legs. Left intertarsal joint with adjacent gastrocnemius tendon was collected and processed for histological examination. The right gastrocnemius tendon's tensile strength and elasticity modulus were analyzed by stressing each tendon to the point of rupture. At 16 weeks of age, gastrocnemius tendons of TARV-infected turkeys showed significantly reduced ($P < 0.05$) tensile strength and modulus of elasticity as compared to those of noninfected control turkeys. Gastrocnemius tendons revealed lymphocytic tendinitis/tenosynovitis beginning at 4 weeks of age, continuing through 8 and 12 weeks, and progressing to fibrosis from 12 to 16 weeks of age. We propose that tendon fibrosis is one of the key features contributing to reduction in tensile strength and elasticity of gastrocnemius tendons in TARV-infected turkeys.

1. Introduction

Turkey reoviruses have often been associated with enteric diseases in turkeys [1–3]. Recently, turkey reoviruses have been isolated from gastrocnemius and digital flexor tendons and synovial fluids of 15-week-old lame turkeys, some of which had ruptured gastrocnemius or digital flexor as well as consistent histological evidence of lymphocytic tenosynovitis. These turkey arthritis reoviruses (TARVs) were found to be genetically distinct from chicken reoviruses (CARVs; [4]).

Experimental inoculation of 1-week-old turkey poults with TARV via oral, intratracheal, and footpad routes resulted in histological lesions of gastrocnemius lymphocytic tenosynovitis at 4 weeks postinoculation (PI). Such lesions were absent in poults inoculated either with turkey enteric reovirus (TERV) or with chicken arthritis reovirus (CARV) [5]. Oral inoculation of TARV in 1-week-old turkey poults induced clinical signs of lameness at 8 weeks of age, which increased in severity by 12 and 16 weeks of age [6].

Avian reoviruses that impact poultry production can result in devastating economic consequences. Avian reovirus (ARV) is ubiquitous in domestic poultry (chickens and turkeys) with >80% of them being nonpathogenic [7]. ARV was first isolated from birds in 1954 [8]. ARV induces tenosynovitis/arthritis in 5–7-week-old chickens resulting in lameness in heavy breeds [9]. Lameness was experimentally reproduced in chickens [10] but trials to reproduce the clinical disease in turkeys were not successful [11].

The aim of this study was to compare the biomechanical properties of gastrocnemius tendons of TARV-infected and noninfected turkeys at 4, 8, 12, and 16 weeks of age. Additionally, histological alterations in the gastrocnemius tendons were described to determine if any difference in biomechanical properties could be associated with morphological

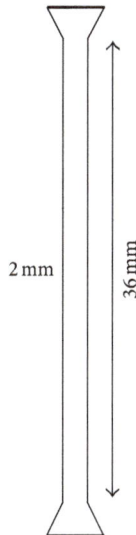

FIGURE 1: Scalloping of the outermost gastrocnemius tendon. The midsection of gastrocnemius tendon was cut as shown to create a predetermined region for measuring tendon failure.

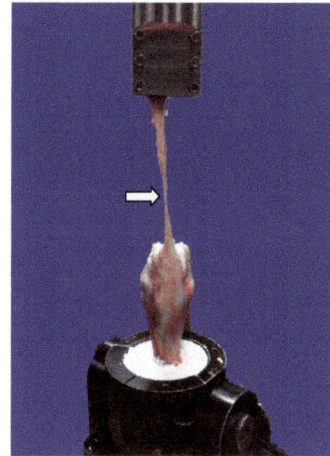

FIGURE 2: Orientation of leg and attached tendon and muscle. The leg of a 4-week-old turkey poult is fixed in the material testing system apparatus. Metatarsus and foot are embedded and fixed at the base of the loading frame and gastrocnemius muscle (with a portion of tendon) is clamped to the upper moveable hydraulic arm. The predetermined point of tendon failure is in the midregion of the exposed tendon (arrow).

changes in the tendons. Establishing a correlation between changes in tendon biomechanical properties with histologic and clinical findings in TARV-infected turkeys is an important aspect of TARV pathogenicity.

2. Materials and Methods

2.1. Samples. Samples were collected from an experimental trial [6] in which male white commercial (Nicholas) poults were divided into two groups; one group was orally inoculated at 1 week of age with 0.2 mL of O'Neil strain of TARV and the noninfected control group was inoculated with virus-free MEM. At 4, 8, 12, and 16 weeks of age, 10 birds from each group were euthanized followed by immediate collection of right intertarsal (hock) joint with gastrocnemius tendon, which was fixed in 10% neutral-buffered formalin for histopathology. The skin of the left leg was removed, wrapped in gauze moistened with phosphate-buffered saline, and kept frozen (−20°C) until subjected to biomechanical testing.

2.2. Histopathology. Formalin fixed intertarsal joint was decalcified in EDTA solution, trimmed, processed, and stained with hematoxylin and eosin (H&E). Slides of stained tissues were examined under an Olympus BX40 microscope and photomicrographs were taken by Olympus DP71 digital microscope camera. Special staining was done by Masson trichrome stain for the detection of collagen, which is indicative of fibrosis.

2.3. Biomechanics. A 36 mm segment of the outer gastrocnemius tendon halfway between the origin (from the gastrocnemius muscle complex) and insertion (to the tarsometatarsus) was trimmed to 2 mm width (Figure 1) using a custom-made dual blade punch. This was done to ensure that the focal point of stress in each tendon (midsection) was of

uniform length and width. The thickness of each tendon at the trimmed midsection was determined by placing the trimmed segment between the pressure plates of a highly sensitive tabletop electromagnetic loading device (Endura TEC, ELF 3200 series, EnduraTEC Systems Corporation, Minnetonka, MN).

The gastrocnemius tendon tensile strength and modulus of elasticity were measured by using MTS 858 Electromagnetic Material Testing System (MTS, MN, USA). The foot and tibiotarsus with attached muscle were embedded in a polyurethane potting compound (Fastcast, Goldenwest MFG, Oak Ridge, CA). The potting cylinder was then anchored to the base of the loading frame of a single pole electromagnetic device and the gastrocnemius tendon (with portion of gastrocnemius muscle) was attached to the upper hydraulic arm of the device with a fixed alligator tooth screw clamp (Figure 2). Force was exerted on each tendon to the point of stretch and complete rupture at the scalloped midsection. The unit used for measurement was megapascals (MPa). Six tendons were analyzed for each experimental group at each time point, and measurements on tendons that did not rupture at the predetermined scalloped midsection were omitted in the final calculation. Tendon rupture in the predetermined scalloped midsection ensured that the measurements of tendon biomechanical characteristics were in the same area in different birds. The software of the device used produced a stress/strain curve for each tendon (Figure 3).

2.4. Statistical Analysis. Significant differences ($P < 0.05$) in tensile strength and elasticity of infected and noninfected groups at 4, 8, 12, and 16 weeks of age were determined by using parametric and nonparametric Student's t-test (NCSS 8 Statistical Software, NCSS LLC, Keysville, UT).

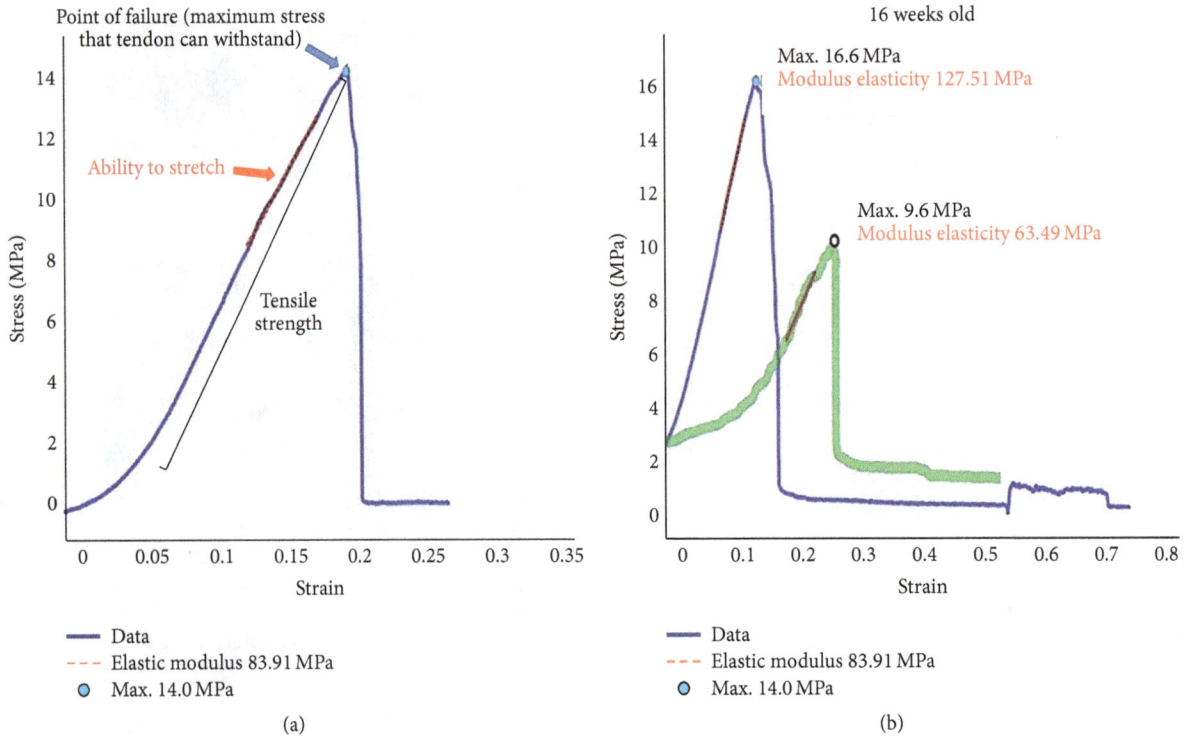

FIGURE 3: Stress/strain curves. (a) Stress/strain curve in 16-week-old turkey. (b) Stress/strain curves of median infected versus noninfected control (16 weeks of age): the blue curve with higher peak of stress refers to the median value of tensile stress in control birds and the green curve with lower peak of stress refers to the median value of tensile strength in infected birds. Unit of measurement in megapascals (MPa).

3. Results

3.1. Lameness and Histopathology. As shown in the previous study [6], turkeys in the infected group displayed lameness first at 8 weeks of age (26%) and the percentage of lame birds increased at 12 and 16 weeks of age to reach 30% and 48%, respectively. At 4 and 8 weeks of age, in TARV-inoculated birds, the gastrocnemius tendon sheath showed prominent lymphocytic infiltration in the subsynovium along with mild synoviocyte hyperplasia. There was also mild subsynovial fibrosis in the gastrocnemius tendon of 8-week-old birds. Lymphocytic infiltration decreased at 12 weeks with increased subsynovial fibrosis which also involved the peritendon and was more prominent in 16-week-old turkeys. Masson trichrome stain revealed a progressive increase in the deposition of collagen in the subsynovium and, in some instances, on the peritendon surface of the gastrocnemius tendon and tendon sheath of 12- and 16-week-old infected turkeys (Figure 4). The tendons histologic inflammation scores were significantly higher in infected birds compared with the noninfected control at all ages [6]. Birds did not display diarrhea. However, body weights of infected birds were significantly lower than of control birds at ages of 12 and 16 weeks [6]. Birds that showed severe lameness, ruptured tendons (only 1 bird at 16 weeks of age), and/or inability to stand were euthanized.

3.2. Biomechanics. Though we had a total of 80 legs, we randomly processed only 48 for biomechanical study due to funding and time constraints. Of the 48 legs examined, we further eliminated 5 gastrocnemius tendons/group because the tendons did not rupture at the predetermined midsection of the tendons. In all instances, the aberrant ruptures occurred at the end or clamped region of the tendon. There were no significant differences between the mean tensile strength and modulus of elasticity of gastrocnemius tendons of infected and noninfected groups at 4, 8, and 12 weeks of age; however, by 16 weeks of age, the gastrocnemius tendons of infected turkeys had a significantly lower ($P < 0.05$) mean tensile strength and modulus of elasticity compared to tendons of noninfected turkeys (Table 1). Interestingly, correlation coefficient between clinical lameness and biomechanical properties (tensile strength and elasticity modulus) showed increased inverse relationship at 16 weeks of age (Figure 5).

4. Discussion

Clinical cases of tendon rupture associated with reovirus infection are generally observed in male turkeys older than 12 weeks of age (David Mills, personal communication). We have found that inoculation of 1-week-old turkey poults with TARV induces histologic tenosynovitis at 4 weeks PI without clinical lameness [5]. However, clinical lameness can be seen at 8 weeks PI, which later progresses at 12 and 16 weeks PI [6]. The aim of the present study was to determine the effect of TARV infection on gastrocnemius tendon tensile strength and modulus of elasticity (resistance to stretch) in turkeys.

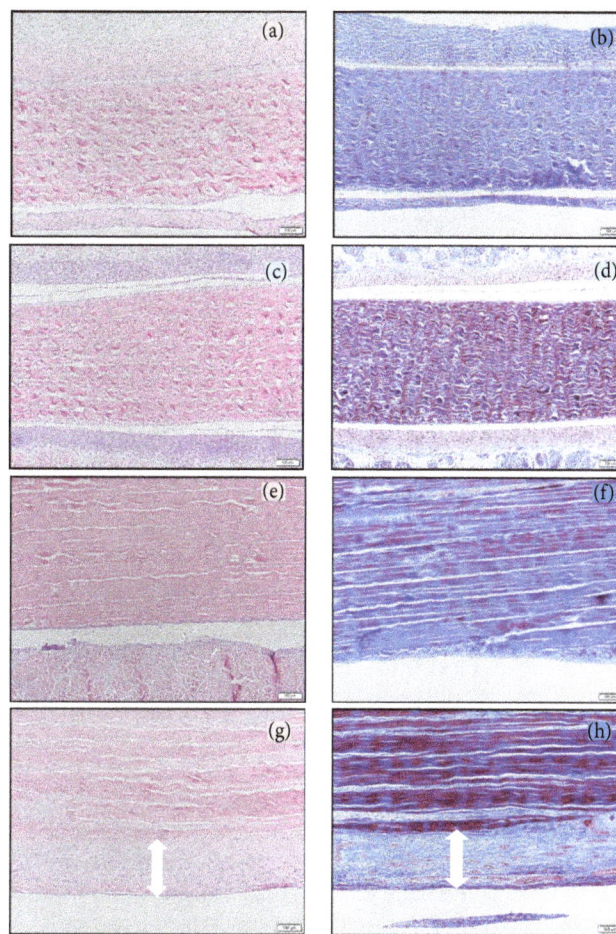

FIGURE 4: Histologic lesions in turkey poults after staining with Masson trichrome (MT) stain: (a) 4-week-old control turkey H&E; (b) 4-week-old control MT; (c) 4-week-old infected H&E; (d) 4-week-old infected MT; (e) 16-week-old control H&E; (f) 16-week-old control MT; (g) 16-week-old infected H&E; (h) 16-week-old infected MT. Inflammatory cells (lymphocytes) in subsynovium in (c) and (d). Collagen (indicative for fibrosis) deposition in the tendon (blue fibrils) in (g) and (h) (double headed white arrows).

TABLE 1: Average tendon tensile strength and elasticity of turkey gastrocnemius tendons at different time points.

Age (weeks)	Group	Number	Tensile strength (MPa) Mean ± SD	Modulus elasticity (MPa) Mean ± SD
4	Control	6	15.4 ± 4.86	75.86 + 29.37
	Infected	6	12.6 ± 11.01	67.10 + 41.51
8	Control	4[+]	9.03[a] ± 2.12	41.45 + 16.54
	Infected	6	12.78 ± 6.70	51.86 + 22.60
12	Control	5	11.76 ± 4.55	57.34 + 2.12
	Infected	6	9.03 ± 5.56	50.76 + 23.08
16	Control	5	19.36 ± 6.59	150.40 + 59.34
	Infected	5	9.84[*] ± 3.75	74.32[*] + 22.15

[*]Significantly lower than control mean at the same age at $P < 0.05$, Mann–Whitney U test.
[a]Significantly lower than control means of other ages at $P < 0.05$, Mann–Whitney U test.
[+]$n = 6$ per group. Tendon measurements were omitted if the tendon did not rupture at the predetermined midsection.
SD: standard deviation.
MPa: megapascals.

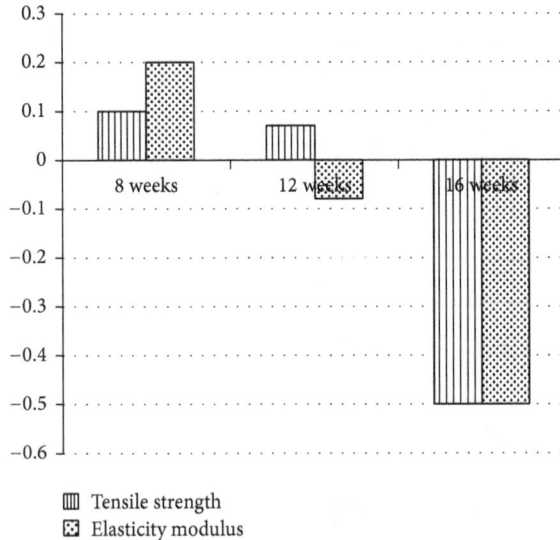

FIGURE 5: Correlation coefficient between lameness and biomechanical properties. Elevated inverse correlation between lameness and tensile strength and elasticity modulus at 16 weeks of age.

Subsynovial fibrosis first developed in 8-week-old turkeys and became predominant by 16 weeks of age. Mean tendon tensile strength and modulus of elasticity were significantly lower ($P < 0.05$) in 16-week-old infected turkeys compared to noninfected turkeys. Mean tendon tensile strength in control turkeys was significantly lower at 8 weeks of age compared with controls of all other time points (Table 1). Perhaps the reduced tensile strength of tendon in 8-week-old control turkeys is spuriously low because only 4 tendons from that group were analyzed as a result of aberrant rupture in two tendons, which were omitted from the study. The means of tendon tensile strength were the same in infected turkeys at all time points ($P < 0.05$). Mean tendon elasticity in control turkeys was the same at 4, 8, and 12 weeks while elasticity was significantly increased in noninfected 16-week-old turkeys ($P < 0.05$) (Table 1). These observations might explain the role of fibrosis in decreasing the tensile strength and modulus of elasticity in infected turkeys.

Previous studies on collagen composition and arrangement in turkey tendons have demonstrated progressive changes in procollagen content and organization as the turkey grows [12]. In our study, induction of substantial inflammation and edema in the gastrocnemius subsynovium and tendon, as well as reovirus replication in these tissues [6], may have altered physiological collagen deposition, ultimately altering tendon tensile strength and elasticity.

A study on gastrocnemius tendon biomechanics in reovirus-infected chickens showed that tendons of chickens infected at one day of age had significantly lower mean tensile strength compared with noninfected chickens at 6, 10, and 18 weeks of age ($P < 0.05$). This work also reported a gradual increase of the mean tendon tensile strength of control birds which was significantly higher only at 18 weeks compared to other time points. Additionally, the mean modulus of elasticity in controls was significantly lower than that of

infected birds only at 18 weeks [13]. Our findings closely parallel those of the chicken study and can improve our understanding of the pathogenesis of TARV [14].

Changes in the biomechanical properties of tendon in the turkeys in our study may be a result of decreased movement of infected lame birds. A previous work showed that immobilized chickens had 10–30% decreased tendon strength and 70% decreased tendon elasticity [15]. These findings were attributed to the decreased organization and diameter of collagen fibers as characterized by electron microscopy.

Finally, the progressive deposition of fibrous connective tissue on and around the tendon of reovirus-infected turkeys as they age combined with the progressive increase in body weight [6] is likely a predisposing factor in inducing lameness and, in some instances, tendon rupture. Increased inverse correlation between clinical lameness and tensile strength and elasticity modulus suggests the possible role of the decreased biomechanical properties values in increasing the clinical lameness at 16 weeks of age. In chickens, it was proposed that fibrosis and adhesions with increased age in heavyweight birds were responsible for gastrocnemius tendon and digital flexor tendon rupture [16].

In conclusion, TARV-infected turkeys developed gastrocnemius lymphocytic tenosynovitis by 4 weeks of age, progressing to fibrosis by 16 weeks of age. Clinical lameness was observed at 8 weeks and was observed in 50% of infected birds at 16 weeks. This lameness was accompanied with tendon rupture in a small percentage of 16-week-old turkeys. The progressive lameness and occasional tendon rupture represent altered tendon function (reduced tensile strength and reduced modulus of elasticity) during infection in a rapidly growing turkey.

Competing Interests

The authors declare that they have no competing interests.

Acknowledgments

The authors thank Dr. Jack Rosenberger for providing TARV-O'Neil for the study. This work was supported in part by the University of Minnesota Rapid Agricultural Research Fund.

References

[1] N. Jindal, D. P. Patnayak, A. F. Ziegler, A. Lago, and S. M. Goyal, "A retrospective study on poult enteritis syndrome in Minnesota," *Avian Diseases*, vol. 53, no. 2, pp. 268–275, 2009.

[2] I. Lojkić, M. Biđin, Z. Biđin, and M. Mikec, "Viral agents associated with poult enteritis in Croatian commercial Turkey flocks," *Acta Veterinaria Brno*, vol. 79, no. 1, pp. 91–98, 2010.

[3] S. K. Mor, T. A. Sharafeldin, M. Abin et al., "The occurrence of enteric viruses in Light Turkey Syndrome," *Avian Pathology*, vol. 42, no. 5, pp. 497–501, 2013.

[4] S. K. Mor, T. A. Sharafeldin, R. E. Porter, A. Ziegler, D. P. Patnayak, and S. M. Goyal, "Isolation and characterization of a Turkey arthritis reovirus," *Avian Diseases*, vol. 57, no. 1, pp. 97–103, 2013.

[5] T. A. Sharafeldin, S. K. Mor, A. Z. Bekele, H. Verma, S. M. Goyal, and R. E. Porter, "The role of avian reoviruses in turkey tenosynovitis/arthritis," *Avian Pathology*, vol. 43, no. 4, pp. 371–378, 2014.

[6] T. A. Sharafeldin, S. K. Mor, A. Z. Bekele et al., "Experimentally induced lameness in turkeys inoculated with a newly emergent turkey reovirus," *Veterinary Research*, vol. 46, article no. 11, 2015.

[7] R. C. Jones, "Reovirus infections," in *Diseases of Poultry*, Y. M. Saif, H. J. Barnes, J. R. Glisson, A. M. Fadly, L. R. McDougald, and D. E. Swayne, Eds., pp. 309–328, Iowa State University Press, Ames, Iowa, USA, 12th edition, 2008.

[8] J. E. Fahey and J. F. Crawley, "Studies on chronic respiratory disease of chickens II. Isolation of a virus," *Canadian Journal of Comparative Medicine*, vol. 18, no. 1, pp. 13–21, 1954.

[9] G. E. Wilcox, M. D. Robertson, and A. D. Lines, "Adaptation and characteristics of replication of a strain of avian reovirus in vero cells," *Avian Pathology*, vol. 14, no. 3, pp. 321–328, 1985.

[10] K. M. Kerr and N. O. Olson, "Pathology of chickens experimentally inoculated or contact-infected with an arthritis-producing virus," *Avian Diseases*, vol. 13, no. 4, pp. 729–745, 1969.

[11] A. A. Afaleq and R. C. Jones, "Pathogenicity of three turkey and three chicken reoviruses for poults and chicks with particular reference to arthritis/tenosynovitis," *Avian Pathology*, vol. 18, no. 3, pp. 433–440, 1989.

[12] L. Knott, J. F. Tarlton, and A. J. Bailey, "Chemistry of collagen cross-linking: biochemical changes in collagen during the partial mineralization of turkey leg tendon," *Biochemical Journal*, vol. 322, no. 2, pp. 535–542, 1997.

[13] F. M. Mohamed, T. L. Foutz, G. N. Rowland, and P. Villegas, "Biomechanical properties of the gastrocnemius tendon in broilers experimentally infected with avian reovirus," *Transactions of the American Society of Agricultural Engineers*, vol. 38, no. 6, pp. 1893–1899, 1995.

[14] T. A. Sharaf Eldin, *Turkey arthritis reovirus: pathogenesis and immune response [Ph.D. thesis]*, University of Minnesota, 2015.

[15] T. L. Foutz, A. K. Griffin, J. T. Halper, and G. N. Rowland, "Effects of activity on avian gastrocnemius tendon," *Poultry Science*, vol. 86, no. 2, pp. 211–218, 2007.

[16] R. C. Jones, "Avian reovirus infections," *Revue Scientifique et Technique de l'OIE*, vol. 19, no. 2, pp. 614–625, 2000.

19

Investigation of *Anaplasma marginale* Seroprevalence in a Traditionally Managed Large California Beef Herd

Thomas R. Tucker III,[1] Sharif S. Aly,[2,3] John Maas,[4] Josh S. Davy,[5] and Janet E. Foley[1]

[1]Departments of Medicine and Epidemiology, School of Veterinary Medicine, University of California, Davis, Davis, CA 95616, USA

[2]Department of Population Health and Reproduction, School of Veterinary Medicine, University of California, Davis, Davis, CA 95616, USA

[3]Veterinary Medicine Teaching and Research Center, School of Veterinary Medicine, University of California, Davis, Tulare, CA 95616, USA

[4]Department of Population Health and Reproduction, University of California, Davis, Davis, CA 95616, USA

[5]Division of Agriculture and Natural Resources, University of California, Davis, Red Bluff, CA 96080, USA

Correspondence should be addressed to Thomas R. Tucker III; thomas.tucker@soc.mil

Academic Editor: Francesca Mancianti

Recent observations by stakeholders suggested that ecosystem changes may be driving an increased incidence of bovine erythrocytic anaplasmosis, resulting in a reemerging cattle disease in California. The objective of this prospective cohort study was to estimate the incidence of *Anaplasma marginale* infection using seroconversion in a northern California beef cattle herd. A total of 143 Black Angus cattle (106 prebreeding heifers and 37 cows) were enrolled in the study. Serum samples were collected to determine *Anaplasma marginale* seroprevalence using a commercially available competitive enzyme-linked immunosorbent assay test kit. Repeat sampling was performed in seronegative animals to determine the incidence density rate from March through September (2013). Seroprevalence of heifers was significantly lower than that of cows at the beginning of the study ($P < 0.001$) but not at study completion ($P = 0.075$). Incidence density rate of *Anaplasma marginale* infection was 8.17 (95% confidence interval: 6.04, 10.81) cases per 1000 cow-days during the study period. Study cattle became *Anaplasma marginale* seropositive and likely carriers protected from severe clinical disease that might have occurred had they been first infected as mature adults. No evidence was found within this herd to suggest increased risk for clinical bovine erythrocytic anaplasmosis.

1. Introduction

Bovine erythrocytic anaplasmosis, caused by *Anaplasma marginale*, creates millions of dollars of annual losses in California alone [1]. Such economic loss makes anaplasmosis prevention a critical component of herd health management for commercial beef cattle producers. All cattle are susceptible to *A. marginale* infection but development of clinical disease is dependent on age at the time of infection as well as factors such as cattle breed, strain virulence, and vector abundance and other factors affecting animal health such as husbandry [2]. When young animals (<6 months of age) are infected, they generally do not develop clinical disease [3]. In contrast,

when mature animals are infected, severe clinical disease may occur, with case-fatality rates reaching 49% in cattle infected after two years of age [4, 5]. Animals surviving infection develop lifelong carrier status and freedom from subsequent clinical anaplasmosis [3, 4, 6].

Bovine anaplasmosis is an endemic vector-borne disease in many parts of California, with tick vectors and both sylvatic (various deer spp.) and livestock reservoirs creating a high risk of infection for naive grazing cattle [7]. Beef cattle managers often move herds of young cattle (<2 years old) to specific pastures throughout the state where high infection prevalence in ticks is thought to occur. The intentional exposure of young cattle to ticks is intended to increase

TABLE 1: Summary of descriptive characteristics for three cattle cohorts from a beef herd in California which were followed up for *Anaplasma marginale* seroconversion.

Age group	Group 1 heifers	Group 2 heifers	Cows
Number sampled	40	66*	37
Age on study day 0	9–12 months	15–17 months	>2 years
Study days sampled	77, 157	0, 70, 193	70, 157
Pastures during study	C (80 days)	A (70 days), B (123 days)	C (80 days)
Study months (2013)	May–August	March–September	May–August

*Sixty-six heifers were sampled on day 0. One heifer was lost to follow-up between day 0 and day 70 and a second heifer was lost to follow-up between day 70 and day 193. These heifers tested negative for *A. marginale* every time they were sampled.

the probability that animals acquire the infection while they are young and attempt to decrease incidence of severe disease when older animals are infected [8]. In California, this management practice should result in high prevalence of young animals with lifelong *A. marginale* carrier status, protected from clinical anaplasmosis [5]. However, over the last three years, ranchers have reported an increased incidence of clinical anaplasmosis which is assumed to be due to a failure of this prophylaxis and high prevalence of *A. marginale* seronegative adult cattle [9]. Ecosystem changes in California have pushed black-tailed deer (*Odocoileus hemionus columbianus*) and mule deer (*Odocoileus hemionus*) from the foothills and into the valleys where they are safer from predation, moving the primary sylvatic reservoir for *A. marginale* to a new region and possibly changing the dynamics of natural exposure to ticks and prevention strategies for clinical anaplasmosis. If true, this would pose a critical herd health challenge of reemergent disease that cattle ranchers and veterinarians must address through new strategic anaplasmosis prophylaxis.

In addition to tick biologic vectors, mechanical vectoring is possible with veterinarians and animal husbandry workers [3, 10]. The organism can be transmitted on drops of blood transferred between animals during vaccination, castration, dehorning, and other routine management practices. Biting flies can also transmit this pathogen if they are interrupted during a blood meal and move from an infected to a naive animal [5, 11–13].

To our knowledge, there are no published studies that report on the true incidence of *A. marginale* infection in California beef cattle herds that are intentionally moved to select pastures for exposure to ticks and prevention of clinical anaplasmosis. The objective of this prospective cohort study was to evaluate the risk of infection in heifers and mature cattle in a large commercial beef cattle herd in California using pasture-based natural infection to prevent clinical anaplasmosis. Comparing seroprevalence between heifers and mature cattle will establish a historic baseline for evaluating efficacy of the natural infection strategy within a herd by determining how many mature cattle were already *A. marginale* carriers and thus resistant to severe disease. We hypothesized that the incidence density rate (IDR) in cows and heifers would be low and would not differ between age classes, supporting claims that adult herds contain high proportions of susceptible animals (>40% [7] *A. marginale* seronegative). Results of this study provide regional insight

into the epidemiology of anaplasmosis in California beef cattle and suggest evidence-based recommendations for anaplasmosis prevention in comparable management systems.

2. Materials and Methods

2.1. Study Population. The study period was from March through September of 2013. A total of 143 animals, part of a commercial herd of Black Angus beef cattle, were enrolled in the study (Table 1). The overall herd had a mean size of 2000 cow/calf pairs and included replacement heifers to maintain a steady population with an approximately 10% cull rate in cows. The home ranch for this herd was in Tehama County, California; however, ranch managers move cattle throughout the state at different times of the year. Cattle were wintered on annual rangeland in Tehama County (6,535 hectares). Summer feed consisted of valley irrigated pasture and mountain meadow irrigated pasture in Tehama County (100 hectares) and Plumas County (975 hectares). The overall herd contained multiple smaller groups of varying numbers. Calves were born on irrigated pastures during midsummer and replacement heifers were selected in the fall. Ranchers managed the herd cattle based on stage of production and pasture carrying capacity by moving animals between groups as necessary for effective management and did not use any anaplasmosis vaccines. Ranchers treated cattle with ivermectin in the fall and doramectin in the spring for internal and external parasites but did not use an acaricide in the herd health program.

Three cohorts were selected for participation based on the likelihood of subsequent accessibility for sample collection and to ensure study events would not interfere with overall herd management. The first cohort (group 2) contained 66 heifers ranging from 15 to 17 months of age at the first sampling date (day 0) and were tested for anaplasmosis from the time they were first placed with the bulls until calving and again two additional times: day 70, just prior to being moved to a second pasture location, and day 193. The ranch manager stated that all of the sites used during this study were thought to contain ticks that were capable of infecting cattle with *A. marginale*. Two additional cohorts (one cohort of heifers and one cohort of cows) were enrolled as they became available to increase sample size and to enable comparison between heifers and mature cows. The two additional cohorts contained 40 heifers (group 1) and 37 cows, respectively, and were enrolled on day 77, at which point they were sampled for anaplasmosis testing and shipped to a second pasture location, where they remained until their final sample collection on day 157. The additional heifer cohort (group 1) ranged from 9 to 12 months of age at day 0. The cows were all >2 years old on day 0. The addition of the second heifer cohort (group 1) and cows allowed comparison of two pasture locations for incidence of anaplasmosis and contrasted the *A. marginale* seroprevalence between cows and heifers.

2.2. Specimen Collection. Blood samples were collected by tail vein venipuncture. Approximately 8 mL of whole blood was collected into serum separator tubes and allowed to sit at ambient temperature until clotted. Samples were then centrifuged and approximately 2 mL of serum was transferred into 2.5 mL cryotubes. Cryotubes were stored on ice packs in an insulated container until the end of the day and subsequently held at −20°C for storage until testing. Animals that were seropositive for *A. marginale* were considered carriers and were not tested again. Each animal was inspected for ticks while being processed through a squeeze chute for blood collection.

2.3. Sample Analysis. Frozen serum samples were thawed and analyzed for the presence of antibodies to *A. marginale* using a commercially produced competitive enzyme-linked immunosorbent assay (cELISA; VMRD, Pullman, Washington). In previous test validation studies, this cELISA had 95% sensitivity and 98% specificity for diagnosis of *A. marginale* infection in cattle raised within *A. marginale* endemic regions [14]. All laboratory testing was performed according to manufacturer instructions. Three positive and two negative controls were included with every 96-well test plate, as per the manufacturer's instructions. Results were determined using a microplate absorbance spectrophotometer with an optical density wavelength of 630 nm. Serological status was determined using percent inhibition cutoffs provided with the test kit (<30% inhibition read as negative and ≥30% inhibition read as positive) for *A. marginale*.

2.4. Statistical Analysis. True prevalence (TP) of anaplasmosis was determined from the measured *A. marginale* seroprevalence using the equation described by Rogan and Gladen [15] using the following formula:

$$TP = \frac{AP + Sp - 1}{Se + Sp - 1}, \qquad (1)$$

where apparent prevalence (AP) was calculated from the serologic results of this study and sensitivity (Se) and specificity (Sp) estimates were those reported by the manufacturer. A 95% confidence interval (CI) for the TP, taking into account diagnostic test Se and Sp studies [14] and the number of animals used in those studies, was approximated using the Reiczigel method (Reiczigel online calculator, http://www2.univet.hu/users/jreiczig/prevalence-with-se-sp.html) [16, 17]. True prevalence was reported except where specifically indicated. The TP and AP of anaplasmosis were compared across cohorts using Pearson's

TABLE 2: Apparent seroprevalence and 95% CI for *Anaplasma marginale* at baseline and final sampling times and *P* values for McNemar's test comparing seroprevalence within groups at baseline and final sampling times for three cattle cohorts from a beef herd in California which were followed up for *A. marginale* seroconversion.

Age group	Baseline sample		Final sample	
	AP (%)	95% CI	AP (%)	95% CI
Group 1 heifers[*]	22.50[a]	(9.56, 35.44)	67.50[c]	(52.98, 82.02)
Group 2 heifers[*†]	42.42[a]	(30.50, 54.35)	89.06[d]	(81.42, 96.71)
Cows[‡]	86.49[b]	(75.47, 97.50)	91.89[d]	(83.10, 100.00)

[a,b,c,d]Within a column, values with different superscript letters are significantly different (*P* < 0.05).
[*]McNemar's test *P* value < 0.001.
[†]Two group 2 heifers were lost to follow-up between the initial and final sample days.
[‡]McNemar's test *P* value *P* = 0.50.

chi-square test. The following procedure was used to determine the number of observed *A. marginale* positive animals within each cohort for the chi-square analysis of TP. The TP, previously calculated for each group, was multiplied by the number of animals in the group. The result of the product was rounded to the nearest whole number and used as the estimate of animals that were *A. marginale* seropositive. The TP and AP of anaplasmosis at the initial and final sampling dates within each cohort were compared using McNemar's test (SPSS, Version 22, IBM, Armonk, NY).

Ninety-five percent CIs for IDR were calculated using the method described by Szklo and Nieto [18] with confidence limit factors for Poisson-distributed variables provided by others [19, 20]. The ratio of two IDRs was calculated to estimate the incidence rate ratio (IRR) as described in Szklo and Nieto [18] and their 95% CIs were calculated as proposed by Ederer and Mantel [20]. An approximate chi-square test with 1 degree of freedom was used to conduct hypothesis testing that the IRR was equal to 1 as described by Szklo and Nieto [18].

The study protocol was reviewed and approved by the Institutional Animal Care and Use Committee at the University of California, Davis, CA 95616. Consent of the animal owner was obtained prior to use of the animals for this research.

3. Results

Mature cows had very high *A. marginale* seropositive AP and TP, from 89.55% at baseline to 95.49% on the final sample days (Tables 2 and 3). By the end of the follow-up period, heifers had also attained a high *A. marginale* carrier status, with TP of 68.68% and 92.38% for group 1 and 2 heifers, respectively. The *A. marginale* seroprevalence was significantly different between each of the study groups at their first sampling day (*P* = 0.045 for group 2 heifers versus group 1 heifers and *P* < 0.0005 for all other comparisons). Over the course of the study, all age groups had an increase in *A. marginale* seroprevalence but this was only statistically

TABLE 3: True seroprevalence and 95% CI for *Anaplasma marginale* at baseline and final sampling times and *P* values for McNemar's test comparing TP within groups at baseline and final sampling for three cattle cohorts from a beef herd in California which were followed up for *Anaplasma marginale* seroconversion.

Age group	Baseline sample		Final sample	
	TP (%)	95% CI	TP (%)[1]	95% CI
Group 1 heifers[*]	19.23[a]	(6.02, 35.92)	68.68[c]	(51.16, 83.06)
Group 2 heifers[*†]	41.13[b]	(27.69, 54.56)	92.38[d]	(80.99, 100.00)
Cows[‡]	89.55[c]	(73.07, 99.57)	95.49[d]	(80.17, 100.00)

[a,b,c,d]Within a column, values with different superscript letters are significantly different ($P < 0.05$).
[*]McNemar's test *P* value < 0.001.
[†]Two group 2 heifers were lost to follow-up between the initial and final sample days.
[‡]McNemar's test *P* value $P = 0.50$.

TABLE 4: Summary of population at risk, incident cases, and time at risk of *Anaplasma marginale* infection for cattle followed up to determine rate of *A. marginale* infection.

Age group	Group 1 heifers	Group 2 heifers[*]		Cows
Pasture	C[§]	A[†]	B[‡]	C[§]
Population at risk	31	37	10	5
Incident cases	18	26	3	2
Days at risk	80	70	123	80

[*]Group 2 heifers were grazed on pasture A for the first 70 study days and on pasture B for the remaining 123 study days.
[†]Annual rangeland pasture, approximately 160 m elevation, Tehama County, CA.
[‡]Valley irrigated pasture, approximately 120 m elevation, Tehama County, CA.
[§]Mountain meadow irrigated pasture, approximately 1060 m elevation, Plumas County, CA.

significant for the heifer groups ($P < 0.0005$). At the end of the follow-up period, *A. marginale* seroprevalence was no longer significantly different between group 2 heifers and the cow group ($P = 0.958$). The seroprevalence of group 2 heifers continued to be higher than the group 1 heifers at study completion ($P = 0.003$). The *A. marginale* seroprevalence (68.68%) of group 1 heifers at the end of the follow-up period was significantly greater than the seroprevalence (41.13%) of group 2 heifers at study onset ($P = 0.014$).

The pasture location, number of animals, and days at risk per pasture as well as incident cases can be found in Table 4. Incidence density rates and their 95% CIs for different groupings of study animals and pasture exposures were calculated using the observed cases (not estimates based on TP calculations) and are presented in Table 5. Group 2 heifers exposed to pasture B had the highest IDR (2.44 cases/1000 heifer-days). The IRR for *A. marginale* infection is presented in Table 6. Incidence rate ratio (group 2 heifers exposed to pasture B as denominator) was the lowest for group 2 heifers exposed to pasture A (4.12) and was significantly greater than the cow group (2.00) ($P = 0.012$) but not significantly greater than group 1 heifers (3.06) ($P = 0.288$). Group 1 heifers also had a significantly higher IRR (3.06) than the cow group

TABLE 5: Summary of incidence density rate (IDR) per 1000 cow-days for three cohorts of California beef cattle followed up for *A. marginale* infection by age group/pasture exposure, age group, and stage of maturity.

Age group	IDR	95% CI
Group 1 heifers, pasture C[*]	7.26	(4.30, 11.47)
Group 2 heifers, pasture A[†]	10.04	(6.56, 14.76)
Group 2 heifers, pasture B[‡]	2.44	(0.50, 7.12)
Group 2 heifers, pasture A + pasture B[§]	9.29	(5.58, 12.00)
Combined heifer groups[‖]	8.39	(6.16, 11.18)
Group 2 heifers, pasture A and group 1 heifers[*]	8.68	(5.81, 12.50)
Cows, pasture C[*]	5.00	(0.61, 18.05)
Combined heifers and cows[¶]	8.17	(6.04, 10.81)

[*]Cows and group 1 heifers were maintained on pasture C throughout their study period.
[†]Group 2 heifers were maintained on pasture A from study day 0 to day 70.
[‡]Group 2 heifers were maintained on pasture B from study day 71 to day 193.
[§]Incident cases and at-risk time combined for all of the group 2 study period.
[‖]Incident cases and at-risk time combined for all of groups 1 and 2 study period.
[¶]Incident cases and at-risk time combined for all study animals throughout the study period.

TABLE 6: Summary of incidence rate ratio (IRR) for three cohorts of California beef cattle followed up for *A. marginale* infection by age group/pasture exposure, age group, and stage of maturity.

Age group	IRR (*P* value) Age group/pasture
Group 1 heifers, pasture C[*]	3.06 (0.048)[a]
Group 2 heifers, pasture A[†]	4.12 (0.012)[a]
Group 2 heifers, pasture B[‡]	Reference
Cows, pasture C[*]	2.00 (0.052)

[*]Cows and group 1 heifers were maintained on pasture C throughout their study period.
[†]Group 2 heifers were maintained on pasture A from study day 0 to day 70.
[‡]Group 2 heifers were maintained on pasture B from study day 71 to day 193.
[a]Relative risk significantly greater for these groups at the 95% confidence level.

(2.00) ($P = 0.048$). No other significant differences were found.

There were significant differences in IDR for animals as seasonal or pasture exposure changed. Group 2 heifers had a significant decrease in infection rate ($P = 0.012$) when they were moved from annual rangeland pasture (March 1, 2013, to May 10, 2013: IDR = 10.04 cases/1000 heifer-days) to valley irrigated pasture (May 10, 2013, Sep. 10, 2013: IDR = 2.44 cases/1000 heifer-days). In contrast to group 2 heifers, during the time period from May 17, 2013, to Aug. 5, 2013, group 1 heifers, on irrigated mountain meadow pasture, had a high infection rate (IDR = 7.26 cases/1000 heifer-days).

No ticks were found on any of the study cattle during the course of the study. No illnesses were reported in any study cattle that corresponded with clinical signs of bovine anaplasmosis. The herd manager regularly observed and treated infectious bovine keratoconjunctivitis but the exact number of treatments was not recorded.

4. Discussion

Cattle in this herd appear to have become *A. marginale* carriers and hence adequately protected from clinical bovine erythrocytic anaplasmosis. Previous literature has suggested that herds with seroprevalence between 1% and 40% would be considered susceptible to new infections from within the herd or from outside the herd via introduction of infected carriers (wildlife reservoirs, introduced cattle) or contaminated fomites (veterinary equipment) [7]. Using 60% seroprevalence against *A. marginale* as a benchmark, the study population well exceeded this threshold.

It is expected that naive animals over a year of age that are infected with *A. marginale* would present with clinical signs. However, there were no observed clinical cases during the course of this study. Several variables may play a role in this including strain and pathogenicity variation as well as animal factors such as health at the time of infection and variation in immune response by this specific breed of livestock. Specifically, one would have expected to see clinical disease in the mature cow that seroconverted during the study. Although it is possible she was infected for the first time during the study, it is also possible that she was a false negative during the initial sampling period.

The difference in IDR across cohorts during similar seasonal periods may be explained by a difference in seasonal vector abundance or feeding activity in various pasture conditions. The high infection rate observed for group 2 pasture A corresponds to a peak of *Dermacentor occidentalis* activity observed at Sierra Foothill Range Field Station in Yuba County, CA, which peaked in March and April in two consecutive years (1987 and 1988) and was largely over by May of those years [21]. The Sierra Foothill Range Field Station is located at 200 m elevation and has similar climate to both of the group 2 heifer pasture exposures. Tick activity decreases dramatically as ambient temperatures increase [21]. The increased elevation of the mountain meadow pasture may have resulted in cooler temperatures in spring and early summer and may have accounted for continued tick activity after group 1 heifers were moved there in May. Another possible contributing factor is that tick vectors in the mountain meadow may have overwintered and passed through early spring with a scarcity of large mammalian hosts but rapidly fed on the cattle herd when the herd was confined to the mountain meadow pasture. Tick vector scenarios are speculative since no ticks were found on cattle to confirm their vector role for *A. marginale* in this study. Mechanical vectors of *A. marginale* infection such as biting flies, vaccinations, and other iatrogenic exposures may also be seasonal and create the results observed in this study.

Additionally, although the midpoint of the age range for group 1 heifers was approximately 5 months younger than the group 2 heifers, the group 1 heifer seroprevalence after 80 days was significantly higher than what was measured for group 2 heifers on day 0. This indicates that in just 80 days group 1 heifers were able to make up for the 5-month age difference (lifetime vector exposure) and cross the benchmark of 60% *A. marginale* seroprevalence, suggesting that pasture exposure at specific critical times is more important than overall exposure

time. Further studies are warranted to identify the level of tick activity and the correlation with *A. marginale* infection incidence for various pastures to assist ranch managers in herd health decision-making processes related to anaplasmosis prevention.

Ticks are the most efficient vector of *A. marginale* transmission [22–24] and are suspected to be the vector in this study despite the inability to collect any during cattle inspection at time of blood sample collection. However, animal temperament, dark colored hides, restraint in a squeeze chute, and cursory examinations may have limited the ability to collect ticks during examination. It is also possible that ticks were present on cattle earlier and were no longer feeding by the time of animal processing and sample collection.

Dermacentor spp. are the most important tick vectors of *A. marginale* in the United States [3]. Of this genus, *D. occidentalis* is known to feed on black-tailed deer (*Odocoileus hemionus columbianus*), mule deer (*O. hemionus hemionus*), and cattle [25]. Host predilection is important given the susceptibility of black-tailed deer to *A. marginale* which may make black-tailed deer the most important wildlife reservoir of *A. marginale* in California and hence the potential source of infections in this study [25]. However, mechanical transmission of *A. marginale* is well documented and biting flies are known vectors of *A. marginale* [5, 11–13] as are veterinarians and husbandry personnel performing procedures such as vaccination or identification using ear tag application or tattooing which may transfer blood from an infected to susceptible animal [3, 10]. Cattle in this study shared vaccine injection needles and ear tag pliers during processing times which is also a potential route of infection.

The IDR for infection measured in the two heifer groups appeared to be adequate to ensure herd seroprevalence of 60% by the time the study cattle were 2 years old. The lower range of the 95% CI for the IDR calculated for heifers during the high infection rate periods was 4.30 cases per 1000 heifer-days (Table 5). Assuming that tick activity is responsible for the infection rates observed in this study and noting that high tick activity was measured over a three-month period in California beef cattle pastures [21], a 77.4% *A. marginale* seroprevalence would be expected without any other exposure during the remaining 9 months of the year:

$$\left(\frac{4.30 \text{ cases}}{1000 \text{ heifer-days}} \right) \times (100 \text{ heifers}) \times \left(\frac{90 \text{ days}}{\text{year}} \right)$$
$$\times (2 \text{ years}) = \frac{77.40 \text{ cases}}{100 \text{ heifers}}. \tag{2}$$

Such an estimate is the low limit for the 95% CI of the IDR and TP values found in this study suggest that a higher *A. marginale* carrier status can be anticipated.

In summary, there was sufficient natural infection of *A. marginale* to prevent an outbreak of bovine erythrocytic anaplasmosis in the study herd; hence, no changes to the herd management protocols to prevent clinical anaplasmosis were warranted. However, cattle ranchers, veterinarians, and livestock advisers should monitor seroprevalence in their herds to ensure that animals continue to become carriers before they become adults to prevent severe disease. The impact of ecosystem change on vector-borne disease is difficult to assess and for this reason continuous monitoring for *A. marginale* infection rates in sentinel herds is recommended to protect California's beef production. Studies with more herds are needed to investigate whether anaplasmosis is a reemerging threat to beef cattle in California before requiring changes to current herd management practices. Additional study of the potential importance for mechanical vectoring as a suitable alternate to biologic exposure is an important future research objective.

Disclosure

This paper represents a portion of a thesis submitted by Dr. Thomas R. Tucker III to the University of California, Davis, School of Veterinary Medicine, as partial fulfillment of the requirements for a Master of Preventive Veterinary Medicine degree.

Competing Interests

The authors declare that they have no competing interests.

Acknowledgments

This study was supported in part by the University of California, Davis, School of Veterinary Medicine. The authors thank Dr. Christie Mayo and Dr. Kristopher Flores, Tom Bengard, Terry Bengard, Jerry Hemsted, and Rogelio Sanchez for technical assistance.

References

[1] W. J. Goodger, T. Carpenter, and H. Riemann, "Estimation of economic loss associated with anaplasmosis in California beef cattle," *Journal of the American Veterinary Medical Association*, vol. 174, no. 12, pp. 1333–1336, 1979.

[2] K. M. Kocan, J. de la Fuente, E. F. Blouin, J. F. Coetzee, and S. A. Ewing, "The natural history of *Anaplasma marginale*," *Veterinary Parasitology*, vol. 167, no. 2–4, pp. 95–107, 2010.

[3] P. Aubry and D. W. Geale, "A review of bovine anaplasmosis," *Transboundary and Emerging Diseases*, vol. 58, no. 1, pp. 1–30, 2011.

[4] E. J. Richey, *Bovine Anaplasmosis*, Proceedings no. 24, American Association of Bovine Practitioners, Stillwater, Okla, USA, 1992.

[5] K. M. Kocan, J. De la Fuente, A. A. Guglielmone, and R. D. Meléndez, "Antigens and alternatives for control of *Anaplasma marginale* infection in cattle," *Clinical Microbiology Reviews*, vol. 16, no. 4, pp. 698–712, 2003.

[6] G. H. Palmer, A. F. Barbet, G. H. Cantor, and T. C. McGuire, "Immunization of cattle with the MSP-1 surface protein complex induces protection against a structurally variant *Anaplasma marginale* isolate," *Infection and Immunity*, vol. 57, no. 11, pp. 3666–3669, 1989.

[7] B. R. Hoar, T. C. Bell, V. Villanueva et al., "Herd-level management and biosecurity factors associated with measures of reproductive success in California beef cow-calf herds," *The Bovine Practitioner*, vol. 42, no. 2, pp. 132–138, 2008.

[8] B. P. Smith, *Large Animal Internal Medicine*, Mosby, Maryland Heights, Mo, USA, 3rd edition, 2002.

[9] J. Maas, *Anaplasmosis: A Re-Emerging Cattle Disease in California*, DROVERS CattleNetwork: University of California, Davis, Calif, USA, 2013.

[10] J. B. Reinbold, J. F. Coetzee, L. C. Hollis et al., "Comparison of iatrogenic transmission of *Anaplasma marginale* in Holstein steers via needle and needle-free injection techniques," *American Journal of Veterinary Research*, vol. 71, no. 10, pp. 1178–1188, 2010.

[11] G. Dikmans, "The transmission of anaplasmosis," *American Journal of Veterinary Research*, vol. 11, pp. 5–16, 1950.

[12] K. M. Kocan, "Development of *Anaplasma marginale* Theiler in ixodid ticks: coordinated development of a rickettsial organism and its tick host," in *Morphology, Physiology, and Behavioral Biology of Ticks*, J. R. Sauer and J. A. Hair, Eds., pp. 472–505, John Wiley and Sons, New York, NY, USA, 1986.

[13] K. M. Kocan, J. de la Fuente, E. F. Blouin, and J. C. Garcia-Garcia, "*Anaplasma marginale* (Rickettsiales: Anaplasmataceae): recent advances in defining host-pathogen adaptations of a tick-borne rickettsia," *Parasitology*, vol. 129, supplement 2, pp. S285–S300, 2004.

[14] S. T. de Echaide, D. P. Knowles, T. C. McGuire, G. H. Palmer, C. E. Suarez, and T. F. McElwain, "Detection of cattle naturally infected with *Anaplasma marginale* in a region of endemicity by nested PCR and a competitive enzyme-linked immunosorbent assay using recombinant major surface protein 5," *Journal of Clinical Microbiology*, vol. 36, no. 3, pp. 777–782, 1998.

[15] W. J. Rogan and B. Gladen, "Estimating prevalence from the results of a screening test," *American Journal of Epidemiology*, vol. 107, no. 1, pp. 71–76, 1978.

[16] Z. Lang and J. Reiczigel, "Confidence limits for prevalence of disease adjusted for estimated sensitivity and specificity," *Preventive Veterinary Medicine*, vol. 113, no. 1, pp. 13–22, 2014.

[17] J. Reiczigel, "Calculator for confidence intervals described," in *Confidence Limits for Prevalence of Disease Adjusted for Estimated Sensitivity and Specificity*, Z. S. Lang and J. Reiczigel, Eds., vol. 113, pp. 13–22, Preventive Veterinary Medicine, 2014.

[18] M. Szklo and F. J. Nieto, *Epidemiology: Beyond the Basics*, Jones & Bartlett, Boston, Mass, USA, 2014.

[19] W. Haenszel, D. B. Loveland, and M. G. Sirken, "Lung-cancer mortality as related to residence and smoking histories. I. White males," *Journal of the National Cancer Institute*, vol. 28, pp. 947–1001, 1962.

[20] F. Ederer and N. Mantel, "Confidence limits on the ratio of two Poisson variables," *American Journal of Epidemiology*, vol. 100, no. 3, pp. 165–167, 1974.

[21] R. Lane, "Seasonal activity of two human-biting ticks," *California Agriculture*, vol. 44, no. 2, pp. 23–25, 1990.

[22] K. M. Kocan, W. L. Goff, D. Stiller et al., "Persistence of *Anaplasma marginale* (Rickettsiales: Anaplasmataceae) in male *Dermacentor andersoni* (Acari: Ixodidae) transferred successively from infected to susceptible calves," *Journal of Medical Entomology*, vol. 29, no. 4, pp. 657–668, 1992.

[23] K. M. Kocan, D. Stiller, W. L. Goff et al., "Development of *Anaplasma marginale* in male *Dermacentor andersoni* transferred from parasitemic to susceptible cattle," *American Journal of Veterinary Research*, vol. 53, no. 4, pp. 499–507, 1992.

[24] G. A. Scoles, A. B. Broce, T. J. Lysyk, and G. H. Palmer, "Relative efficiency of biological transmission of *Anaplasma marginale* (Rickettsiales: Anaplasmataceae) by Dermacentor andersoni (Acari: Ixodidae) compared with mechanical transmission by *Stomoxys calcitrans* (Diptera: Muscidae)," *Journal of Medical Entomology*, vol. 42, no. 4, pp. 668–675, 2005.

[25] K. L. Kuttler, "*Anaplasma* infections in wild and domestic ruminants: a review," *Journal of Wildlife Diseases*, vol. 20, no. 1, pp. 12–20, 1984.

20

Identification of *bap*A in Strains of *Salmonella enterica* subsp. *enterica* Isolated from Wild Animals Kept in Captivity in Sinaloa, Mexico

Gabriela Silva-Hidalgo,[1] **Martin López-Valenzuela,**[1] **Nora Cárcamo-Aréchiga,**[1] **Silvia Cota-Guajardo,**[1] **Mayra López-Salazar,**[1] **and Edith Montiel-Vázquez**[2]

[1]*Pathology Laboratory, Faculty of Veterinary Medicine and Animal Husbandry, Autonomous University of Sinaloa, Boulevard San Ángel s/n, Fraccionamiento San Benito, 80246 Culiacán, SIN, Mexico*
[2]*Enteric Bacteriology Laboratory, Institute of Epidemiological Diagnosis and Reference, Francisco de P. Miranda 177, Lomas de Plateros, Álvaro Obregón, 01480 Mexico City, DF, Mexico*

Correspondence should be addressed to Gabriela Silva-Hidalgo; gabsilhid@uas.edu.mx

Academic Editor: Remo Lobetti

*bap*A, previously named *stm2689*, encodes the BapA protein, which, along with cellulose and fimbriae, constitutes biofilms. Biofilms are communities of microorganisms that grow in a matrix of exopolysaccharides and may adhere to living tissues or inert surfaces. Biofilm formation is associated with the ability to persist in different environments, which contributes to the pathogenicity of several species. We analyzed the presence of *bap*A in 83 strains belonging to 17 serovars of *Salmonella enterica* subsp. *enterica* from wildlife in captivity at Culiacan's Zoo and Mazatlán's Aquarium. Each isolate amplified a product of 667 bp, which corresponds to the expected size of the *bap*A initiator, with no observed variation between different serovars analyzed. *bap*A gene was found to be highly conserved in *Salmonella* and can be targeted for the genus-specific detection of this organism from different sources. Since *bap*A expression improves bacterial proliferation outside of the host and facilitates resistance to disinfectants and desiccation, the survival of *Salmonella* in natural habitats may be favored. Thus, the risk of bacterial contamination from these animals is increased.

1. Introduction

Biofilms, composed of cellulose, fimbriae, and biofilm-associated protein A (BapA, encoded by *bap*A), are communities of microorganisms that grow in a matrix of exopolysaccharides and can adhere to inert surfaces or living tissues [1]. Biofilm formation is associated with the ability to persist in different environments [2], which contributes to the pathogenicity of several species [3]. It has been shown that bacteria growing in biofilms are more resistant to antimicrobial agents than those growing in planktonic cultures due to their physical structure and the formation of multilayer biofilms [4]. Whereas acute bacterial infections can be eliminated after a brief antibiotic treatment, infections by biofilm-producing bacteria normally fail to be completely eliminated and lead to recurrent infections, which can only be resolved by replacing the initial antibiotic therapy [3].

Salmonella are rod-shaped bacteria commonly found in biofilms [5]. This genus includes flagellated, Gram-negative bacteria without spores that thrive in animals' digestive tracts and environments that facilitate long periods of survival, which makes elimination difficult [6].

Fimbriae, or pili, are important for biofilm formation by *Salmonella* [7]. These protein structures recognize a wide range of molecular targets, allowing the bacteria to interact with various surfaces and adhere to specific tissues in the host [8]. For example, type 1 fimbriae are thin, rigid, adhesive structures that express FimH adhesins, which promote bacterial adhesion to and invasion of epithelial cells [9]. Type 1 fimbriae also mediate interactions with abiotic surfaces [9].

TABLE 1: List of *Salmonella* serovars used in the study.

Identification number	Serovar	Source (# of isolates)
1	Typhimurium	Reference strain
2	Albany	*Leopardus pardalis* (f)[a], *Panthera leo* (f), *Felis concolor* (f), *Panthera tigris sumatrae* (f), *Panthera tigris tigris* (f), *Lynx rufus* (f), *Ursus americanus* (f), *Hippopotamus amphibius* (f), *Ara macao* (f), *Carassius auratus* (w)[b], aquatic birds (f), aquatic bird (s)[c], *Rattus* spp. (f), *Periplaneta americana* (i)[d], *Musca domestica* (i), raw chicken (F)[e]
3	3, 10, H: r:-	*Hippopotamus amphibius* (f), *Bassariscus astutus* (f), aquatic birds (f), aquatic birds (w), *Cebus apella* (f)
4	San Diego	Aquatic birds (f), aquatic birds (s), *Python regius* (h)[f], *Rattus* spp. (f)
5	Braenderup	*Mephitis macroura* (f), *Felis concolor* (f), *Panthera tigris* (f), *Procyon lotor* (f), *Ateles geoffroyi* (f)
6	Weltevreden	*Columba flavirostris* (f), *Columba fasciata* (f), *Sus scrofa domestica* (f), aquatic birds (f), aquatic birds (s)
7	Derby	*Cebus apella* (f), *Panthera onca* (f), *Panthera tigris* (f), *Rattus* spp. (f)
8	Oranienburg	*Urocyon cinereoargenteus* (f), *Saimiri sciureus* (f)
9	6, 7, H: en x:-	*Hippopotamus amphibius* (w), *Crocodylus acutus* (w)
10	Poona	Psittaciformes birds (f), *Rattus* spp. (f)
11	Saint Paul	Aquatic birds (f)
12	Panama	*Crocodylus acutus* (w), *Rana* spp. (f)
13	Pomona	*Ramphastos sulfuratus* (f), biological filter
14	Newport	Aquatic birds (f)
15	Enteritidis	Psittaciformes birds (f)
16	Javiana	*Rana* spp. (f)
17	Give	*Iguana iguana* (f)
18	Agona	*Ara* spp. (f)

[a]Feces. [b]Water. [c]Soil. [d]Insect. [e]Food. [f]Rectal *Hyssopus*.

Salmonella biofilm matrices are composed of cellulose, fimbriae, and BapA. The exopolysaccharide cellulose is a major component of these matrices and plays an important role in the resistance to desiccation, disinfectants, and UV light. Cellulose production is regulated by the union of the cyclic nucleotide c-di-GMP, whose synthesis depends on a family of GGDEF domain-containing proteins [10].

After a *Salmonella* infection, continued elimination of the bacteria in stool gives rise to a chronic asymptomatic carrier. Once excreted into the environment, *Salmonella* can resist dehydration for long periods of time in both stool and food for human or animal consumption [11, 12]. Due to its ability to adhere to many surfaces and resist the action of common disinfectants, the presence of this bacterium in the environment is a public health concern because salmonellosis is a zoonotic disease [13]. Additionally, bacteria in biofilms have greater resistance to antibiotics due to several factors. For example, these bacteria present replicative and metabolic heterogeneity, which affects the action of the antibiotic and the structure of the biofilm, thereby impeding the action of the antimicrobial agent [10].

Understanding the capacity of biofilm formation in this bacterial genus will allow us to establish preventive measures to prevent outbreaks of disease in both animals and humans, particularly those in close contact with infected animals. Identifying the genes involved in bacterial resistance will determine the type of antibiotic therapy necessary to treat animal health problems. Thus, the objective of this study was

to detect the presence of *bap*A in *Salmonella* strains isolated from wild animals in captivity.

2. Material and Methods

2.1. Strains. Eighty-three strains of *Salmonella* spp. belonging to 17 different serovars (Table 1) obtained from enclosures, food, and feces from zoo and aquarium animals in captivity in Culiacan and Mazatlán, Sinaloa, Mexico, were used in the study. All isolates were confirmed through biochemical and serological methods by the Enteric Bacteriology Laboratory, Institute of Epidemiological Diagnosis and Reference (InDRE), DF, Mexico, and maintained on nutrient freezing medium until being tested. *Salmonella* Typhimurium 14028S from the American Type Culture Collection (ATCC) was used as a reference control strain.

2.2. Recovery and Purity Verification of Strains. *Salmonella* strains were recovered from preservation medium containing soy broth-glycerol (freezing medium), transferred to trypticase soy broth, and incubated at 37°C for 18 h. The bacterial suspensions obtained were plated on MacConkey and XLT4 agar to confirm the negative reaction of *Salmonella* strains to lactose and to visually analyze the purity of the strains grown at 37°C for 24 h. Inclined tubes containing blood agar base (BAB) were inoculated with confirmed strains until further use.

2.3. Bacterial DNA Extraction. DNA was extracted from isolated bacterial strains with a commercial matrix (InstaGene Matrix, Bio-Rad®).

2.4. PCR Identification of bapA. The oligonucleotide primers for PCR were synthesized according to the published DNA sequences of the *bapA* gene [10] and have, respectively, the following nucleotide sequence: forward, 5′-GCCATGGTGCTGGAAGGCCTGGCGGTT-3′; reverse, 5′-GGTCGACGGGAAGGGTAAAATGACCTTC-3′. Amplification was carried out in a thermocycler (Bio-Rad, MJ Mini Personal Thermal Cycler) with a reaction mixture of 25 μL, which contained 5 μL of template DNA, 1 μL (10 pmol L^{-1}) of each of the forward and reverse primers, 12.5 μL PCR SuperMix (22 mM Tris-HCl, 55 mM KCl, 1.65 mM MgCl$_2$, 220 μM dGTP, 220 μM dATP, 220 μM dTTP, 220 μM dCTP, and 22 U/mL recombinant Taq DNA Polymerase), and 1.5 μL MgCl$_2$ (50 mM). The final volume was prepared with nuclease-free water. The PCR program included an initial denaturation step at 94°C for 5 min followed by 30 cycles of denaturation (94°C for 1 min), annealing (50°C for 45 s), and extension (72°C for 1 min). Final extension was carried out at 72°C for 5 min. Amplification products were separated by submarine gel electrophoresis on 1.5% agarose gel with prestained GelRed (solution at 1 : 10,000) in 0.5x Tris-EDTA electrophoresis buffer. A 100 bp DNA ladder (Bio-Rad) was used as a molecular weight marker. The gels were visualized in Gel Documentation System™ EZ GelDoc and photographed for analysis.

2.5. Statistical Analysis. The frequency of the presence of *bapA* was determined according to the previously reported formula [14]. To determine whether there were significant statistical differences among the different serovars examined, chi-square tests were performed using the epidemiological data analysis program, Epidat 3.1.

3. Results and Discussion

PCR reactions of the 83 isolates belonging to 17 different serovars with oligonucleotides to *bapA* amplified a product of 667 bp, which corresponds to the expected size of the *bapA* initiator (Figure 1). Importantly, there were no differences detected in this initiator element between different serovars tested. Of the strains analyzed, 65 were isolated from animal feces (mammals, birds, and reptiles), 6 were isolated from *American cockroach* and *Musca domestica*, 2 were isolated from food, 1 was isolated from a biological filter, and 4 and 5 were isolated from enclosures of water and soil, respectively.

All serovars amplified *bapA*, consistent with previous results [10], which suggests that *bapA* is a very conserved gene both between and within different serovars with a high degree of identity (99%) [15]. This conservation offers diagnostic advantages because the presence of *bapA* can be used to identify the *Salmonella* genus in different environments [16].

BapA belongs to a family of large surface proteins involved in bacterial adhesion to various surfaces and maturation of biofilms [17]. The protein, which was previously

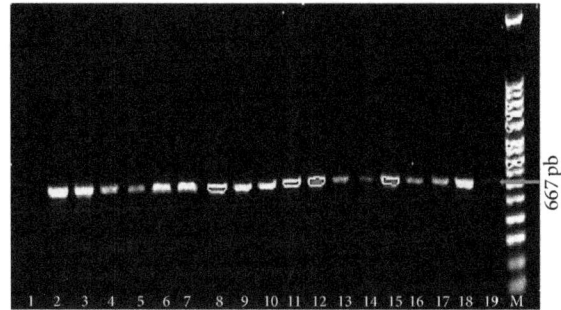

FIGURE 1: PCR results for the detection of *bapA* from different *Salmonella* serovars. Lane 1: nontemplate control; Lane 2: *Salmonella* Albany; Lane 3: *Salmonella* 3, 10, H: r:-; Lane 4: *Salmonella* San Diego; Lane 5: *Salmonella* Braenderup; Lane 6: *Salmonella* Weltevreden; Lane 7: *Salmonella* Derby; Lane 8: *Salmonella* Oranienburg; Lane 9: *Salmonella* 6, 7, H: en x:-; Lane 10: *Salmonella* Poona; Lane 11: *Salmonella* Saint Paul; Lane 12: *Salmonella* Panama; Lane 13: *Salmonella* Pomona; Lane 14: *Salmonella* Newport; Lane 15: *Salmonella* Enteritidis; Lane 16: *Salmonella* Javiana; Lane 17: *Salmonella* Give; Lane 18: *Salmonella* Agona; Lane 19: *Salmonella* Typhimurium reference strain (ATCC 14028S); Lane M: 100 bp ladder. Thick arrow identifies the 667 bp band of interest.

named Stm2689, plays an important role in the mouse model of intestinal colonization as well as bacterial spread to other organs [18]. In this study, strains were isolated from the stool of wild animals lacking gastroenteric disorders, which suggests that intestinal colonization in these animals is associated, in part, with the presence of the *bapA* gene. Supporting this notion, previous research compared the propensities of *Salmonella* strains with or without *bapA* to colonize the intestine and demonstrated that mutated strains exhibited lower colonization rates than those with wild-type *bapA* [19].

The mechanisms that allow these pathogens to persist in animals' digestive tracts are poorly understood. However, the intestinal persistence of *Salmonella* spp. observed in clinically healthy animals increases the risk of bacterial contamination because *bapA* expression ensures that more bacteria survive outside of the host and retain their infective ability. This allows the bacteria to resist desiccation and the action of the disinfectants; thus, the survival of *Salmonella* in natural habitats may be favored [20, 21]. Further understanding of the mechanisms involved in bacterial intestinal persistence will facilitate the development of innovative strategies that safeguard the public population against salmonellosis, a natural zoonotic disease.

4. Conclusions

bapA was identified in all 83 strains belonging to 17 different serovars isolated from wildlife in captivity which suggests that it is a highly conserved gene in *Salmonella* and can be targeted for the genus-specific detection of this organism from different sources and diagnostic potentials, which need to be explored. Additionally, most animals that tested positive were asymptomatic carriers. This poses a challenge for professionals in the health care area to overcome, because the capacity of *Salmonella* to survive in many environments suggests that its dissemination will likely continue to increase in the future.

Competing Interests

The authors declare that there are no competing interests regarding the publication of this paper.

Acknowledgments

The authors thank the 2011 Programa de Fomento y Apoyo a Proyectos de Investigatción (PROFAPI, translated as Program of Incentives and Support for Research Projects) for funding.

References

[1] A. P. White, D. L. Gibson, G. A. Grassl et al., "Aggregation via the red, dry, and rough morphotype is not a virulence adaptation in *Salmonella enterica* serovar typhimurium," *Infection and Immunity*, vol. 76, no. 3, pp. 1048–1058, 2008.

[2] N. Gruzdev, R. Pinto, and S. Sela, "Effect of desiccation on tolerance of *Salmonella enterica* to multiple stresses," *Applied and Environmental Microbiology*, vol. 77, no. 5, pp. 1667–1673, 2011.

[3] T.-F. C. Mah and G. A. O'Toole, "Mechanisms of biofilm resistance to antimicrobial agents," *Trends in Microbiology*, vol. 9, no. 1, pp. 34–39, 2001.

[4] R. M. Donlan and J. W. Costerton, "Biofilms: survival mechanisms of clinically relevant microorganisms," *Clinical Microbiology Reviews*, vol. 15, no. 2, pp. 167–193, 2002.

[5] M. Malcova, H. Hradecka, R. Karpiskova, and I. Rychlik, "Biofilm formation in field strains of *Salmonella enterica* serovar Typhimurium: identification of a new colony morphology type and the role of SGI1 in biofilm formation," *Veterinary Microbiology*, vol. 129, no. 3-4, pp. 360–366, 2008.

[6] E. B. Solomon, B. A. Niemira, G. M. Sapers, and B. A. Annous, "Biofilm formation, cellulose production, and curli biosynthesis by *Salmonella* originating from produce, animal, and clinical sources," *Journal of Food Protection*, vol. 68, no. 5, pp. 906–912, 2005.

[7] J. W. Austin, G. Sanders, W. W. Kay, and S. K. Collinson, "Thin aggregative fimbriae enhance *Salmonella* enteritidis biofilm formation," *FEMS Microbiology Letters*, vol. 162, no. 2, pp. 295–301, 1998.

[8] P. Klemm and M. A. Schembri, "Bacterial adhesins: function and structure," *International Journal of Medical Microbiology*, vol. 290, no. 1, pp. 27–35, 2000.

[9] C. Solano, B. García, J. Valle et al., "Genetic analysis of *Salmonella enteritidis* biofilm formation: critical role of cellulose," *Molecular Microbiology*, vol. 43, no. 3, pp. 793–808, 2002.

[10] R. Biswas, R. K. Agarwal, K. N. Bhilegaonkar et al., "Cloning and sequencing of biofilm-associated protein (BapA) gene and its occurrence in different serotypes of *Salmonella*," *Letters in Applied Microbiology*, vol. 52, no. 2, pp. 138–143, 2011.

[11] D. A. Pegues, M. E. Ohl, and S. I. Miller, "*Salmonella*, including *Salmonella* Typhi," in *Infections of the Gastrointestinal Tract*, pp. 669–697, Lippincott Williams & Wilkins, Philadelphia, Pa, USA, 2nd edition, 2002.

[12] H. Steenackers, K. Hermans, J. Vanderleyden, and S. C. J. De Keersmaecker, "*Salmonella* biofilms: an overview on occurrence, structure, regulation and eradication," *Food Research International*, vol. 45, no. 2, pp. 502–531, 2012.

[13] O. Habimana, K. Steenkeste, M.-P. Fontaine-Aupart, M.-N. Bellon-Fontaine, S. Kulakauskas, and R. Briandet, "Diffusion of nanoparticles in biofilms is altered by bacterial cell wall hydrophobicity," *Applied and Environmental Microbiology*, vol. 77, no. 1, pp. 367–368, 2011.

[14] M. Thursfield, "Measures of disease occurrence," in *Veterinary Epidemiology*, pp. 53–55, Wiley-Blackwell, Hoboken, NJ, USA, 3rd edition, 2007.

[15] C. Latasa, A. Roux, A. Toledo-Arana et al., "BapA, a large secreted protein required for biofilm formation and host colonization of *Salmonella enterica* serovar Enteritidis," *Molecular Microbiology*, vol. 58, no. 5, pp. 1322–1339, 2005.

[16] M. Díez-García, R. Capita, and C. Alonso-Calleja, "Influence of serotype on the growth kinetics and the ability to form biofilms of *Salmonella* isolates from poultry," *Food Microbiology*, vol. 31, no. 2, pp. 173–180, 2012.

[17] C. Latasa, C. Solano, J. R. Penadés, and I. Lasa, "Biofilm-associated proteins," *Comptes Rendus—Biologies*, vol. 329, no. 11, pp. 849–857, 2006.

[18] C. B. García-Calderón, J. Casadesús, and F. Ramos-Morales, "Rcs and PhoPQ regulatory overlap in the control of *Salmonella enterica* virulence," *Journal of Bacteriology*, vol. 189, no. 18, pp. 6635–6644, 2007.

[19] C. Latasa, B. García, M. Echeverz et al., "*Salmonella* biofilm development depends on the phosphorylation status of RcsB," *Journal of Bacteriology*, vol. 194, no. 14, pp. 3708–3722, 2012.

[20] A. Bridier, R. Briandet, V. Thomas, and F. Dubois-Brissonnet, "Resistance of bacterial biofilms to disinfectants: a review," *Biofouling*, vol. 27, no. 9, pp. 1017–1032, 2011.

[21] A. P. White and M. G. Surette, "Comparative genetics of the rdar morphotype in *Salmonella*," *Journal of Bacteriology*, vol. 188, no. 24, pp. 8395–8406, 2006.

21

Prevalence of Needlestick Injury and Its Potential Risk among Veterinarians in Nigeria

Philip Paul Mshelbwala,[1] J. Scott Weese,[2] and Jibrin Manu Idris[3]

[1]*Department of Veterinary Medicine, Faculty of Veterinary Medicine, University of Abuja, Abuja, Nigeria*
[2]*Department of Pathobiology, Ontario Veterinary College, University of Guelph, Guelph, ON, Canada*
[3]*African Field Epidemiology Network, Abuja, Nigeria*

Correspondence should be addressed to Philip Paul Mshelbwala; philbwala@yahoo.com

Academic Editor: William Ravis

A cross sectional study using multistage sampling method by means of structured interviewer administered questionnaire was designed to estimate the rate of occurrence of needlestick injuries among veterinarians involved in clinical practice and to evaluate needle handling practices and risk factors. The study was carried out during the months of August–November 2015. Out of the 215 veterinarians that participated in the survey, 171 (79.5%) reported to have suffered needlestick injuries (NSIs). In the multivariable model, only male sex (OR 2.8, 95% CI 1.4–6.0, and $P = 0.006$) and working with poultry daily (OR 2.4, 95% CI 1.1–6.2, and $P = 0.036$) were significantly associated with NSI. Most (111, 64.9%) veterinarians had discomfort including pain, headache, fever, worry, and local numbness from NSIs; however, none was hospitalised. Only 1 (0.6%) had lost time at work. The approach to needlestick injury avoidance was poor and most (98.8%) NSIs were not reported. The findings of this research call for comprehensive health and injection safety programs for veterinarians involved in clinical practice.

1. Introduction

Accidental puncture of the skin by a needle, otherwise known as "needlestick" or "needlestick injury" (NSI), can occur before, during, and after a procedure, before, during, and after improper needle disposal (e.g., leaving needles in a laboratory coat with subsequent needlestick injury to laundry worker [1]), or at any other time in the process where a needle is handled. Needlestick injuries pose risks from injection of contents, exposure to pathogens, and physical trauma. Infectious disease risks include exposure to blood-borne pathogens, organisms from the animal's or person's skin (*Staphylococcus* spp.) or from fine-needle aspirates (*Pasteurella* spp., *Staphylococcus* spp., *Streptococcus* spp., and *Blastomyces*), or modified live vaccines [1]. Severe laceration such as an NSI occurring during animal movement during injection or blood collection can be significant. Even limited trauma can result in potentially serious consequences in some locations, such as injuries associated with joints, nerves, tendons, and bone. Exposure to medications and vaccines also poses potential risk of reaction to the medication, including typical drug effects (e.g., sedatives), allergic effects (e.g., penicillin allergy), toxic effects (e.g., tilmicosin exposure), and idiosyncratic effects.

In human medicine, considerable time, effort, and resources have been put in place to reduce the incidence of NSIs largely driven by the infection of healthcare workers (HCWs) with infectious agents such as hepatitis B virus, hepatitis C virus, and human immunodeficiency virus (HIV) [2]. However, in veterinary medicine, a similar proactive approach towards NSIs is lacking; this is likely due to poorly developed culture of concern regarding occupational health and safety in the profession and because serious blood-borne zoonotic pathogens of domestic animals are not recognised as important problems in most regions. There are over five thousand registered veterinarians in Nigeria [3]. Needlestick injuries are considered to be very common types of injuries among healthcare workers; however, the quality of available data is variable and it is believed that there is significant underreporting [4]. The incidence of NSIs might be higher in veterinary medicine given the potential laxity in sharps handling practices because of fewer identified blood-borne pathogens risks. There have been few studies of the incidence of NSIs in veterinary medicine when compared with human medicine, but available data indicate concerningly high rates [1]. For example, in a study conducted among female veterinarians, 64% reported one or more NSIs in their career, with vaccines accounting for 50% of the incidents [5]. In study conducted by Ansa et al. [6], in three health institutions from South West Nigeria, they observed that basic protective equipment supplies were grossly inadequate in all the health institutions and safety practices were not adhered to; all these could increase the risk of contracting blood-borne infections. About three million healthcare workers are estimated to experience percutaneous exposure to blood-borne pathogens annually [7]. The majority of the cases occur in developing countries in Africa, probably due to poor injection safety practices and lack of basic supplies. The prevalence of NSI in Africa among healthcare workers varies from 31% to 68%; it is 30.9% in Southern Ethiopia, 52.9% in Tanzania, 67.9% in Alexandria in Egypt, and 68% among gynaecologists in Nigeria [8]. However, in Nigeria and other developing countries of Africa, corresponding data are lacking among veterinarians. Understanding NSI rates and risk factors is important for identifying education and intervention needs to reduce the incidence and impact of NSIs among veterinary personnel. This study was designed to estimate the rate of occurrence of NSIs among veterinarians involved in clinical practice in Nigeria and to evaluate needle handling practices and identify factors associated with NSIs. Inferences drawn from this study will be used in the development of effective risk reduction strategies.

2. Materials and Method

A cross sectional study using multistage purposive sampling method was performed by means of self-administered structured interviewer questionnaire (available in the Supplementary Material online at http://dx.doi.org/10.1155/2016/7639598). The questionnaire was developed and pretested among 32 veterinarians involved in clinical practice in two veterinary teaching hospitals in Nigeria. The questionnaire was thereafter administered to veterinarians who were willing to participate in the study across six veterinary teaching hospitals in the country and during the 52nd annual conference of the Nigerian Veterinary Medical Association (NVMA), Rivers States University of Science and Technology, Diobu area of Port Harcourt, Rivers State, Nigeria, 16–20 November 2015. The theme was "Providing Holistic Solutions to the Staggering Nigerian Economy: Challenges and Opportunities for Veterinarians." Veterinarians who attended the conference came from all the states of the federation and from different universities. The questionnaire was administered to all volunteers that were involved in clinical practice. Respondents were briefed on the purpose of the study and their consent was sought. The questionnaire covered various aspects of demographics, practice type, qualification, years in practice, NSIs, and injury reporting. Multiple choice and open-ended questions were included. Retrospective incidence data were

TABLE 1: Number of needlestick injuries reported by veterinarians.

Number of needlestick injuries	Number of veterinarians
1–4	51 (29.8%)
5–8	34 (19.9%)
8–10	50 (29.2%)
>10	36 (21.1%)

collected by asking questions related to activity over past week, month, and year and over career. Respondents were at liberty to skip questions they did not want to answer. Data were analysed using Statistical Package For Social Science (SPSS) Version 17. Univariable logistic regression models were constructed to estimate the association between having experienced an NSI and a variety of independent variables. Continuous independent variables were assessed to determine whether there was a linear relationship between the variable and the log odds of the outcome, with continuous data transformed if required. All significant variables based on a liberal P value (i.e., $P < 0.25$) in the univariable analysis were considered for inclusion in the multivariable model. The multivariable model was fitted using a backwards stepwise approach to create a main effects model using a significance level of $\alpha = 0.10$ while retaining confounding variables regardless of statistical significance. Confounding was assessed by examining the change in the coefficients for the remaining significant variables after removal of the potentially confounding variable. If the coefficient for one of these variables changed more than 20%, the removed variable was considered a confounder and was retained in the model. A P value of <0.05 was considered significant. Model fit was assessed after completion of the final multivariable model.

3. Results

Two hundred and fifteen veterinarians completed the questionnaire; 159 (74%) were male and 65 (26%) female. This represented 49% (197/404) from the conference attendees and 18 from the teaching hospitals. One hundred and twenty (55.8%) had Doctor of Veterinary Medicine (DVM) degree, 77 (35.8%) had M.S. degree, and 18 (8.4%) had a Ph.D. degree. Needlestick injuries were very common, with 171 (79.5%) reporting at least one NSI during their career. Most veterinarians had experienced numerous NSIs (Table 1). A total of 216 NSIs were estimated to have occurred, with more cases among those who handled poultry and dogs. Univariable data are reported in Table 2. In the multivariable model, only male sex (OR 2.8, 95% CI 1.4–6.0, and $P = 0.006$) and working with poultry daily (OR 2.4, 95% CI 1.1–6.2, and $P = 0.036$) were significant. Model fit testing indicated that the data fit the model ($P = 0.80$).

Veterinarians were carrying out various tasks during the last NSIs, with recapping of needle (50, 29.2%) being the main reason for NSIs (Table 3).

Various reasons were implicated by veterinarians as causative factors for NSIs (Table 4) with poor restraint as the major cause (42.7%). A variety of substances were present in

TABLE 2: Univariable logistic regression results for variables that entered the model based on a $P \leq 0.25$.

Variable	Referent	Category	Odds ratio (95% CI)	P value
Sex	Female	Male	3.1 (1.6–6.3)	0.002
Frequency of treating dogs	Never	Daily	8.3 (2.3–35.8)	0.001
		Weekly	4.4 (1.2–16.4)	0.022
		Greater than weekly	3.2 (1.0–10.4)	0.049
Frequency of treating horses	Never	Greater than weekly	2.6 (1.2–5.5)	0.01
Frequency of treating poultry	Never	Daily	4.5 (1.2–16.9)	0.03
Frequency of treating goats	Never	Daily	3.3 (1.1–10.8)	0.036
		Weekly	5.7 (1.8–20.0)	0.002
Frequency of treating sheep	Never	Daily	4.1 (1.2–16.2)	0.02
		Weekly	4.6 (1.5–16.0)	0.007
Frequency of treating cattle	Never	Daily	5.5 (1.3–37.8)	0.019
		Weekly	4.1 (1.4–12.9)	0.008
		Greater than weekly	3.1 (1.4–7.1)	0.006
Temporary placement of syringes in laboratory coat following use	Yes	No	2.1 (0.88–5.3)	0.11
Work type	Government or university	Private practice	1.7 (0.75–4.6)	0.023

TABLE 3: Activity carried out during the last needlestick injury ($n = 171$).

Activity	
Withdrawing drug	14 (8.2%)
Collecting blood sample	14 (8.2%)
Manipulating needle in patient	37 (21.6%)
Handling garbage	5 (5.9%)
Handling uncooperative patient	26 (15.2%)
Recapping of needle	50 (29.2%)
Taking off cap	3 (1.8%)
Other	6 (3.5%)
No response	1 (0.6)

TABLE 4: Reasons for needlestick injury ($n = 171$).

Factor	
Long working hours	12 (7.0%)
Inappropriate environment	12 (7.0%)
Stress	24 (14.0%)
Inappropriate training	6 (3.5%)
Poor lightning	22 (12.9)
Poor restraint	73 (42.7%)
Other	11 (6.4%)
No response	11 (6.4%)

TABLE 5: What was contained in the syringe ($n = 171$)?

Content	
Killed vaccine	26 (15.2%)
Live vaccine	6 (3.5%)
Antibiotic	99 (57%)
Multivitamin and other	32 (18.8%)

TABLE 6: What do you do with used syringe and needle?

Place in sharp container after recapping	121 (56%)
Sometime place in sharp container	14 (6.5%)
Do not have sharp container	45 (20.9%)
Always place in sharp container without recapping	17 (7.9%)

syringes associated with NSIs, with antibiotics (57.9%), killed vaccines (15.2%), and modified live vaccines (3.5%) being the most common (Table 5). Most (111, 64.9%) respondents had experienced discomfort from the NSI, including pain, headache, fever, worry, and local numbness; however, none was hospitalised. Only 2 (1.2%) sought medical care. The majority (148, 86.5%) applied antiseptic at the site, while 14 (8.2%) did nothing. Information on needle handling practices indicated that most veterinarians do not have sharp containers in their clinics. The majority of respondents (128, 59.5%) reported not having access to a sharps container in their clinic, with only 66 (30.7%) responding to a sharps container and 21 (9.8%) declining to respond. Most respondents place used syringes in sharp container after recapping (Table 6). The majority of respondents (195, 90.7%) knew NSIs can transmit diseases and 171 (79.5%) indicated they needed injection safety training.

4. Discussion

The high incidence of NSIs was concerning but consistent with previous veterinary studies [4, 9, 10] as well as a study of gynaecologists in Nigeria [11]. This high occurrence of NSIs raises concerns because of the potential for adverse effects and the deficiencies in preventive and reporting practices that potentiate the risk of NSIs and hamper understanding of the problem.

Various factors were associated with increased odds of NSI in the univariable analysis, but only being male and working with poultry daily remained significant in the final multivariable model. The increased odds of NSI among male veterinarians is interesting and should prompt consideration of why this occurs. It may be due to behavioural differences and less care when handling sharps; however, those details were not possible to investigate in this study.

The association with poultry practice, but not other clinical practices, was interesting and has not been previously reported. This could be associated with a larger number of NSI opportunities, through handling and injection of larger numbers of animals, compared with work on other species. This finding indicates a need to target poultry practitioners for education campaigns regarding sharps handling practices and NSI avoidance.

A variety of practices are recommended to reduce the incidence of NSIs. These include not recapping needles by hand, disposing of needles directly into an approved sharps container, never leaving uncapped needles on a surface, never leaving needles in laundry, and ensuring good restraint [12]. Poor compliance with these recommendations was identified in this study, something that has been identified in previous surveys and an observational study in veterinary medicine [9, 13]. Recapping was the most common event associated with NSI, something that is avoidable but common in veterinary medicine; this agrees with the report of Anderson and Weese [9]. Manual recapping is a leading cause of NSIs through missing the cap and puncturing a finger or driving the needle through the side of the cap and into a finger. This is a modifiable activity and reducing recapping would probably have a profound impact on NSI rates. Poor restraint was also commonly implicated as a cause of NSI. Poor restraint can create risk of self-puncture when injecting a struggling animal or when the veterinarian is distracted by the poorly restrained animal. Improvements in patient handling along with associated aspects such as avoiding rushing and ensuring adequate restraint prior to injection can probably impact NSI risk. Stress and fatigue were other reported factors, both of which could lead to decreased attention, decreased care, and rushing to inject in the absence of proper restraint. In human medicine, there is increasing use of "safety engineered devices" such as retracting needles or capping systems to reduce any chance of NSI [14]. The added cost and decreased attention to NSIs in veterinary medicine likely account for limited use of these approaches, particularly in developing countries.

Poor compliance is a common problem with many infection control practices, including needle handling. Various reasons can be present, including lack of education, lack of motivation, inadequate supervision, inadequate time, and a lack of supplies or infrastructure. All these could play a role in the results of this study. Only 56% of participants reported placing their used syringes in a sharps container after recapping, indicating a lack of education or motivation about the risks of recapping. The lack of ready access to proper sharps disposal containers, something that would preclude safe needle handling, was another problem, with 20.9% of veterinarians not having a sharps disposal container in the clinic. This lack of basic supplies precludes safe needle handling; this is similar to the report of Ansa et al. [6] who carried out a study in three health institutions from South West Nigeria. They observed that basic protective equipment supplies were grossly inadequate in all the health institutions and safety practices were not adhered to, factors that could increase the risk of contracting blood-borne infections. Some clinicians (30.7%) placed their used syringe and needle in their laboratory coat temporally following use, a high risk practice as either the veterinarian or laundry personnel is likely to sustain an NSI during wearing of the coat or laundering, exposing both the clinician and other personnel to risk.

Education is an important aspect of infection control and occupational health. While needles are handled very regularly, knowledge about optimal handling practices may be variable. This perception may indicate a lack of understanding given the widespread inadequacy. Veterinarians were exposed to a variety of substances (Table 5) from NSIs. Antibiotics were the most common. The high rates of exposure to antibiotics is of great concern due to the potential problems from the direct effects of drugs and allergic reactions [15].

The very low reporting rate of NSIs (1.2%) was perhaps unsurprising but nonetheless concerning. Reporting rates were slightly higher but still shockingly low (9.2%) in a study of gynaecologists in Nigeria [11], highlighting a gap in education about the importance of NSIs and the need for reporting. Reporting of NSIs is important to ensure that any indicated prophylactic care is provided and to collect accurate NSI data. While medical care was rarely sought, the majority of participants reported applying an antiseptic following the injury. However, while antiseptics may be useful to reduce the risk of infection, they do not eliminate that risk or address other relevant issues such as local inflammation and systemic reactions.

While NSI rates among veterinarians are high, limited information is available about the incidence of infectious diseases associated with NSIs. While anecdotal, two respondents reported to have known veterinarians who came down with brucellosis and trypanosomiasis as a result of NSIs, while 9 (0.04%) had themselves developed conjunctivitis following exposure to Newcastle Disease Vaccine. Considering the limited reporting of NSIs and the lack of mandatory reporting system for NSI associated infections, unreported infections almost certainly occur. There was no association between the incidence of NSIs among veterinarians in private practice and those working with the veterinary teaching hospitals.

This study has demonstrated that NSIs are very common among veterinarians involved in clinical practice in Nigeria and that potentially unsafe practices are widespread. The frequency of injuries and the poor approach to needlestick avoidance call for comprehensive health and injection safety programs for veterinarians involved in clinical practice. The major limitations of this study are lack of data about wearing gloves, the localization of NSI, and the occurrence of observable NSI through regular visits to various practice fronts.

Competing Interests

The authors declare that there is no conflict of interests regarding the publication of this paper.

Acknowledgments

The authors wish to express their sincere gratitude to all veterinarians who completed the questionnaire and Drs. Chigozie Ukwueze, Victor Erondo, and Namu Amos who assisted in administering the questionnaire. The first author wishes to express his sincere gratitude to the management of the African Field Epidemiology Network (AFENET), Abuja, Nigeria, for numerous thematic training he enjoyed on injection safety which stimulated him to design this study.

References

[1] J. S. Weese and D. C. Jack, "Needlestick injuries in veterinary medicine," *Canadian Veterinary Journal*, vol. 49, no. 8, pp. 780–784, 2008.

[2] D. J. Haiduven, S. M. Simpkins, E. S. Phillips, and D. A. Stevens, "A survey of percutaneous/mucocutaneous injury reporting in a public teaching hospital," *Journal of Hospital Infection*, vol. 41, no. 2, pp. 151–154, 1999.

[3] Nigerian Veterinary Medical Association, 2016, http://nvma.org.ng/.

[4] A. Elder and C. Paterson, "Sharps injuries in UK health care: a review of injury rates, viral transmission and potential efficacy of safety devices," *Occupational Medicine*, vol. 56, no. 8, pp. 566–574, 2006.

[5] J. R. Wilkins III and M. E. Bowman, "Needlestick injuries among female veterinarians: frequency, syringe contents and side-effects," *Occupational Medicine*, vol. 47, no. 8, pp. 451–457, 1997.

[6] V. O. Ansa, E. J. Udoma, M. S. Umoh, and M. U. Anah, "Occupational risk of infection by human immunodeficiency and hepatitis B viruses among health workers in South-eastern Nigeria," *East African Medical Journal*, vol. 79, no. 5, pp. 254–256, 2002.

[7] WHO, *Secretariat of the Safe Injection Global Network. Health Care Worker Safety*, World Health Organization, Geneva, Switzerland, 2015, http://www.injectionsafety.org.

[8] C. O. Amira and J. O. Awobusuyi, "Needle-stick injury among health care workers in hemodialysis units in Nigeria: a multi-center study," *International Journal of Occupational and Environmental Medicine*, vol. 5, no. 1, pp. 1–8, 2014.

[9] M. E. C. Anderson and J. S. Weese, "Video observation of sharps handling and infection control practices during routine companion animal appointments," *BMC Veterinary Research*, vol. 11, article 185, 2015.

[10] A. M. Mansour, "Which physicians are at high risk for needlestick injuries?" *American Journal of Infection Control*, vol. 18, no. 3, pp. 208–210, 1990.

[11] E. R. Efetie and H. A. Salami, "Prevalence of, and attitude towards, needle-stick injuries by Nigerian gynaecological surgeons," *Nigerian Journal of Clinical Practice*, vol. 12, no. 1, pp. 34–36, 2009.

[12] A. Castella, A. Vallino, P. A. Argentero, and C. M. Zotti, "Preventability of percutaneous injuries in healthcare workers: a year-long survey in Italy," *Journal of Hospital Infection*, vol. 55, no. 4, pp. 290–294, 2003.

[13] B. L. Cullen, F. Genasi, I. Symington et al., "Potential for reported needlestick injury prevention among healthcare workers through safety device usage and improvement of guideline adherence: expert panel assessment," *Journal of Hospital Infection*, vol. 63, no. 4, pp. 445–451, 2006.

[14] J. C. Trim and T. S. J. Elliott, "A review of sharps injuries and preventative strategies," *Journal of Hospital Infection*, vol. 53, no. 4, pp. 237–242, 2003.

[15] C. Georgios, "Adverse outcome of using tilmicosin in a lamb with multiple ventricular septal defects," *Canadian Veterinary Journal*, vol. 50, no. 1, pp. 61–63, 2009.

22

A Homemade Snare: An Alternative Method for Mechanical Removal of *Dirofilaria immitis* in Dogs

Ana Margarida Alho,[1] António Fiarresga,[2] Miguel Landum,[1] Clara Lima,[3] Óscar Gamboa,[3] José Meireles,[1] José Sales Luís,[1,3] and Luís Madeira de Carvalho[1]

[1]CIISA, Faculty of Veterinary Medicine, ULisboa, Avenida da Universidade Técnica, 1300-477 Lisboa, Portugal
[2]Cardiology Unit, Hospital de Santa Marta, Centro Hospitalar de Lisboa Central, EPE, Rua de Santa Marta 50, 1169-024 Lisboa, Portugal
[3]Small Animal Teaching Hospital, Faculty of Veterinary Medicine, ULisboa, Avenida da Universidade Técnica, 1300-477 Lisboa, Portugal

Correspondence should be addressed to Ana Margarida Alho; margaridaalho@fmv.ulisboa.pt

Academic Editor: Sumanta Nandi

Canine dirofilariosis is a life-threatening parasitic disease that is increasingly reported worldwide. Once diagnosed the main treatment goals are to improve the animal's clinical condition and to eliminate all life stages of the parasite with minimal posttreatment side effects. This can be achieved through mechanical, surgical, or chemotherapeutical approaches. Currently, manual extraction is the preferred method to remove adult heartworms due to its diminished invasiveness, reduced damage to the vascular endothelium, and shortened anaesthesia duration. However, it remains an expensive technique that can be highly traumatic. To address this issue, a nontraumatic homemade catheter-guided snare was developed for heartworm removal by adapting and folding a 0.014-inch coronary wire (BMW, Abbott Vascular). Transvenous heartworm extraction was performed on a dog severely infected with adult heartworms by inserting the modified snare into a 6-F Judkins right coronary guiding catheter BMW (Cordis) and advancing it into the right ventricle under fluoroscopic guidance. Fifteen adult specimens of *Dirofilaria immitis* were successfully extracted from the pulmonary artery and right ventricle without complications. To assure the death of both larvae and adults, postoperative treatment was successfully managed using ivermectin, doxycycline, and melarsomine, with no recurrence after surgery.

1. Introduction

Canine dirofilariosis is a severe canine vector-borne disease with potentially fatal consequences. It is widely distributed throughout the world, with an increasing incidence in previously nonendemic areas [1, 2]. The main treatment goals are to improve the animal's clinical condition and to eliminate all forms of the parasite (microfilariae, larval stages, juveniles, and adults) with minimal complications. This can be achieved pharmacologically by combining melarsomine dihydrochloride, macrocyclic lactones, and doxycycline [3]. However, this approach can lead to several complications and adverse effects including pulmonary thromboembolism due to the worm death and anaphylactic shock secondary to the sudden death of high microfilariae counts [4]. For this reason, either mechanical or surgical heartworm removal is generally preferred as a means to eliminate as many adult worms as possible before pharmacological treatment is initiated. Manual extraction is the preferred method due to its diminished invasiveness, reduced damage to the vascular endothelium, and shortened anaesthesia duration [4, 5]. However, it remains an expensive technique out of the reach of many owners. Additionally, some of the available devices are also traumatic. To address these issues a nontraumatic intravascular snare was developed by adapting an economical coronary wire (commonly used in human patients) to attempt heartworm removal.

2. Materials and Methods

2.1. Case Presentation. A senior unneutered mixed-breed male dog (body weight: 6.1 kg) was presented to the Small Animal Teaching Hospital of the Faculty of Veterinary Medicine, ULisboa, with a history of severe cough, weakness, dyspnoea, exercise intolerance, and syncope. The owner reported a recent episode of hind limb weakness and temporary loss of balance which lasted for approximately 40 seconds. The dog was adopted from a shelter one month prior to presentation and his age was unknown (10 years old approximately). During the intervening period between adoption and presentation at the hospital no prophylactic treatment was initiated by the owner. On physical examination the dog had normal weight and was alert and responsive, but it was tachypnoeic and slightly dyspnoeic. Mucous membranes were pink with a capillary refill time of less than two seconds. Thoracic auscultation revealed an increased respiratory effort associated with mild crackles. A loud systolic regurgitant heart murmur (grade III approximately) was audible on the right side of the thorax, more significantly over the tricuspid valve and near the right side of the heart apex. The remainder of the physical examination was unremarkable.

2.2. Diagnostic Methods. Blood was collected from the cephalic vein and direct smears were performed. Under light microscopy, several microfilariae were observed. These were identified as *Dirofilaria immitis* using Knott modified test based on their morphometric characteristics [6]. The commercial WITNESS® Dirofilaria kit (Synbiotics Corp., Europe) was also used, supporting the previous diagnosis. A complete blood count was performed [white blood cell count, $11.3 \times 10^3/\mu L$ ($6-17 \times 10^3/\mu L$); red blood cell count, $6.2 \times 10^6/\mu L$ ($5.5-8.5 \times 10^6/\mu L$); platelet count, $347 \times 10^3/\mu L$ ($200-500 \times 10^3/\mu L$); haemoglobin, 14.1 g/dL (12-18 g/dL); haematocrit, 46.8% (37-55%); eosinophils, $1.4 \times 10^3/\mu L$ ($0.1-1.3 \times 10^3/\mu L$)], revealing a mild eosinophilia. Routine serum biochemistry profile was also performed [glucose, 107 mg/dL (60-125 mg/dL); total protein, 9.0 g/dL (5.1-7.8 g/dL); creatinine, 0.7 mg/dL (0.4-1.8 mg/dL); alkaline phosphatase, 116 $\mu l/L$ (10-150 $\mu l/L$)]. Prerenal azotaemia [blood urea nitrogen, 52.3 mg/dL (7-27 mg/dL)] and moderately increased hepatic enzymes, alanine transaminase (ALT) [240 $\mu l/L$ (5-60 $\mu l/L$)] and aspartate transaminase (AST) [96.6 $\mu l/L$ (5-55 $\mu l/L$)], were found, possibly explained by passive liver congestion due to right cardiac overload.

To assess the severity of heartworm cardiopulmonary disease, lateral and ventrodorsal radiographic projections of the thorax were made at full inspiration, revealing slight dilation of the right ventricle and bulging of the pulmonary arteries. Vertebral heart score was 9.8 (8.7-10.7) and there was no evidence of lung inflammation in the areas surrounding the pulmonary arteries. Further transthoracic echocardiography revealed the presence of linear, mobile, parallel hyperechoic

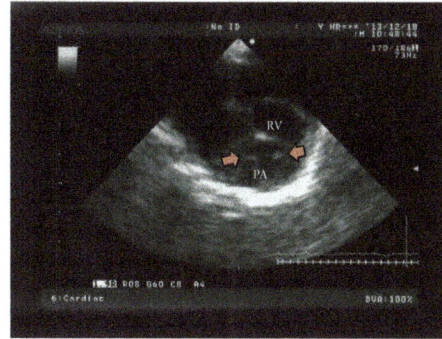

FIGURE 1: An echocardiographic image of the right ventricle (RV) and pulmonary artery (PA), in a short axis view, right parasternal section, in a right lateral decubitus. Note the presence of linear, parallel hyperechoic structures corresponding to adult worms (arrows) within the pulmonary artery.

structures (short parallel-sided images with the appearance of "equal signs") within the right ventricle outflow tract and main pulmonary artery, consistent with the presence of heartworms (Figure 1). Spectral Doppler echocardiography showed mild tricuspid regurgitation (velocity of 2.3 meters per second). Additionally, slight dilation of the right ventricle was noticed without increase of the pulmonary flow velocity or abnormal tricuspid relation between E wave and A wave [E : A ratio]. No heartworms were visualized within the tricuspid orifice or posterior vena cava, excluding the diagnosis of caval syndrome.

Considering the clinical signs exhibited by the dog (coughing, exercise intolerance, weakness, dyspnoea, and syncope), the abnormal findings on the thoracic radiography, and the visualization of hyperechoic structures consistent with parasites within the right ventricle and pulmonary artery, it was concluded that the dog was severely infected with heartworms [3] and was at high risk for thromboembolic complications. As overall survival is significantly improved in animals that undertake mechanical heartworm removal (prior to the adulticide therapy) [3], and as the echocardiography showed worms in accessible locations to be percutaneously removed, heartworm removal procedure was proposed using a homemade snare. Owner's informed consent was given and heartworm removal was scheduled.

2.3. Transvenous Heartworm Extraction Procedure. Two weeks prior to surgery the dog was stabilized with furosemide (1 mg/kg, per os [PO], twice a day [BID]) and enalapril (0.5 mg/kg, PO, once a day [SID]) to minimize cardiac overload. Also doxycycline (10 mg/kg, PO, BID) was prescribed at the same time. In order to reduce the thromboembolic risk associated with heart catheterization and adult worm death, the dog was also started on prednisolone (0.5 mg/kg, PO, BID) and cetirizine (1 mg/kg, PO, SID) one week prior to the procedure.

On the day of the procedure, the dog was premedicated with heparin (100 U/kg, subcutaneously [SC]) and an association of amoxicillin and clavulanic acid (20 mg/kg, BID, intramuscularly [IM]). Anaesthesia was induced with

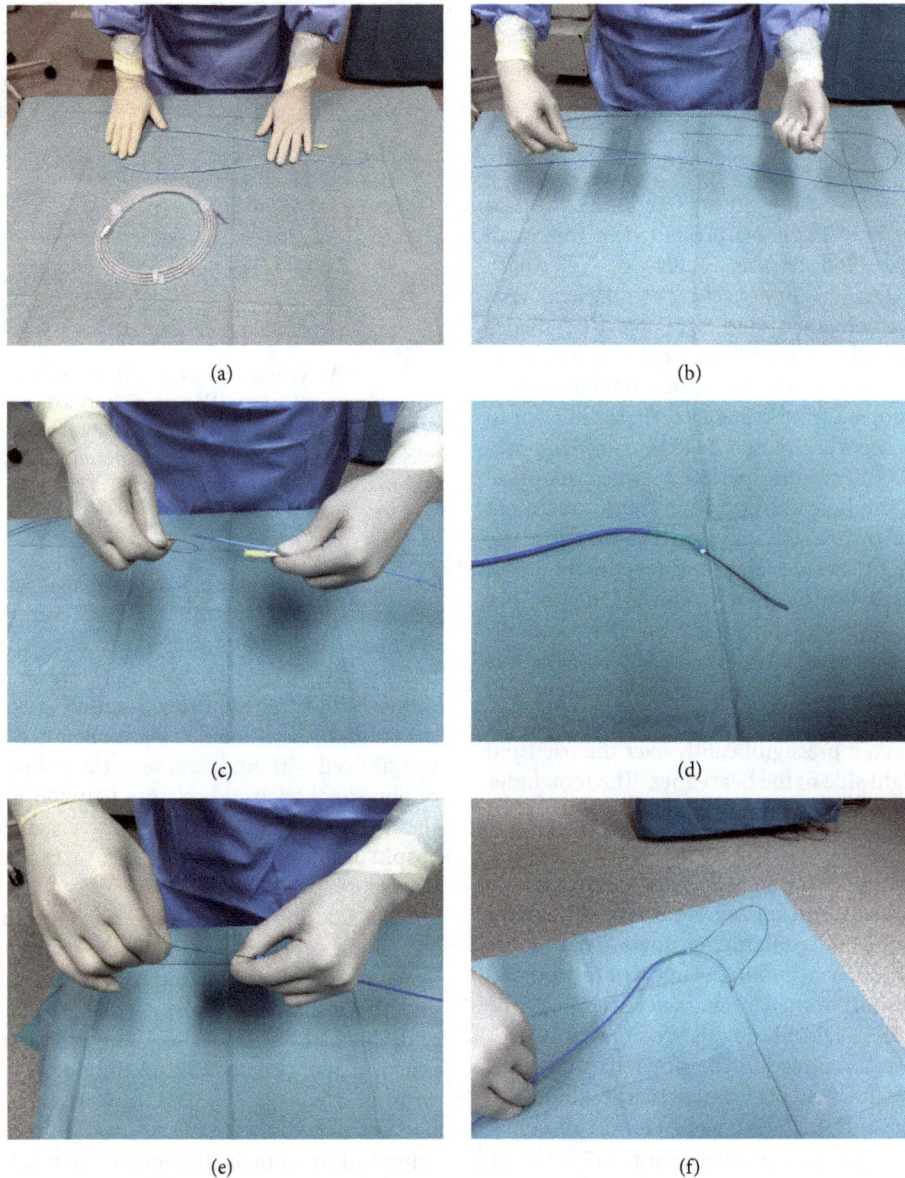

FIGURE 2: Mechanical heartworm removal device used during the procedure. (a) A snare introducer, a 6-F plastic sheath, inserted via the right external jugular vein. (b) A specific carrier, a 6-F Judkins right coronary guiding catheter BMW (Cordis). ((c), (d), and (e)) A 0.014-inch coronary wire (Boston Scientific) that was folded and pushed through the coronary guiding catheter. (f) Final aspect of the homemade snare.

propofol (4 mg/kg, intravenously [IV]) and maintained with isoflurane (2–2.5% concentration) after tracheal intubation. The dog was kept in left lateral recumbence and the right side of the cervical region was prepared. Venous puncture was performed using the Seldinger technique and a 6-F plastic sheath was introduced via the right external jugular vein. Anticoagulation was enhanced with intravenous heparin (100 U/kg). Under fluoroscopic guidance, a 6-F Judkins right coronary guiding catheter BMW (Cordis) was introduced and moved towards the cranial vena cava, right atrium, and right ventricle. A homemade snare was created by folding a 0.014-inch coronary wire (Boston Scientific) (Figure 2). This

device was subsequently inserted into the guiding catheter keeping both distal parts exteriorized. The operator fixed one of the wire extremities with one hand and moved the other end forward, adapting the size and shape of the loop according to the number and location of the worms (Figure 3). To retract the worms through the catheter, both extremities of the wire were gently withdrawn at the same time.

Since navigation into the pulmonary artery was difficult with the 8-F guiding catheter, it was downsized to a 6-F model. For this reason, a smaller device was created using 0.014-inch coronary wire (BMW, Abbott Vascular), which

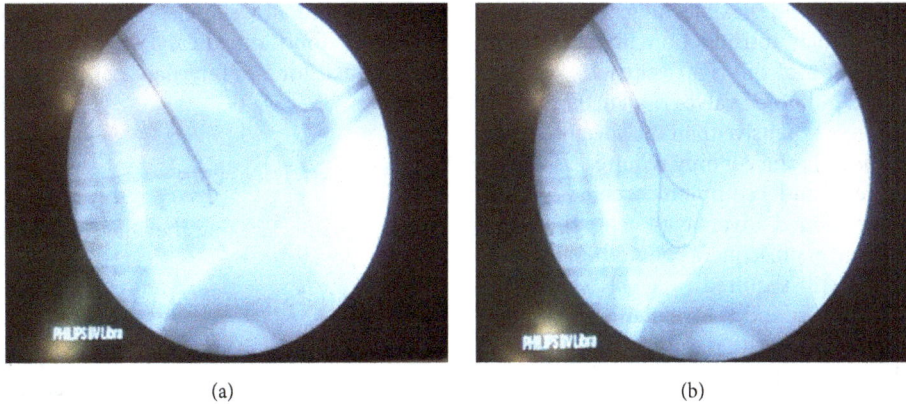

(a)   (b)

FIGURE 3: Heartworm surgical extraction under fluoroscopy guidance. (a) A 6-F Judkins guiding catheter BMW (Cordis) and the loop wire, placed at the right ventricle. (b) Increasing the size of the loop wire in order to snare the heartworms, followed by gentle retraction of the snare.

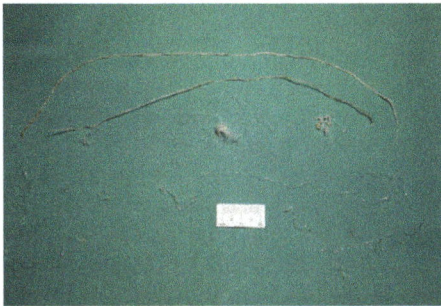

FIGURE 4: Retracted worms. Note the 15 specimens of *Dirofilaria immitis* extracted with the homemade snare from the right side of the heart and pulmonary artery.

was folded using the same method described previously. This homemade snare was then used to pull out the remaining heartworms through the sheath.

3. Results

In total, fifteen adult specimens of *Dirofilaria immitis* were caught and gently retracted through the catheter from the right ventricle and proximal portion of the pulmonary artery (Figure 4). Considering the risks of cardiac arrest and potential heart and vascular lesions due to continued catheter manipulation as well as the prolonged duration of the anaesthesia, the catheter was retracted and no further attempts were made. Haemostasis was achieved with manual compression and the dog was sent to the intensive care unit after the procedure was completed. Recovery occurred without complications and the dog was discharged after careful evaluation with amoxicillin and clavulanic acid (20 mg/kg, BID, PO) and with instructions for the owner to restrict exercise.

A postoperative reevaluation was scheduled seven days after the procedure. Once the dog was recovering well, treatment with ivermectin (10 μg/kg, PO) was initiated to prevent potential residual infection. Doxycycline (10 mg/kg, PO, for 28 days, BID) was also restarted. The first melarsomine

injection was performed 60 days after surgery (2.5 mg/kg, IM). The second and third consecutive treatments were performed 90 and 91 days after surgery, as recommended by the American Heartworm Society [3]. Exercise restriction was imposed during the entire treatment regimen.

Three months after surgery, the dog was reevaluated. Clinical signs relating to the presence of heartworms were resolved and no murmurs were auscultated. The owner reported that the dog had a good appetite and energy levels but still coughed occasionally. Routine heartworm prevention on a monthly basis was recommended. Eight months after surgery, the dog was very alert and active and no coughing was reported. An additional commercial antigen, WITNESS Dirofilaria kit, was performed, testing negative for *D. immitis* infection.

4. Discussion and Conclusion

In order to offer an affordable and safe treatment to every owner, in cases where mechanical heartworm removal is the most appropriate treatment, a catheter-guided technique using a homemade snare for adult heartworms retrieval was developed.

In general, mechanical extraction is a far less invasive and painful method when compared to cardiothoracic surgery, allowing a faster recovery and reducing the risk of infection. The snare is a safer technique when compared with forceps or the horsehair brush, since it minimizes accidental intracardiac and vascular damage, frequently associated with blind grasping [7]. The snare is also advantageous in comparison with the basket retrieval device, since the operator can control the degree of closure of the snare and thus reduce the risk of traumatizing or breaking the ensnared worms [7]. The snare's loop can also be manipulated to adopt the size, shape, or angle intended by the practitioner, increasing the likelihood of worm retrieval. In addition, since venotomy is not required to access the jugular vein, surgical closure is not necessary and the subsequent bleeding associated with catheter insertion is practically insignificant. The snare also appears to be more effective over previously described heartworm extraction methods, namely, Ishihara and flexible alligator forceps, whose size only permits their introduction into the right atrium and proximal portion of the right ventricle and not through the tricuspid and pulmonic valves [7]. Furthermore, this homemade snare is less expensive than the specific snare usually employed for this task, since it only requires a sheath, a coronary guiding catheter, and a common coronary wire.

Despite the abovementioned advantages, general anaesthesia, fluoroscopic guidance, subsequent chemotherapy, and a skilled practitioner are still required [4, 7]. Besides, the potential risk for cardiac arrest and ventricular arrhythmias caused by snare manipulation in the right ventricle or even the risk of transecting an adult heartworm still remains. Without direct visualization of the worms, the success of percutaneous heartworm extraction will always rely upon the operator's ability to ensnare the worms, which is dependent on their anatomical location and burden and the size of the parasites. To accomplish a more efficacious heartworm extraction, care must be taken to move one of the snare tips while the other is maintained in a fixed position, in order to achieve the necessary loop size.

Scant data is currently available in the literature regarding transvenous procedures for adult heartworm retrieval in companion animals. The most common reported devices used are Ishihara forceps, Jones forceps, the horsehair brush, tripod forceps [8], basket forceps [8, 9], alligator forceps [10–13], endoscopic grasping forceps, flexible three wires nail tipped forceps [14], and the gooseneck snare [7]. More sophisticated commercial snares, which include the nitinol gooseneck snare, have total and reproducible memory allowing the loop to return to a specific shape and diameter, a considerable advantage over the homemade snare. But, evidently, these are more expensive and thus are not a viable alternative for low-cost surgery [15].

Further surgical transvenous interventions need to be done to validate and improve the efficiency of this technique. Nevertheless, we believe that the possible cost reductions and less traumatic damage induced by this snare, when compared to existing alternatives, will allow adult heartworm extraction to be more affordable and consequently widespread, thereby promoting the treatment of a larger number of animals, enhancing a specific chemotherapy with higher safety.

Abbreviations

ALT: Alanine transaminase
AST: Aspartate transaminase
BID: Twice a day
E : A ratio: Relation between E wave and A wave
IM: Intramuscularly
IV: Intravenously
PO: Per os
SC: Subcutaneously
SID: Once a day.

Ethical Approval

All technical procedures were in accordance with National (DL 276/2001 and DL 314/2003) and European Legislation

regarding animal welfare and met the International Guiding Principles for Biomedical Research Involving Animals by the Council for the International Organizations of Medical Sciences.

Conflict of Interests

The authors declare that they have no competing interests.

Acknowledgments

This work was supported by Fundação para a Ciência e a Tecnologia (FCT) through the research grants reference UID/CVT/00276/2013 (CIISA, Faculty of Veterinary Medicine, ULisboa) and SFRH/BD/85427/2012. This work was done under the frame of European Network for Neglected Vectors and Vector-Borne Infections, COST Action TD1303.

References

[1] R. Morchón, E. Carretón, J. González-Miguel, and I. Mellado-Hernández, "Heartworm disease (*Dirofilaria immitis*) and their vectors in Europe—new distribution trends," *Frontiers in Physiology*, vol. 3, article 196, 2012.

[2] F. Simón, M. Siles-Lucas, R. Morchón et al., "Human and animal dirofilariasis: the emergence of a zoonotic mosaic," *Clinical Microbiology Reviews*, vol. 25, no. 3, pp. 507–544, 2012.

[3] C. T. Nelson, J. W. McCall, and D. Carithers, *Current Canine Guidelines for the Diagnosis, Prevention, and Management of Heartworm (Dirofilaria immitis) Infection in Dogs*, American Heartworm Society, 2014, https://www.heartwormsociety.org/.

[4] C. Atkins, "Canine heartworm disease," in *Textbook of Veterinary Internal Medicine: Diseases of the Dog and Cat*, S. Ettinger and E. Feldman, Eds., pp. 1353–1381, Saunders Elsevier, St. Louis, Mo, USA, 2010.

[5] C. M. Bové, S. G. Gordon, A. B. Saunders et al., "Outcome of minimally invasive surgical treatment of heartworm caval syndrome in dogs: 42 cases (1999–2007)," *Journal of the American Veterinary Medical Association*, vol. 236, no. 2, pp. 187–192, 2010.

[6] J. Magnis, S. Lorentz, L. Guardone et al., "Morphometric analyses of canine blood microfilariae isolated by the Knott's test enables *Dirofilaria immitis* and *D. repens* species-specific and *Acanthocheilonema* (syn. *Dipetalonema*) genus-specific diagnosis," *Parasites and Vectors*, vol. 6, article 48, 2013.

[7] M. T. Small, C. E. Atkins, S. G. Gordon et al., "Use of a nitinol gooseneck snare catheter for removal of adult *Dirofilaria immitis* in two cats," *Journal of the American Veterinary Medical Association*, vol. 233, no. 9, pp. 1441–1445, 2008.

[8] W. K. Yoon, R. Choi, S. G. Lee, and C. Hyun, "Comparison of 2 retrieval devices for heartworm removal in 52 dogs with heavy worm burden," *Journal of Veterinary Internal Medicine*, vol. 27, no. 3, pp. 469–473, 2013.

[9] W.-K. Yoon, D. Han, and C. Hyun, "Catheter-guided percutaneous heartworm removal using a nitinol basket in dogs with caval syndrome," *Journal of Veterinary Science*, vol. 12, no. 2, pp. 199–201, 2011.

[10] N. Arita, I. Yamane, and N. Takemura, "Comparison of canine heartworm removal rates using flexible alligator forceps guided by transesophageal echocardiography and fluoroscopy," *Journal of Veterinary Medical Science*, vol. 65, no. 2, pp. 259–261, 2003.

[11] Y. Sasaki, H. Kitagawa, K. Ishihara, and T. Masegi, "Improvement in pulmonary arterial lesions after heartworm removal using flexible alligator forceps," *Nippon Juigaku Zasshi*, vol. 52, no. 4, pp. 743–752, 1990.

[12] R. B. Atwell and A. L. Litster, "Surgical extraction of transplanted adult *Dirofilaria immitis* in cats," *Veterinary Research Communications*, vol. 26, no. 4, pp. 301–308, 2002.

[13] H. Y. Yoon, S. W. Jeong, J. Y. Kim et al., "The efficacy of surgical treatment with flexible alligator forceps in dogs with heartworm infection," *Journal of Veterinary Clinics*, vol. 22, pp. 309–313, 2005.

[14] S.-G. Lee, H.-S. Moon, and C. Hyun, "Percutaneous heartworm removal from dogs with severe heart worm (*Dirofilaria immitis*) infestation," *Journal of Veterinary Science*, vol. 9, no. 2, pp. 197–202, 2008.

[15] C. Mullins, "Foreign body removal," in *Cardiac Catheterization in Congenital Heart Disease: Pediatric and Adult*, pp. 359–360, Blackwell Publishing, Oxford, UK, 2006.

23

Subsequent Fertility of Goats with Prenatal Mortality Diagnosed by Ultrasound and Treated by $PGF_{2\alpha}$ and Oxytetracycline

A. S. Aban,[1] **R. M. Abdelghafar,**[2] **M. E. Badawi,**[2] **and A. M. Almubarak**[2]

[1]*Department of Surgery and Gynecology, Faculty of Veterinary Medicine, Upper Nile University, Malakal, South Sudan*
[2]*Department of Veterinary Medicine and Surgery, College of Veterinary Medicine, Sudan University of Science and Technology, Khartoum, Sudan*

Correspondence should be addressed to R. M. Abdelghafar; rehabeen@gmail.com

Academic Editor: Francesca Mancianti

Thirteen Saanen and Saanen crossbred female goats, between the ages of 6 months and 7, years were presented to the clinic, College of Veterinary Medicine, Sudan University of Science and Technology, for sonographic pregnancy diagnosis. Transabdominal ultrasound was performed using 3.5 MHz probe which revealed non-viable fetuses as judged by absence of heart beats and movements. Twelve goats were given single i/m injection of $PGF_{2\alpha}$ analogue and 5% oxytetracycline. Ten goats responded to the treatment and six of them became pregnant and gave birth within the normal gestational period. One goat was diagnosed as non-pregnant, one goat developed hydrometra, and the subsequent fertility of two goats was unknown. Two full-term goats did not respond to treatment. Another dose of $PGF_{2\alpha}$ was administered to them and again they did not respond. Manual attempts were done to deliver the full-term goat with dilated cervix and they were unsuccessful. Cesarean section and hysterectomy were then performed for the three full-term goats with unfavorable outcome. It can be concluded that ultrasound is a rapid, reliable, and nonhazardous procedure for the diagnosis of fetal mortality in goats and $PGF_{2\alpha}$ treatment in conjunction with oxytetracycline is an efficient treatment.

1. Introduction

Sudan possesses about 31 million goats [1]. Small ruminants, especially goats, are very important in rural economy and have potentially been used as a tool for poverty alleviation [2]. Fetal death is defined as cessation of heart beats and absence of fetal movement [3, 4]. Embryonic and fetal mortality contribute to large economic loss [5]. Economic losses resulting from fetal death are substantial since they include not only the loss of offspring but also a prolonged open period for the dam leading to increased culling rates [4]. The high rate of embryonic loss (25–40%) in domestic species during early pregnancy may result in false positive diagnosis [6]. The causes of fetal death are multifactorial and can be divided broadly into infectious and non-infectious origin with the most frequently detected infectious agents being bacteria, viruses, fungi, and parasites. Non-infectious causes of fetal death include malnutrition, stress, maternal endocrine imbalance, and ambient temperature [7–9]. Several infectious agents that cause fetal death and abortion are zoonotic, for example, *Brucella, Listeria, Coxiella, Chlamydia,* and *Toxoplasma* [7].

Early and accurate diagnosis of pregnancy, determination of litter size, and estimation of gestational age in livestock are crucial for improving efficiency of reproduction in goats [10–13]. Ultrasound technique has become an essential tool in veterinary medicine for the evaluation of intrauterine life of the fetus [14]. Lack of echogenicity of amniotic fluid, the proper amount of fluid for the gestational stage, and normal fetal posture and movement are signs of a healthy fetus [15].

Fetal size incompatible with the expected gestational age may indicate earlier fetal death. Absence of heart beats and movements, increased fluid echogenicity, collapsed fetal posture, and hyperechogenicity of the cotyledons are a common finding in a non-viable pregnancy [7, 15]. If fetal degeneration occurs, sonographic image will demonstrate an undifferentiated image of the uterine content with anechoic to hyperechoic structure [16]. The exact outcome of antenatal death is unpredictable and is influenced by several factors, including the cause of fetal mortality, differences in pregnancy between species, stage of gestation at fetal death, and number of fetuses [17]. Early embryonic death with the loss of corpus luteum produces a subsequent return to estrus following resorption of the embryonic material [15]. However, the outcome in case of failure of the corpus luteum to undergo luteolysis may be prolonged gestation, pyometra, or fetal mummification [18, 19]. In cases of abortion and fetal maceration, the hormonal support of pregnancy is lost [20]. Major infectious agents of abortion in goats are *Chlamydia, Toxoplasma, Leptospira, Brucella, Coxiella burnetii,* and *Listeria.* Non-infectious causes of abortion may be genetic, chromosomal, hormonal, and nutritional. Nutritional factors include plant toxins, such as broom weed or locoweed poisoning; dietary deficiencies of copper, selenium, vitamin A, and magnesium; certain drugs such as estrogen, glucocorticoids, phenothiazine, carbon tetrachloride, and levamisole in late gestation [3, 20].

Prostaglandins are secreted by almost all body tissues. $PGF_{2\alpha}$ is the natural luteolytic agent that terminates the luteal phase of the oestrous cycle and allows for the initiation of a new one in the absence of fertilization, and it is particularly potent in terminating early pregnancy [3].

Administration of prostaglandin $F_{2\alpha}$ and its agonist cloprostenol is an efficient treatment of fetal death in does [21]. It has been concerned in the changes that occur in the connective tissue of the cervix at labor onset and stimulates contractions of the uterus [3, 22]. Unlike other ruminants where placenta-derived progesterone becomes significant, the goat depends on corpus-luteum-derived progesterone throughout pregnancy and is thus susceptible to luteolytic agents, including prostaglandins, throughout the whole period of pregnancy [15].

To the best of the authors' knowledge, few case reports have been published in the Sudan regarding diagnosis of fetal death in goats using ultrasound technique [23, 24]; however, treatment, follow-up, and subsequent reproductive performance were not reported. Thus, the aim of the current research was to report sonographic diagnosis of antenatal mortality, treatment, and consequent reproductive performance in goats for the first time.

2. Materials and Methods

2.1. Animals. Two nulliparous and 11 pluriparous ($n = 13$) Saanen and Saanen crossbred female goats were included in the present study. Their ages were between 6 months and 7 years. The goats were presented to the Veterinary Teaching Hospital, College of Veterinary Medicine, Sudan University of Science and Technology (SUST), during the period of March 2015-2016 for sonographic pregnancy diagnosis. Ten goats presented for routine pregnancy diagnosis because of absence of estrus and three goats were presented because they did not give birth at the estimated gestational age as determined early by ultrasonography.

2.2. Methods

2.2.1. Clinical Examination. Full clinical examination was done for all goats. Ten goats were alert, in a good condition and all physiological parameters were within the normal range. Regarding the three full-term goats, one of them had a hard palpable immobile abdominal mass, the os cervix was closed, respiratory and heart beats were normal, and the general condition of the goat was not altered. The second goat had dilated cervix and fetid bloody stained vaginal discharge was realized. The general condition of the goat was poor with greatly increased heart beats and respiratory rate. The 3rd goat had a closed cervix.

2.3. Ultrasound Scanning

2.3.1. Animal Preparations. Animals were deprived from food for 12 hours prior to the scanning to avoid accumulation of gases into the gastrointestinal tract. Area of scanning which extends across the width of the abdomen, passing from one side of the udder, a cross the abdomen in front of the udder, to the other side and 15 cm anterior to the udder [25] was clipped and shaved carefully using manual clippers (Super-Max, Green, Feltham, London TW13 7LR, UK). A copious amount of ultrasonic gel (Aquasonic, Parker Laboratories, Inc., Fairfield, NJ 07004, USA) was applied to the ventral abdomen prior to scanning.

2.3.2. Animal Positioning. Animals were turned on their backs (dorsal decubitus) and well restrained on especially designed table.

2.3.3. Machine and Image Recording. Transabdominal ultrasonography was performed using a real-time ultrasound scanner (Pie Medical, Esaote, Netherlands) equipped with dual frequency (3.5–5) MHz convex transducer. Sagittal, parasagittal, and cross sections were taken to ascertain accurate diagnosis. Images were stored in a memory card attached to the scanner and later were printed in thermal papers (Sony Corporation, type 1, Normal, UPP-110S, 1-7-1, Konan, Minato-ku, Tokyo, Japan) using video graphic printer UP-895EC (Sony, Japan).

3. Results

3.1. Ultrasound Scanning. Ultrasonographic examination of the thirteen goats revealed non-viable fetuses characterized by absence of heart beats and fetal movements. Regarding the full-term goats with dead fetuses, fetal fluids were greatly diminished and distal acoustic shadowing was clearly realized. Out of thirteen goats, two were diagnosed as having dead twins (Figure 1) and 11 were diagnosed as having single dead fetus (Figure 2). Three goats were diagnosed at gestational age of about 60 days, three at about 40 days, four at about 120 days, and three goats at full term.

3.2. Treatment and Consequent Fertility. Twelve goats were treated using intramuscular injection of $PGF_{2\alpha}$ analogue

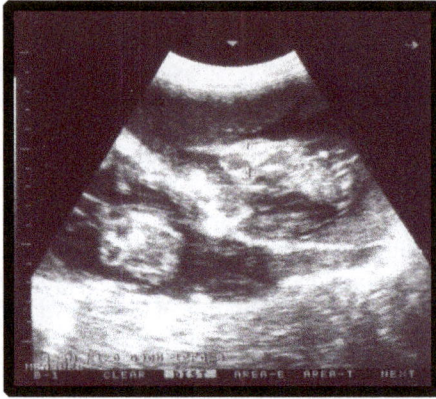

FIGURE 1: Dead twins at 60 days of gestation (arrows).

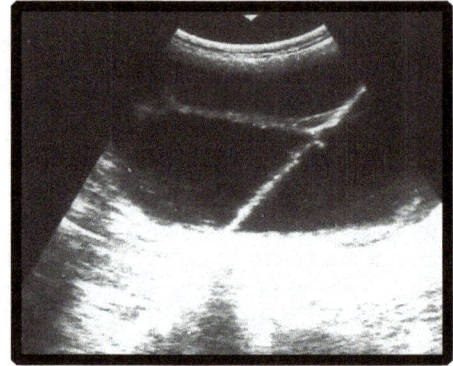

FIGURE 2: Single dead fetus at 120 days of gestation (arrow).

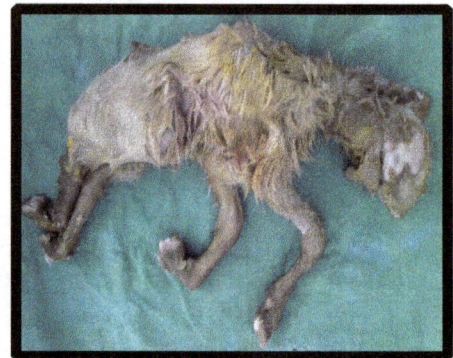

FIGURE 3: Hydrometra.

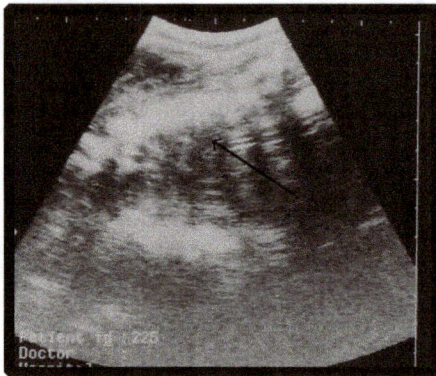

FIGURE 4: Full-term dead fetus removed by cesarean section.

(Estrumate 125 μg i/m, Schering-Plough Animals Health, Germany) and oxytetracycline (5%) with a dose rate of 0.5 mL and 5 mL (for five consecutive days), respectively. After treatment, ten goats responded successfully to the treatment as judged by dilatation of the cervix, abortion of fetuses after 48–96 hours. The animals returned to estrus and the animals' owners were advised to breed their goats at the next coming oestrus cycle. Six out of ten goats were diagnosed later as pregnant as confirmed by ultrasonography and gave birth at the normal gestational period. Two goats were not mated and thus the subsequent fertility was unknown. One goat was diagnosed as non-pregnant and one goat developed hydrometra (Figure 3). Two full-term goats did not respond to the treatment and another dose of PGF$_{2\alpha}$ was administered. The goats did not respond to the treatment for the second time and hence were referred to surgery. Regarding the third full-term goat with dilated cervix, more than a few attempts were made to deliver the goat, but all attempts were unsuccessful. Supportive treatment and broad-spectrum antibiotic injection was administered to the goat and also referred to surgery. Cesarean section and hysterectomy were performed for the three full-term goats and fetuses were removed (Figure 4) with unfavorable outcome.

4. Discussion

Pregnancy diagnosis can be performed accurately using real-time ultrasonography. Transabdominal ultrasound can detect the embryo with its heart beat by day 27 of gestation [26]. Fertilization rate in domestic animals is generally very high; however, as many as 65% are lost during embryonic and fetal development [19].

The most serious curtailment of efficient animal production and herd profitability is pregnancy loss [27]. Reproductive efficiency was affected by fertilization failure and embryonic mortality with the latter being the more significant [28]. Prenatal death is divided into embryonic and fetal death [3]. Embryonic mortality denotes the death of fertilized ova and embryos up to the end of implantation [29].

In early pregnancy stages, dying embryos usually undergo a partial degeneration process before being expelled [30]. Several factors have been implicated in embryo and fetal loss and are normally categorized as those of genetic, physiological, endocrine, and environmental origin [31]. Results of the current study revealed that death can occur at any time during gestation; however, the exact outcome of fetal mortality is unpredictable and influenced by several factors, such as the cause of the death, stage of gestational age, and number of fetuses [17]. Results showed that fetal death occurring during 2–4 months had excellent consequence; however, fetal death at full-term gestation had unfavorable outcome. It was concluded that real-time ultrasonography is a rapid, accurate, and nondisruptive method for diagnosis of antenatal death and prostaglandin $F_{2\alpha}$ and oxytetracycline proved to be efficient treatment for fetal death during 2–4 months of gestation.

Competing Interests

The authors declared that there are no competing interests regarding this manuscript.

Acknowledgments

This study was kindly funded by the Scientific Research Council (SRC), Sudan University of Science and Technology (Grant no. RP 07-010).

References

[1] MOAR, "Ministry of animal resources, estimate of animal population," in *Statistical Bulletin for Animal Resources*, vol. 23, Information Center, Khartoum, Sudan, 2015.

[2] A. Aziz, "Present status of the world goat populations and their productivity," *Lohmann Information*, vol. 45, no. 2, pp. 42–52, 2010.

[3] B. Hafez and E. S. E. Hafez, *Reproduction in farm animals*, Lippincott Williams & Wilkins, Baltimore, Maryland, USA, 7th edition, 2000.

[4] H. Samir, A. Karen, T. Ashmawy, M. Abo-Ahmed, M. El-Sayed, and G. Watanabe, "Monitoring of embryonic and fetal losses in different breeds of goats using real-time B-mode ultrasonography," *Theriogenology*, vol. 85, no. 2, pp. 207–215, 2016.

[5] A. B. Dixon, M. Knights, J. L. Winkler et al., "Patterns of late embryonic and fetal mortality and association with several factors in sheep," *Journal of Animal Science*, vol. 85, no. 5, pp. 1274–1284, 2007.

[6] E. P. B. X. Moraes, L. M. Freitas Neto, C. R. Aguiar Filho et al., "Mortality determination and gender identification of conceptuses in pregnancies of Santa Ines ovine by ultrasound," *South African Journal of Animal Sciences*, vol. 39, no. 4, pp. 307–312, 2009.

[7] F. H. Jonker, "Fetal death: comparative aspects in large domestic animals," *Animal Reproduction Science*, vol. 82-83, pp. 415–430, 2004.

[8] I. F. M. Marai, A. A. El-Darawany, A. Fadiel, and M. A. M. Abdel-Hafez, "Physiological traits as affected by heat stress in sheep: a review," *Small Ruminant Research*, vol. 71, no. 1–3, pp. 1–12, 2007.

[9] A. Orman, C. Kara, E. Topal, and E. Carkungoz, "Effects of supplementary nutrition in yearling saanen kids on sexual behaviors and reproductive traits," *Journal of Animal and Veterinary Advances*, vol. 9, no. 24, pp. 3098–3103, 2010.

[10] S. Yotov, "Diagnostics of early pregnancy in Stara Zagora dairy sheep breed," *Bulgarian Journal of Veterinary Medicine*, vol. 8, pp. 41–45, 2005.

[11] H. Oral, S. M. Pancarci, O. Gungor, and C. Kacar, "Determination of gestational age by measuring fetal heart diameter with transrectal ultrasonograph in sheep," *Medycyna Weterynaryjna*, vol. 63, no. 12, pp. 1558–1560, 2007.

[12] M. Anwar, A. Riaz, N. Ullah, and M. Rafig, "Use of ultrasonography for pregnancy diagnosis in Balkhi sheep," *Pakistan Veterinary Journal*, vol. 28, pp. 144–146, 2008.

[13] K. Suguna, S. Mehrotra, S. K. Agarwal et al., "Early pregnancy diagnosis and embryonic and fetal development using real time B mode ultrasound in goats," *Small Ruminant Research*, vol. 80, no. 1–3, pp. 80–86, 2008.

[14] G. Serin, Ö. Gökdal, T. Tarimcilar, and O. Atay, "Umbilical artery doppler sonography in Saanen goat fetuses during singleton and multiple pregnancies," *Theriogenology*, vol. 74, no. 6, pp. 1082–1087, 2010.

[15] J. Matthews, *Diseases of the Goat*, Blackwell, 3rd edition, 2009.

[16] J. W. Hesselink and M. A. Taverne, "Ultrasonography of the uterus of the goat," *Veterinary Quarterly*, vol. 16, no. 1, pp. 41–45, 1994.

[17] R. C. Lefebvre, É. Saint-Hilaire, I. Morin, G. B. Couto, D. Francoz, and M. Babkine, "Retrospective case study of fetal mummification in cows that did not respond to prostaglandin $F_{2\alpha}$ treatment," *Canadian Veterinary Journal*, vol. 50, no. 1, pp. 71–76, 2009.

[18] P. Chauhan, P. Kapadiya, T. Sutaria, H. Nakhashi, and V. Sharma, "Retention of mummified fetus due to uterine inertia after kidding in doe," *Veterinary Clinical Science*, vol. 2, no. 4, pp. 64–66, 2014.

[19] D. E. Noakes, T. J. Parkinson, and G. C. England, *Veterinary Reproduction and Obstetrics*, W. B. Saunders, Elsevier, New York, NY, USA, 9th edition, 2009.

[20] S. Aiello and M. Moses, *Prolonged Gestation Associated with Fetal Death*, The Merck Veterinary Manual, Kenilworth, UK, 11th edition, 2012.

[21] A. Ali, "Causes and management of dystocia in small ruminants in Saudia Arabia," *Journal of Agricultural and Veterinary Sciences*, vol. 4, no. 2, pp. 95–108, 2011.

[22] H. K. Palliser, J. J. Hirst, G. E. Rice et al., "Labor-associated regulation of prostaglandin E and F synthesis and action in the ovine amnion and cervix," *Journal of the Society for Gynecologic Investigation*, vol. 13, no. 1, pp. 19–24, 2006.

[23] R. M. Abdelghafar, "Ultrasonography as a diagnostic tool for fetal mortality in goats (Capra hircus) in the Sudan (two case reports)," *Assiut Veterinary Medical Journal*, vol. 56, no. 127, pp. 316–322, 2010.

[24] R. M. Abdelghafar, "Fetal death in Saanen goats: case reports," *Ruminant Science*, vol. 4, no. 2, pp. 231–233, 2015.

[25] P. J. Goddard, *Veterinary Ultrasonography*, Cab International, Wallingford, UK, 1995.

[26] G. R. Padilla-Rivas, B. Sohnrey, and W. Holtz, "Early pregnancy detection by real-time ultrasonography in Boer goats," *Small Ruminant Research*, vol. 58, no. 1, pp. 87–92, 2005.

[27] G. P. Allen, "The pregnancy that doesn't stay—lessons from 25 years of observation," *Veterinary journal (London, England : 1997)*, vol. 153, no. 3, pp. 239–244, 1997.

[28] N. Bajaj, M. Panchal, I. Kalyani, and V. Kavani, "Bacterial isolates and antibiotic sensitivity spectrum of cervico-vaginal mucus of endometritic buffaloes," *JNKVV Research Journal*, vol. 40, pp. 91–95, 2006.

[29] N. K. Bajaj and N. Sharma, "Endocrine causes of early embryonic death: an overview," *Current Research in Dairy Sciences*, vol. 3, no. 1, pp. 1–24, 2011.

[30] O. J. Ginther, "Embryonic loss in mares: incidence, time of occurrence, and hormonal involvement," *Theriogenology*, vol. 23, no. 1, pp. 77–89, 1985.

[31] M. G. Diskin and D. G. Morris, "Embryonic and early foetal losses in cattle and other ruminants," *Reproduction in Domestic Animals*, vol. 43, supplement 2, pp. 260–267, 2008.

24

Prevalence and Antimicrobial Susceptibility Pattern of *E. coli* O157:H7 Isolated from Traditionally Marketed Raw Cow Milk in and around Asosa Town, Western Ethiopia

Nigatu Disassa,[1] **Berhanu Sibhat,**[2] **Shimelis Mengistu,**[2] **Yimer Muktar,**[2] **and Dinaol Belina**[2]

[1]*Assosa University, P.O. Box 18, Assosa, Ethiopia*
[2]*Haramaya University College of Veterinary Medicine, P.O. Box 138, Dire Dawa, Ethiopia*

Correspondence should be addressed to Shimelis Mengistu; shimemenge@yahoo.com

Academic Editor: William Ravis

A cross-sectional study was conducted from October 2014 to July 2015 to determine the prevalence and populations of *E. coli* as well as the prevalence and antimicrobial susceptibility of *E. coli* O157:H7 isolated from raw milk. Biochemical and serological tests methods were used to confirm *E. coli* and *E. coli* O157:H7 and isolates were subjected to antimicrobial susceptibility test using the agar disc diffusion method. Out of 380 raw milk samples examined, 129 (33.9%) and 11 (2.9%) were contaminated with *E. coli* and *E. coli* O157:H7, respectively. The highest prevalence was recorded in samples obtained from vendors (39.1%, $4.978 \pm 0.180 \log_{10}$/ml) compared with samples from farmers (28.1%, $3.93 \pm 0.01 \log_{10}$/ml) with significant differences ($P = 0.02$). The frequency of contamination was higher in the samples collected from milk that was stored and transported in plastic containers (39.4%) than in the containers made of stainless steel (23.0%) ($P = 0.002$). The antimicrobial susceptibility profile showed that *E. coli* O157:H7 were resistant to tetracycline (81.8%), streptomycin (81.8%), and kanamycin (63.6%). Milk samples were produced and handled under poor hygienic conditions, stored, and transported in inappropriate containers and under temperature abuse conditions leading to high health risk to the consumers. Additional studies would be needed to establish association between the occurrences of *E. coli* O157:H7 in raw milk and all the risk factors involved in and around Asosa town.

1. Introduction

Escherichia coli is a normal inhabitant of the intestines of animals and humans; its recovery from food may be of public health concern due to the possible presence of enteropathogenic and/or toxigenic strains which lead to sever gastrointestinal disturbance. It is among many pathogenic microorganisms which can get access to milk and dairy products and is considered as a reliable indicator of contamination by manure, soil, and contaminated water [1, 2].

Outbreaks of VTEC infections involving serogroup O157 have been reported from different countries of the world including United States, Canada, Asia, Australia, Europe, and Africa through various sources of infection and different case fatality [3]. In southern Africa and Swaziland in 1992 an outbreak of *E. coli* O157:H7 affecting thousands was attributed to contamination of surface water with cattle dung and animal carcasses. Dairy products (milk and cheese), both unpasteurized and pasteurized, of bovine and ovine origin have been implicated in VTEC infections. This has included a number of outbreaks among children that have been attributed to the consumption of raw milk and dairy products. Antibiotic use in VTEC infections is controversial because of the potential to increase production and secretion of Shiga toxins. However, increase in antibiotic resistance has been noted over the last 20 years [4–7].

Food borne diseases are common in developing countries, including Ethiopia, because of the prevailing poor food handling and sanitation practices, inadequate food safety laws, weak regulatory systems, lack of financial resources to invest in safer equipment, and lack of education for food-handlers. The National Hygiene and Sanitation Strategy program reported that about 60% of the disease burden was related to poor hygiene and sanitation in Ethiopia. Unsafe sources, contaminated raw food items, improper food storage, poor personal hygiene during food preparation, inadequate cooling and reheating of food items, and a prolonged time lapse between preparing and consuming food items have been identified as contributing factors for outbreaks of food borne diseases [8, 9].

The consumption of raw milk and its derivatives is common in Ethiopia, which is not safe from a consumer health point of view as it may lead to the transmission of various diseases [10]. The ability of raw or processed milk to support the growth of several spoilage or pathogenic microorganisms can lead to spoilage of the product or infections and intoxications in consumers. The most commonly known bacterial pathogens still of concern today in raw milk and other dairy products include *Bacillus cereus*, *Listeria monocytogenes*, *Yersinia enterocolitica*, *Salmonella* spp., *Escherichia coli*, and *Campylobacter jejuni*, among which *E. coli* O157:H7 was the focus of this study [1, 11, 12].

Even though milk represents an important food in consumers' nutrition as well as in the nutrition and income of producers, there is limited work so far undertaken regarding the assessment of the bacteriological quality and safety of raw cow milk in western Ethiopia, in general, and in Assosa town, in particular. Therefore, the aim of the present study was to determine the prevalence and antimicrobial susceptibility pattern of *E. coli* and *E. coli* O157:H7 and to evaluate the hygienic condition of raw cow milk at two different points that are considered as critical points (farmers and vendors) in the value chain in Asosa of western Ethiopia.

2. Materials and Methods

2.1. Description of the Study Area. Asosa is a town found in Asosa zone in western Ethiopia and the capital of the Benishangul-Gumuz Regional State, Ethiopia. The town is located at latitude and longitude of 10°04′N 34°31′E, with an elevation of 1570 meters, at 476 km distance from the capital city of the country, Addis Ababa. In this area, the mixed farming system is dominant, in which about 92.5% of the population is engaged in agriculture as a major means of subsistence. The region is bordered with the Sudan in the west, Amhara Regional State in the east and north, Oromia Regional State in the east and south east, and Gambella Regional State in the south. Three administrative zones, one special woreda, 19 woredas, and 425 kebeles exist in the region. It covers a total area of about 5,038,100 hectares. Plain undulating slopes and mountains characterize the topography of the region. The agroclimatic zone of the region is categorized as 75% "*kola*," 24% "*woinadega*," and 1% "*dega*."

The rainfall distribution pattern is monomodal, commencing towards the end of April and ending in October. The topography of the woreda is mainly plain [13].

2.2. Study Design. A cross-sectional study was conducted from October 2014 to July 2015 to determine the prevalence and populations of *E. coli* with emphasis on *E. coli* O157:H7 in bovine milk and to determine the antimicrobial sensitivity of the *E. coli* O157:H7 isolates.

2.3. Sample Size Determination. The prevalence of the selected bacteria at the study area was not known; hence, the required sample size was calculated considering a previously published prevalence estimate of 44.4% [10] reported from a study on the microbial quality of milk in Mekelle town. Accordingly, a total of 380 (178 from farmers and 202 from venders) raw cow milk samples, each consisting of 25 ml, were collected at weekly intervals.

2.4. Sampling Methods and Procedures. First, a baseline survey was conducted to identify the total number of farms, farm size, farming system, and the status and number of vendors in and around the Asosa town. According to the results of the survey all farms were at the household/smallholder level, with farm size not more than 4 cows per farm. Then, a total of 60 small farms and 25 small vendors were identified as main sources of milk for consumers in and around the town and included in the study using stratified sampling methods. A simple random sampling technique was applied to collect raw milk samples from each group of vendors. Then all individuals involved directly or indirectly in milk production and marketing were communicated to allow us permission to obtain samples and provide us with relevant information. After that, 178 milk samples were collected aseptically using sterile test tubes from milking buckets immediately after milking and 202 raw milk samples were collected from vendors' containers. The samples were transported to the Asosa Regional Veterinary Research Laboratory under refrigeration (using ice boxes) for bacteriological analysis. The examination of milk samples was conducted within 4 hours after collection. Isolation and identification of *E. coli* O157:H7 were also conducted in the laboratory and antimicrobial sensitivity test was undertaken for *E. coli* O157:H7 isolates.

In addition to this, questionnaires and observation check lists were used as a tool to gather information (data) on the hygienic practices during milking, handling, storage, transportation, duration of transportation, and storage of the milk by the stakeholders and their knowledge regarding diseases associated with milk, in order to assess the associated risks.

3. Study Methodologies

3.1. Isolation and Identification of E. coli and E. coli O157:H7. Each raw cow milk sample was enriched using EC-broth at 37°C for 24 hours, inoculated on MacConkey agar, and then incubated at 37°C for 24 hours. Typical colonies on MacConkey agar (pink, due to their ability to ferment lactose) were stained using gram stain and observed for their staining and morphological characteristics and transferred to eosin-methylene-blue (EMB) agar. The colonies with metallic sheen on EMB agar which is typical feature of *E. coli* were transferred to sorbitol MacConkey agar to check the presence of *E. coli* O157:H7 phenotype (inability to ferment sorbitol). Then the confirmed pure cultures considered as *E. coli* positive were transferred to nutrient agar to be used for additional confirmatory biochemical tests (IMViC tests) and serological tests as described below [14]

TABLE 1: Prevalence of *E. coli* in the study samples in different conditions.

	Tested samples	Presence of *E. coli*		Presence of *E. coli* O157:H7	
		Negative	Positive	Negative	Positive
Farm	178 (46.8%)	128 (71.9%)	50 (28.1%)	177 (99.4%)	1 (0.6%)
Vendor	202 (53.2%)	123 (60.9%)	79 (39.1%)	192 (95.0%)	10 (5%)
X^2		5.12		6.48	
P value		0.02		0.01	
Good*	150 (39.5%)	112 (74.7%)	38 (25.3%)	149 (99.3%)	1 (0.7%)
Poor**	230 (60.5%)	139 (60.4%)	91 (39.6%)	220 (95.7%)	10 (4.3%)
X^2		8.20		4.38	
P value		0.004		0.04	
Plastic***	234 (66.2%)	154 (60.6%)	100 (39.4%)	245 (96.5%)	9 (3.5%)
Steel****	126 (33.2%)	97 (77.0%)	29 (23.0%)	124 (98.4%)	2 (1.6%)
X^2		10.05		1.15	
P value		0.002		0.28	
<1 hour	197 (51.8%)	136 (69.0%)	61 (31.0%)	195 (99%)	2 (1%)
1–4 hours	96 (25.3%)	43 (44.8%)	26 (27.1%)	93 (96.9%)	3 (3.1%)
>4 hours	87 (22.9%)	45 (51.7%)	42 (48.3%)	81 (93.1%)	6 (6.9%)
X^2		13.2		4.81	
P value		0.001		0.09	
Total	380 (100%)	251 (66.1%)	129 (33.9%)	369 (97.1%)	11 (2.9%)

*Milk containers are usually cleaned properly before and after milking using quality water with help of detergent and using of containers made of stainless steel.
**The condition that does not fulfill or partially fulfill the first case.
***Samples collected from raw cow milk held in containers made of plastic.
****Samples collected from raw cow milk held in container made of stainless steel.

3.2. Serological Test.
The *E. coli*-sorbitol-negative colonies were serologically confirmed by using *E. coli* O157:H7 latex agglutination assay containing latex particles coated with antibodies specific for the *E. coli* O157 and the *E. coli* H7 antigen. Identification of *E. coli* O157:H7 was carried out following the manufacturer's instructions; hence colonies that agglutinated were considered to be *E. coli* O157:H7.

3.3. Enumeration of E. coli.
Milk samples (25 ml) were diluted in buffered peptone saline water (225 ml); serial dilution of 10^{-1}, 10^{-2}, and 10^{-3} was applied in order to quantify this microbial group. Most probable number (MPN) method was used after serial dilutions to estimate the populations of *E. coli*. *E. coli* was enumerated by growing each serial dilution in 3 test tubes in *Escherichia coli* broth (EC-broth) after 24/48 hours of incubation at 45°C as stated in [14].

3.4. Antimicrobial Susceptibility Testing.
Mueller-Hinton agar media were used for susceptibility testing according to the criteria of the National Committee for Clinical Laboratory Standards [15]. The isolated *E. coli* O157:H7 strains were tested for sensitivity to the most commonly used antimicrobials including, cefoxitin (CF) (5 μg), gentamicin (GCN) (10 μg), kanamycin (K) (30 μg), norfloxacin (NOR) (10 μg), streptomycin (S) (10 μg), trimethoprim-sulfamethoxazole (SXT) (25 μg), and tetracycline (TE) (30 μg).

3.5. Data Analysis.
The data obtained was coded and entered in Excel 2010 for storage and then entered in to data editor view of SPSS (Version 20) for statistical analysis. Cross tabulation was used to calculate the frequencies of the parameters of the variables. In some cases, the chi-square statistic was used to test for significant difference in prevalence of *E. coli* in raw milk samples collected from raw milks managed in different conditions considered as risk factors. The level of significance was set at 0.05. The microbiological count data per milliliter of sample was transformed to logarithm of base ten (log counts ml^{-1}) before statistical analysis and the results are presented as the geometric means.

4. Results and Discussion

4.1. Microbiological Isolation and Identification.
Out of the 380 raw cow milk samples collected in the present study, *E. coli* was isolated from 129 (33.9%) of the samples based on morphological and cultural characteristics and also biochemical tests (Table 1). This prevalence is lower when compared to reports of [10] from Mekelle town, [16] from Britain, [17] from South India, and [18] from Malaysia who reported prevalence of *E. coli* from raw milk of 44.4%, 63%, 70%, and 65%, respectively. On the other hand, [19] reported a 38.0% prevalence from India.

The variation that was seen in prevalence in different studies may be due to difference in sample size, farming

TABLE 2: Mean (±SE) count ($\log_{10}$/ml) of *E. coli* in raw cow milk from two different sources collected under different conditions.

	Range	Mean	95% CI for mean value		SE
			Lower	Upper	
Sources					
Farmer	1.10–7.00	4.720	4.312	5.127	0.203
Vendors	1.10–7.00	4.978	4.620	5.336	0.180
Hygienic condition					
Good	1.10–7.00	4.556	3.983	5.111	0.278
Poor	1.81–7.00	5.016	4.416	5.316	0.151
Containers					
Plastic	1.10–7.00	4.926	4.615	5.238	0.157
Stainless steel	1.10–6.13	4.710	4.170	5.250	0.264
Time ranges					
<1 hour	1.10–7.00	4.258	4.214	4.902	0.173
1-2 hours	5.35–7.00	4.425	3.336	5.513	0.481
2:01–4 hours	1.81–6.13	5.779	5.028	6.529	0.354
4:01–5 hours	1.81–7.00	6.161	4.103	8.218	0.478
>5 hours	1.81–7.00	5.239	4.626	5.853	0.297

system, farm size, milking equipment, milking technique, geography, ecology, duration of milk transportation, and hygienic conditions [20]. The presence of *E. coli* may not necessarily indicate a direct fecal contamination of milk but is an indicator of poor hygiene and unsanitary practices during milking and further handling of milk and presents a potential hazard for people consuming such products [21].

The frequency of contamination of *E. coli* was significantly higher ($P = 0.02$) in raw milk samples collected from vendors (39.1%) than from different farms (28.1%) and also significantly increased ($P = 0.001$) as the time required for the milk to reach the market increased. The container in which milk was collected was evaluated and a higher rate of contamination was detected in the samples collected from milk held in plastic containers than stainless steel. The observed differences are probably due to the longer time taken for the milk to reach the market at ambient temperature under poor hygienic conditions which support the growth of the bacteria in the milk samples taken from the vendors.

In this study, the methods of production, transportation, handling, and sale of milk are prone to contamination. Hence, milk can be easily contaminated from different sources including the contaminated udder, milk handlers with poor personal hygiene, water of poor quality, and inappropriately cleaned and/or sanitized containers, all of which contribute to milk contamination [16, 18, 21].

In the current study, the overall prevalence of *E. coli* O157:H7 was found to be 2.9% (11/380). According to the results indicated in Table 1, a greater prevalence was observed in the milk samples collected from milk venders (5.0%) compared to those collected from the farmers (0.6%) and also in milk samples collected in containers managed under poor hygienic condition (4.3%) than from properly cleaned containers (0.7%) (Table 1). In both cases, the observed differences were statistically significant ($P < 0.05$). The containers made of plastic were identified to be more prone

to be contaminated by *E. coli* O157:H7 than stainless steel, but the difference was not statistically significant. There are a number of studies from different countries of the world concerning the prevalence of *E. coli* O157 in raw milk. Arafa and Soliman [21] reported that of raw milk and fresh cream examined in Egypt 2.6% and 1% were contaminated with *E. coli* O157:H7, respectively. Allerberger et al. [22] reported 3% of the milk samples tested in Austria to be positive for *E. coli* O157:H7, Klie et al. [23] found that 3.9% of the raw milk analyzed in Germany was contaminated with *E. coli* O157:H7, and Chye et al. [18] detected *E. coli* O157:H7 in 33.5% of raw milk samples in Malaysia. This might be due to differences in animal management, milking system, and milk handling practices among different regions.

4.2. Enumeration of E. coli. Most probable number (MPN) is one of the most commonly used methods to estimate the microbial load from milk and milk products. The mean MPN value of *E. coli* in raw milk samples was calculated with respect to different conditions that were considered as risk factors. Slightly higher mean MPN values ($\log_{10}$) were obtained in samples collected from vendors (4.978 ± 0.180/ml) than in milk collected from farmers (4.720 ± 0.203/ml), whereas milk held in plastic containers had a higher mean *E. coli* count (4.926 ± 0.157/ml) than the milk held in stainless steel (4.710 ± 0.264/ml). Similarly, samples collected from milk managed under poor hygienic conditions had a higher mean count (5.016 ± 0.151/ml) than the samples collected from milk managed under good hygienic condition (4.556 ± 0.278/ml). At the same time the load of *E. coli* increased with time, with the highest mean value (6.161 ± 0.478/ml) detected in the samples collected from the milk that had taken 4:01–5 hours to reach the market (Table 2).

According to an earlier report, the *E. coli* count in milk samples obtained from vendors was significantly higher (3.64 ± 0.776 cfu/ml) than milk samples obtained from dairy

TABLE 3: Antimicrobial resistance profile of E. coli O157:O7 isolates.

	Susceptible	Intermediate	Resistant
Streptomycin	0 (0%)	2 (18.2%)	9 (81.8%)
Trimethoprim-sulfamethoxazole	2 (18.2%)	6 (54.5%)	3 (27.3%)
Cefoxitin	1 (9.1%)	4 (36.4%)	6 (54.5%)
Kanamycin	0 (%)	4 (36.4%)	7 (63.6%)
Gentamycine	4 (36.4%)	3 (27.3%)	4 (36.4%)
Tetracycline	0 (0%)	2 (18.2%)	9 (81.8%)
Norfloxacin	1 (9.1%)	4 (36.4%)	6 (54.5%)

farms (3.93 ± 0.01 cfu/ml) [24], suggesting that allowing the milk samples' temperature to stay in the environmental temperature zone will favour the growth of E. coli and could be responsible for the high observed counts. There are several reasons for these variations, such as differences in hygienic practices during milking, differences in geographic location, and differences in seasonal trends [21].

In the study area, milking animals were kept with the rest of the stock in a shade or enclosure during the night. Milking was done in the shaded grazing field in front of the homestead, or under trees. However, as these areas were not generally kept clean enough, cows usually become soiled with dung and urine. Moreover, cleaning of the udder and of the hind quarters of the cows was not a common practice among milkers. This, coupled with the unhygienic cleaning and handling of milk containers, resulted in microbial contamination of milk [25, 26].

The bacterial counts in milk probably reveal the general conditions of sanitation and temperature control under which milk was produced, handled, and held [21]. In earlier studies, E. coli was detected as the most abundantly isolated species in raw milk sampled from smallholder producers in the central highlands of Ethiopia [12, 27], which is a good indicator of fecal contamination [28]. E. coli are often used as indicator microorganisms, and high populations of E. coli imply a risk that other enteric pathogens may be present in the sample [21].

Possible reasons for the high counts could be due to infected udders of the cows, use of unclean equipment, poor personal hygiene, lack of cooling after milking, and lack of heat treatment, which contribute to the poor hygienic quality of raw milk. Therefore, training and guidance in general milking hygiene practices and in keeping milk at low temperature should be given to the farmers to avoid microbial growth and lengthen the shelf life of milk [29].

The average values (ranging from 4.258 to 6.161, Table 3) in the present study indicated that the milk for consumers was of inferior quality and should be considered as unsafe. Since E. coli are indicator organisms for fecal pollution and E. coli O157:H7 often coexists with other coliform pathogens, the high enumerated levels of E. coli might be enough to say the milk is unsafe for consumers.

4.3. Antimicrobial Resistance Pattern of E. coli O157:H7. The susceptibility of the E. coli O157:H7 isolates against seven commonly used antimicrobials was tested and the isolates ($n = 11$) were characterized as susceptible, intermediate, and resistant based on the size of zone of inhibition [15]. According to the test results most of the E. coli O157:H7 ($\geq 50\%$) isolates were resistant to tetracycline (81.8%), streptomycin (81.8%), kanamycin (63.6%), cefoxitin (54.5%), and norfloxacin (54.5%) (Table 3). Development of antibiotic resistance among bacteria such as E. coli poses an important public health concern. Effectiveness of treatments and ability to control infectious diseases in both animals and humans may be severely hampered [19]. The currently recommended management of an infection mainly relies on supportive therapy and hydration [30].

4.4. Questionnaire Data and Its Interpretation. A total of 125 respondents were included in the study to collect relevant information regarding their knowledge about keeping the quality of the milk, the hygienic status, the type of milk containers, and the elapsed time for the milk to reach the market. Respondents were categorized into 4 groups including farmers (32.0%) (40), venders (32.0%) (40), cafeteria (12.0%) (15), and household consumers (24.0%) (30).

According to the findings summarized in Table 4 most of milk supplied to consumers in the town was originated from village around the town which was transported for a longer time to reach the market and managed by people with mostly unsatisfactory knowledge on the keeping quality of milk in plastic containers. Similarly, the sources of water for sanitation were underground water wells, pipes, or both wells and pipes with poor frequency of sanitation (Table 4). All these conditions favour the introduction and multiplication of pathogenic bacteria in the milk. These bacteria will reach the consumer through consumption of improperly cooked/ boiled milk and improperly treated/prepared "ergo" or cheese since milk is also consumed through both of these forms.

5. Conclusion

Most of the milk supplied to the consumer in the town was managed under poor hygienic conditions at ambient temperatures with poor levels of sanitation in plastic containers. Most of the stakeholders were managing the raw milk with limited awareness and knowledge on milk contamination and on the public health impact of milk-borne pathogens. The sources of E. coli in the raw cow milk may be from contaminated udders, contaminated water, poor sanitation practices, contaminated containers, and milk handlers themselves. Since the milk is managed at an ambient temperature, high microbial populations can be reached within short period of time. In this study, the presence and populations of E. coli as an indicator organisms and E. coli O157:H7 as pathogenic organisms in raw cow milk samples showed that the produced milk is of poor microbiological quality and of public health risk to the consumer. E. coli O157:H7 can cause infection as well as toxic infection at a very low infective dose like < 100 cells. In the study area, there is no standard hygienic conditions followed by producers during milk production. The hygienic conditions are different according to the

Table 4: Summary of questionnaire data.

Risk factors	Cafeteria ($n = 15$)	Household ($n = 30$)	Vender ($n = 40$)	Farmer ($n = 40$)	Total ($n = 125$)
Knowledge about keeping quality of milk					
Nonsatisfactory*	12 (80.0%)	24 (80.0%)	37 (92.3%)	38 (95.0%)	111 (88.8%)
Satisfactory**	3 (20.0%)	6 (20.0%)	3 (7.7%)	2 (5.0%)	14 (11.2%)
Water for sanitation					
Well	2 (10.0%)	0 (0%)	13 (65.0%)	5 (25.0%)	20 (16.0%)
Pipe	10 (73.4%)	13 (77.5%)	20 (30%)	14 (45%)	57 (45.6%)
Both	3 (6.20%)	17 (35.4%)	7 (14.6)	21 (43.8)	48 (38.4%)
Frequency of sanitation					
Usually	10 (67.5%)	12 (40.0%)	19 (47.5%)	16 (40.0%)	57 (45.6%)
Sometimes	5 (33.5%)	18 (60.0%)	21 (52.5%)	24 (60.0%)	68 (54.4%)
Washing equipment					
Only water	4 (26.7%)	12 (86.7%)	23 (82.5%)	24 (87.5%)	63 (50.4%)
Water & detergents	11 (17.7%)	18 (29.0%)	17 (27.4%)	16 (25.8%)	62 (49.6%)
Containers					
Plastic container	10 (11.5%)	24 (27.6%)	24 (27.6%)	29 (33.3%)	87 (70.7%)
Stainless steel	5 (13.2%)	6 (15.8%)	16 (42.1%)	11 (28.9%)	28 (29.3%)
Sources of milk					
Town	3 (5.1%)	16 (27.1%)	0 (0%)	40 (67.8%)	59 (47.2%)
Village***	12 (18.2%)	14 (21.2%)	40 (60.6%)	0 (0%)	66 (52.8%)
Knowledge of keeping quality of milk gained					
From parents	3 (33.3%)	11 (53.3%)	15 (27.5%)	17 (57.5%)	46 (36.8%)
Observations	8 (14.0%)	11 (19.3%)	22 (38.6%)	16 (28.1%)	57 (45.6%)
Formal training	4 (13.4%)	8 (10%)	3 (12.5%)	7 (7.5%)	22 (17.6%)
Time required to reach the market					
≤1 hour	2 (4.0%)	7 (14.0%)	6 (12.0%)	35 (70.0%)	50 (40.0%)
1-2 hours	4 (16.7%)	6 (25.0%)	9 (37.5%)	5 (20.8%)	24 (19.2%)
2:01–5 hours	4 (15.4%)	14 (53.8%)	8 (30.8%)	0 (0%)	26 (20.8%)
>5 hours	5 (20.0%)	3 (12.0%)	17 (68.0%)	0 (0%)	25 (20.0%)

*Lack of awareness and knowledge about sources and detection of contamination, public health impacts of contaminated milk, and necessary steps to control pathogens. **With awareness and knowledge about sources of contamination, public health impacts of contaminated milk and necessary steps to control pathogens. ***Sources of the milk from where milk was transported on foot and took more than an hour.

production system, adapted practices, level of awareness, and availability of resources. In most of the cases under smallholder condition, the common hygienic measures taken during milk production especially during milking are limited to letting the calf to suckle for few minutes and/or washing the udder before milking. The quality of the water used for cleaning purposes (to wash the udder, milk equipment, and hands), however, is not secured. The study also indicated that the E. coli O157:H7 isolates were resistant to most of the antimicrobials used at the study area, which may exacerbate E. coli infections in the future.

Competing Interests

The authors declare that there is no conflict of interests.

Acknowledgments

The authors would like to extend sincere thanks to Asosa regional research laboratory for their kind cooperation and willingness to support the study providing laboratory materials and equipment. The authors also like to thank Asosa administrative, agricultural sector for their assistance in gathering farm data/information during baseline survey including facilitation of sample collection.

References

[1] S. P. Oliver, K. J. Boor, S. C. Murphy, and S. E. Murinda, "Food safety hazards associated with consumption of raw milk," Foodborne Pathogens and Disease, vol. 6, no. 7, pp. 793–806, 2009.

[2] WHO, "A response to the need for comprehensive, consistent and comparable information on diseases and injuries at global and regional level," The Global Burden of Disease, World Health Organization, 2004.

[3] G. Duffy, "Emerging pathogenic E. coli," in Emerging Foodboren Pathogens, M. Yasmine and A. Martin, Eds., pp. 253–272, CRC Press, London, UK, 1st edition, 2006.

[4] X. Zhang, A. D. McDaniel, L. E. Wolf, G. T. Keusch, M. K. Waldor, and D. W. K. Acheson, "Quinolone antibiotics induce Shiga toxin-encoding bacteriophages, toxin production, and death in mice," Journal of Infectious Diseases, vol. 181, no. 2, pp. 664–670, 2000.

[5] A. Mora, J. E. Blanco, M. Blanco et al., "Antimicrobial resistance of Shiga toxin (verotoxin)-producing Escherichia coli O157:H7 and non-O157 strains isolated from humans, cattle, sheep and food in Spain," Research in Microbiology, vol. 156, no. 7, pp. 793–806, 2005.

[6] M. A. Raji, U. Minga, and R. Machangu, "Current epidemiological status of enterohaemorrhagic Escherichia coli O157:H7 in Africa," Chinese Medical Journal, vol. 119, no. 3, pp. 217–222, 2006.

[7] C. Walsh, G. Duffy, R. O'Mahony, S. Fanning, I. S. Blair, and D. A. McDowell, "Antimicrobial resistance in Irish isolates of verocytotoxigenic Escherichia coli (E. coli)-VTEC," International Journal of Food Microbiology, vol. 109, no. 3, pp. 173–178, 2006.

[8] FAO and WHO, "Code of hygienic practice for milk and milk products," AC/RCP 57, Codex limentarius, Rome, Italy, 2004, http://www.codexalimentarius.org.

[9] S. P. Oliver, B. M. Jayarao, and R. A. Almeida, "Foodborne pathogens in milk and the dairy farm environment: food safety and public health implications," Foodborne Pathogens and Disease, vol. 2, no. 2, pp. 115–129, 2005.

[10] D. Shunda, T. Habtamu, and B. Endale, "Assessment of bacteriological quality of raw cow milk at different critical points in Mekelle, Ethiopia," International Journal of Livestock Research, vol. 3, no. 4, pp. 42–48, 2013.

[11] L. Abera, Study on milk production and traditional dairy handling practices in east Shoa zone, Ethiopia [M.S. thesis], Faculty of Veterinary Medicine, Addis Ababa University, 2008.

[12] Z. Yilma and B. Faye, "Handling and microbial load of cow's milk and Irgo-fermented milk collectedfrom different shops and producers in Central Highlands of Ethiopia," Ethiopian Journal of Animal Production, vol. 6, no. 2, pp. 67–82, 2006.

[13] MoARD, "Horn of Africa consultations of food security," Country Report, Ministry of Agriculture and Rural Development, Government of Ethiopia, Addis Ababa, Ethiopia, 2007.

[14] P. J. Quinn, M. E. Carter, B. Markey, and G. R. Carter, Clinical Veterinary Microbiology, Mosby, Internal Ltd, London, UK, 2002.

[15] National Committee for Clinical Laboratory Standards (NCCLS), "Performance standards for antimicrobial susceptibility testing," 14th Informational Supplement, Approved Standard M100-S14, NCCLS, 2004.

[16] A. A. Ali, "Incidence of Escherichia coli in raw cow's milk in Khartoum State," British Journal of Dairy Science, vol. 2, no. 1, pp. 23–26, 2011.

[17] S. Lingathurai and P. Vellathurai, "Bacteriological quality and safety of raw cow milk in Madurai (South India)," Bangladesh Journal of Scientific and Industrial Research, vol. 48, no. 2, pp. 109–114, 2013.

[18] F. Y. Chye, A. Abdullah, and M. K. Ayob, "Bacteriological quality and safety of raw milk in Malaysia," Food Microbiology, vol. 21, no. 5, pp. 535–541, 2004.

[19] H. C. Thaker, M. N. Brahmbhatt, and J. B. Nayak, "Study on occurrence and antibiogram pattern of Escherichia coli from raw milk samples in Anand, Gujarat, India," Veterinary World, vol. 5, no. 9, pp. 556–559, 2012.

[20] A. H. Soomro, M. A. Arain, M. Khaskheli, and B. Bhutto, "Isolation of Escherichia coli from raw milk and milk products in relation to public health sold under market conditions at Tandojam," Pakistan Journal of Nutrition, vol. 1, no. 3, pp. 151–152, 2002.

[21] M. Arafa and M. Soliman, "Bacteriological quality and safety of raw cow's milk and fresh cream," Slovenian Veterinary Research, vol. 50, no. 1, pp. 21–30, 2013.

[22] F. Allerberger, M. Wagner, P. Schweiger et al., "Escherichia coli O157 infections and unpasteurised milk," Euro surveillance, vol. 6, no. 10, pp. 147–151, 2001.

[23] H. Klie, M. Timm, H. Richter, P. Gallien, K. W. Perlberg, and H. Steinruck, "Detection and occurrence of verotoxin forming and/or shigatoxin producing Eschericia coli (VTEC and/or STEC) in milk," Berliner und Münchener tierärztliche Wochenschrift, vol. 110, pp. 337–341, 1997.

[24] T. Teklemichael, K. Ameha, and S. Eyassu, "Quality and safety of cow milk produced and marketed in Dire Dawa Town, Eastern Ethiopia," International Journal of Integrative Sciences, Innovation and Technology, vol. 2, no. 6, pp. 1–5, 2013.

[25] A. Gonfa, H. A. Foster, and W. H. Holzapfel, "Field survey and literature review on traditional fermented milk products of Ethiopia," International Journal of Food Microbiology, vol. 68, no. 3, pp. 173–186, 2001.

[26] A. Tola, Traditional milk and milk products handling practices and raw milk quality in Eastern Wollega [M.S. thesis], Alemaya University, Alemaya, Ethiopia, 2002.

[27] Z. Yilma, G. Loiseau, and B. Faye, "Manufacturing efficiencies and microbial properties of butter and Ayib—Ethiopian cottage cheese," Livestock Research for Rural Development, vol. 19, no. 7, 2007.

[28] T. Bintsis and A. S. L. Angelidis, Psoni, Some Modern Laboratory Practices- Analysis of Dairy Products, Advanced Dairy Technology, Blackwell Publishing Ltd, Oxford, UK, 2008.

[29] P. Singh and A. Prakash, "Isolation of Escherichia coli, Staphylococcus aureus and Listeria monocytogenes from milk products sold under market conditions at Agra region," Acta Agriculturae Slovenica, vol. 92, no. 1, pp. 83–88, 2008.

[30] C. M. Thorpe, "Shiga toxin-producing Escherichia coli infection," Clinical Infectious Diseases, vol. 38, no. 9, pp. 1298–1303, 2004.

25

Microscopic and Molecular Detection of Camel Piroplasmosis in Gadarif State, Sudan

Abdalla Mohamed Ibrahim,[1,2] **Ahmed A. H. Kadle,**[3] **and Hamisi Said Nyingilili**[4]

[1]*Abrar Research and Training Centre, Abrar University, Mogadishu, Somalia*
[2]*College of Veterinary Medicine, University of Bahri, Khartoum, Sudan*
[3]*ICRC, Mogadishu, Somalia*
[4]*Vector and Vector Borne Diseases Institute, Tanga, Tanzania*

Correspondence should be addressed to Abdalla Mohamed Ibrahim; abdallami73@gmail.com

Academic Editor: Remo Lobetti

The socioeconomic importance of camels (*Camelus dromedarius*) could not be neglected in the Sudan. The present study was planned to confirm the presence of piroplasmosis in camels from the Eastern region of the Sudan (Gedarif State) using microscopical (blood film) and molecular technique (PCR). A total of 55 camels of different sexes (34 females and 21 males) were sampled from four localities of the state between January 2011 and January 2012. The prevalence rates using parasitological and molecular examinations were 43.6% and 74.5%, respectively. The prevalence rates significantly vary between the localities ($p = 0.011$) but not between the different sexes ($p = 0.515$). PCR technique showed higher sensitivity than microscopy. The present paper was to be the first report investigating camel piroplasmosis using both parasitological and molecular methods in the Eastern region of the Sudan. Further studies in the phylogenetic sequencing are to be continued for parasite speciation. Moreover, studies on the clinical and economic consequences of camel piroplasmosis are recommended.

1. Introduction

Sudan has the second largest camel population in the world, estimated at nearly 4,000,000, and owns 17% of the total world camel population [1]. Camels in the Sudan are receiving more attention, as they constitute a major component of livestock export to the neighboring countries. The camel "district" zone in the Sudan runs from the Eastern frontiers where camels come in contact with Ethiopian and Eritrean camel's herds to the Western frontiers where they can mix with the Chadian herds.

Causing serious economic losses tick and tick borne diseases (T and TBDs) still remain to be a major threat to animal's industry in the Sudan [2, 3] (El hussein et al., 2004; Hassan, and Salih 2009). The role of biting flies in the epidemiology of animal piroplasmosis was also discussed in the Sudan [4]. The most prevalent tick species affecting camels in the Sudan is *Hyalomma dromedary* in addition to

other *Hyalomma* sp., *Amblyomma* sp., and *Rhipicephalus* sp. (Hassan, and Salih 2009).

Very few camel piroplasmosis reports are available recently in the one-humped camel zone, such as Egypt [5], Iraq [6], and Iran [7]. With the exception of Abdelrahim et al. [8], there is not any report available on camel's TBDs from the Sudan.

Babesia caballi was molecularly detected from Sudanese camel [8] using Reverse Line Block (RLB). Both *Babesia caballi* and *Theileria equi* were molecularly confirmed in camels from Iraq [6] using PCR. Therefore, equines are supposed to play an important role in the epidemiology of camel piroplasmosis because they are usually found to be infected with the same piroplasms species [9, 10].

Clinical, haematological, and biochemical changes induced by naturally occurring babesiosis in dromedary camels were described by [11] in Kingdom of Saudi Arabia (KSA).

Among the few common diseases affecting camels, camel TBDs are usually neglected in the Sudan (Hassan, and Salih 2009) [12]. Many old and unpublished reports stated that camels are not susceptible to TBDs, although Shommein and Osman [13] earlier suspected that theileriosis, ehrlichiosis, and babesiosis may also be responsible for morbidity and mortality rates in camels. The economic impact of tick and tick borne diseases (T and TBDs) has inspired researchers to investigate TBDs in many animal species. However, in Sudan in spite of having the second largest counts of camels, data on camel piroplasmosis is not available. The present study was designed to determine the presence of piroplasms in one-humped camel in the Eastern region of the country using parasitological (microscopic) and molecular (PCR) techniques.

2. Materials and Methods

2.1. Study Area. Al Gadarif is one of the 18 states of the Sudan and one of the three states of Eastern region of the country. It shares an international border with Ethiopia to the East. The state shares borders with four Sudanese states including, Kassala and Khartoum States to the north, Al-Jazira State to the west, and Sennar to the south (Figure 1). It is located between longitudes 33° 30 and 36° 30 East, and latitudes 12° 40 and 15° 46 North. It has an area of 75,263 km^2 and an estimated population of approximately 1,400,000 (2000). It is one of the best agricultural (farms and livestock) areas in the Sudan. Four out of the ten localities of the state were included in this study, namely, Gadarif, Butana, Rahad, and Gala'alnahal.

2.2. Animals. Dromedary camels (*Camelus dromedarius*) were sampled among other animal's species for blood parasite investigation including piroplasms. These camels were sampled during area wide project entitled Survey for Epizootic Diseases. The project was designed by Ministry of Livestock, Fisheries and Range Lands (MLFRL), Sudan, in the year 2011. A total of 55 apparently healthy camels (34 females and 21 males) were included in this study.

2.3. Blood Samples. Fifty-five heparinized camel's blood samples (34 females and 21 males) were collected from jugular vein. Thin dried fixed blood smears and blood spot on Whatman No. 4 filter paper were prepared at the sample site. These samples were transported to Khartoum and submitted for further laboratory work in Laboratory of Parasitology, College of Veterinary Medicine, Sudan University of Science and Technology (SUST), Sudan. The thin dried fixed blood smears were stained using Giemsa's protocol and examined microscopically for presence of any blood parasites including piroplasms. The dried blood spots on filter paper were stored in −20°C until shipped to Vector and Vector Borne Diseases Institute (VVBDI), Tanga, Tanzania. These samples were investigated molecularly for presence of camel piroplasmosis in VVBDI using Polymerase Chain Reaction (PCR).

2.4. Extraction of the DNA. More than 10 micropunches of 1.2 mm each were taken from the preserved dry spot of whole blood on the filter paper. To reduce the chances of missing out piroplasm DNA punches were done randomly and kept on sterile 1.5 μL Eppendorf tube. The well cleaned Harris 1.2 mm micropunch (Whatman Biosciences Ltd.) was used. To prevent contamination between samples, the punches were cleaned after every sample using a 70% ethanol; then punches were used to cut a clean filter paper before using it on the next sample.

Total DNA was isolated by fastest version of the chelex extraction technique. Briefly 200 μL volume of solution with Chelex 100 (Sigma-Aldrich, St. Louis, USA) (final concentration 20%) was added to the 1.5 μL Eppendorf tube with samples boiled for 10 min and preserved in −20°C and were spanned at 13000 rpm for 3 minutes before using 2 μL of supernatant for PCR.

2.5. Polymerase Chain Reaction (PCR). Extracted DNA samples were subjected to Internal Transcribed Spacers (ITS1) Polymerase Chain Reaction (PCR) amplification. Presence of piroplasms was characterized by PCR using the primers Bab-sp-F (GTTTCTGCCCCATCAGCTTGAC) and Bab-sp-R (CAAGACAAAAGTCTGCTTGAAAC) which were used as the forward and reverse primers, respectively [7, 14]. Both primers were supplied by Bioneer Corporation. The PCR amplifications were performed in a total reaction volume of 25 μL containing 0.5 μL of 10 pM of each primer, 12.5 μL of one 2x master mix (BioLab. new England), 9.5 μL of PCR water, and 2 μL of each DNA template. PCR amplifications were performed with a thermal cycler (Gene Amp 9700 PCR system, Applied Biosystems). Amplification condition was initial denaturation at 94°C for 1 min and 30 seconds, followed by 45 cycles of 94°C for 20 s, 65°C for 30 s, followed by 68°C for 30 min, and final extension at 68°C for 10 min.

To ensure that results were not biased by false positives during repeated PCRs, negative controls in which DNA templates were replaced with sterile water as well as positive control DNA were included in all PCR reactions. The amplified PCR product was electrophoresed on a 1.5% agarose gel in 1x TBE. Quick loading 100 bp DNA ladder (BioLab, New England) was included on each gel, stained by ethidium bromide, run at 100–120 V for 60 min, and final visualized in Uvidock (Cambridge, UK).

The DNA template of a clear positive sample microscopically showing the characteristic pyriform and single amoebic form of *Babesia* sp. was firstly extracted and checked repeatedly by PCR to be used as positive control.

2.6. Data Management and Analysis. Data were stored in a Microsoft® Excel spread sheet for Windows® 2007 before being transferred to SPSS sheet for Windows version 20. The differences were considered statistically significant when $p \leq 0.05$.

Photos of the detected parasites were captured directly from microscope eye piece using digital camera (Sony, 16.1 MP) and stored in computer.

Survey of Epizootic Diseases in Gadarif
State_June 2011

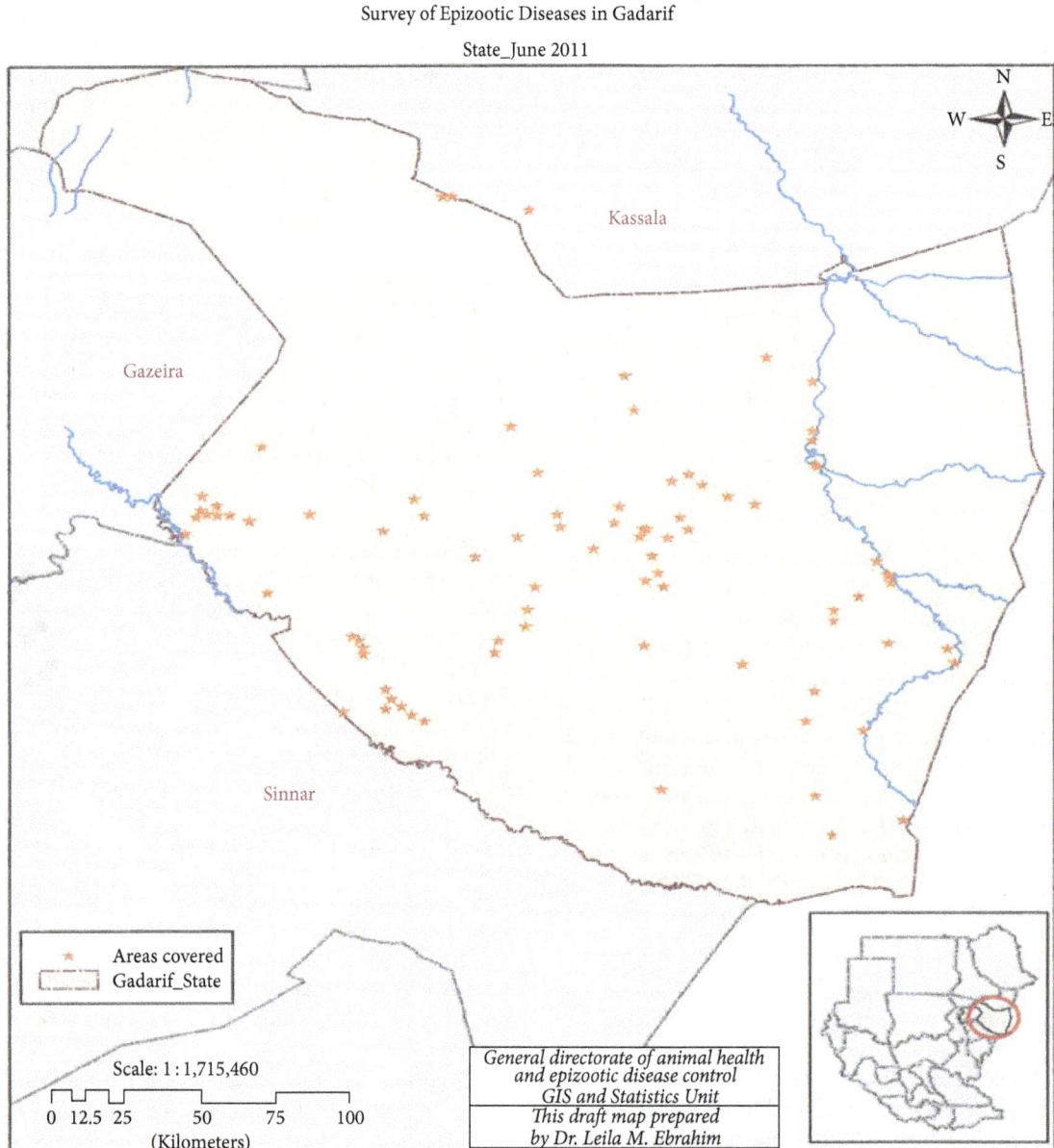

FIGURE 1: The sampled site in the study area (Gadarif State).

3. Results

3.1. Microscopic Prevalence of Camel Piroplasmosis. Piroplasms were detected microscopically in Giemsa's stained blood films of 43.6% of the examined camels. The different shapes of detected parasites were presented in Figure 2 (arrows). Rahad locality revealed the highest microscopical prevalence rate (68.2%) with highly statistically significant ($p = 0.011$) variation from Gadarif (42.9%) and Gala'alnahal (28.6%) localities (Table 1). No piroplasm (0.0%) was detected microscopically in Butana locality.

3.2. Molecular Prevalence of Camel Piroplasmosis. Babesia DNA was detected molecularly in the extracted blood of 74.5% of the examined camels. The bands of the positive and

negative Babesia DNA product were presented in Figure 3. Without any statistical significance ($p = 0.328$), Gadarif locality revealed the highest molecular prevalence rate (100%) followed by Gala'alnahal (76.2%) and Rahad (68.2%) localities (Table 1). Piroplasm DNA with prevalence rate of 60% was detected molecularly in Butana locality.

3.3. Prevalence of Camel Piroplasmosis in Different Sexes. Using both microscopical or molecular examination, there was not any statistically significant ($p = 0.515$ or 0.391) variation between male and female camels in the susceptibility of piroplasms infection. However, when male revealed higher susceptibility molecularly, female showed higher prevalence rate microscopically (Table 2).

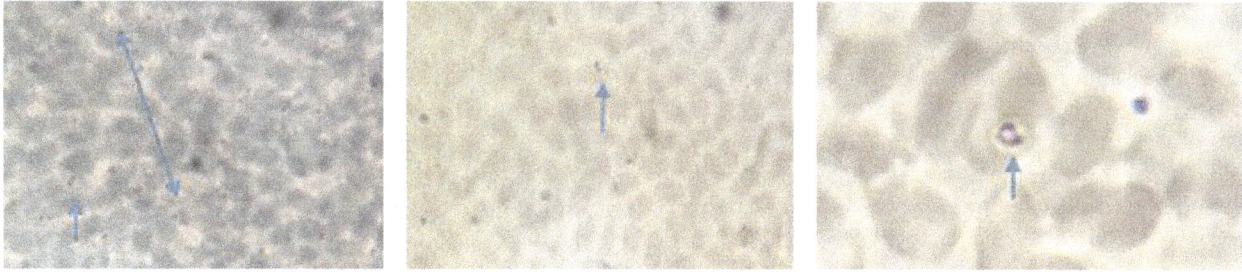

FIGURE 2: Piroplasms with different shapes (arrows) in Giemsa's stained blood.

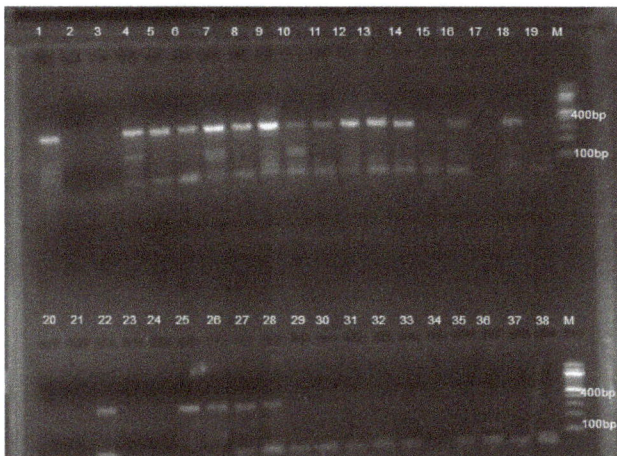

FIGURE 3: Agarose gel (1.5%) electrophoresis of amplified DNA from *Babesia*. Lane M: DNA ladder (100 bp). Lane 1: positive control and Lane 20: negative control. Positive product showed clear band in 400 bp (e.g., Lanes 4, 5, 6, 7, 8, 9, 12, 13, 14, 18, 22, 25).

TABLE 1: Prevalence of camel piroplasmosis in the investigated localities.

Locality	N	Prevalence n (%)	
		Parasitological	PCR
Butana	5	0 (0.0)	3 (60)
Gadarif	7	3 (42.9)	7 (100)
Gala'anahal	21	6 (28.6)	16 (76.2)
Rahad	22	15 (68.2)	15 (68.2)
Total	55	24 (43.6)	41 (74.5)
p value		0.011	0.328

3.4. *Level of Agreement between Microscopical and Molecular Tests.* PCR technique detected more infection (74.5%) than microscopical one (43.6%). PCR technique detected 22 (71.0%) and 19 (79.2%) out of the 31 negative and 24 positive samples microscopically, respectively (Table 3). The level of agreement between the two techniques is very poor (Kappa = 0.076).

4. Discussion

The socioeconomic value of Sudanese camels is well recognized nationally, regionally, and internationally. The most

TABLE 2: Prevalence of camel piroplasmosis in different sexes.

Sex	N	Prevalence n (%)	
		Parasitological	PCR
Male	21	8 (38.1)	17 (81.0)
Female	34	16 (47.1)	24 (70.6)
Total	55	24 (43.6)	41 (74.5)
p value		0.515	0.391

TABLE 3: The level of agreement between the two techniques using Kappa test.

		Molecular (PCR)		Total
		N−ve	P+ve	
Microscopic (BF)	N−ve	9 (29.0)	22 (71.0)	**31 (100)**
	P+ve	5 (20.8)	19 (79.2)	**24 (100)**
Total		14 (25.5)	41 (74.5)	**55 (100)**
Kappa value		**0.076**		

important pathogenic and epidemic diseases affecting camels in the Sudan are of parasitic origin. There are very few and sporadic serious diseases of viral and bacterial origin. With the exception of the single case of molecular camel babesiosis [8], there is not any report on camel's TBDs available from the Sudan.

The present study revealed that more than two-thirds (74.5%) of camels of the investigated area were found to be infected with piroplasmosis. The prevalence of camel piroplasmosis using microscopical examination in this study was higher than that reported in KSA [11], Egypt [5], and Iraq [6]. This could be attributed to the higher prevalence rate of ticks and biting flies infesting camel in the investigated area of the Sudan [2] (Hassan, and Salih 2009). This was clearly confirmed when the molecular results of the present study were found to be also higher than that recorded by Khamesipour et al. [7] in Iran and Jasim et al. [6] in Iraq. Only one camel (0.5%) sample out of 200 samples from Western region of the Sudan showed *Babesia caballi* DNA [8] using the Reverse Line Block (RLB). It is incomparable with the present results and that is may be only due to the different molecular technique (ITS1-PCR) used in this study.

The results of this study revealed that PCR is more sensitive for detection of camel piroplasmosis than microscopy. Similar observations were reported in camels from Iran [7] and Iraq [6].

In this study, about 75% of the investigated camels were found to be positive for piroplasmosis. However, no pathognomonic clinical signs of piroplasmosis (e.g., haemoglobinurea) were recorded during sampling. Swelum et al. [11] reported some clinical, haematological, and biochemical changes due to natural infection of babesiosis in dromedary camels in Kingdom of Saudi Arabia (KSA). Camel is known to be tolerant to many diseases. However, from the present results, the effect of piroplasmosis in degree of anaemia as well as production and the productivity of camel need to be investigated in depth. Additionally, when mix-infection of protozoan parasites causing immunosuppression is present, the impact of the disease will be higher [3, 15]. Based on the present results, camel could be a source of infection for the coherded equines and vice versa, because camels are found to be infected by equine piroplasms including *Babesia caballi* and *Theileria equi* [6, 8]. Thus, camels should be considered in the epidemiology of equine piroplasmosis [9, 10].

From the results of the present study, female camels showed more acute infection when more parasitaemia was detected microscopically than males, although sex has no significant effect ($p > 0.05$) in the susceptibility of infection.

Ticks are widespread in camel-raising habitats in the Sudan [2] (El hussein et al., 2004; Hassan, and Salih 2009). They cause serious adverse effects such as anaemia, dermatitis, mastitis, reduced meat and milk production, and low quality hides. The high prevalence of piroplasmosis revealed in this study could explain that TBDs may seriously affect the production and the productivity of camels in the Sudan. Moreover, the present results come to support the earlier suggestion of Shommein and Osman [13] that TBDs could be responsible for morbidity and mortality rate of Sudanese camels. Therefore, we come to conclude that to improve camel production and productivity in the Sudan, it is high time to monitor camels from tick borne diseases and to implement prophylaxis and treatment. Further study in the phylogenetic sequence of these DNA templates is recommended for parasite speciation.

Competing Interests

The authors declare that they have no conflict of interests regarding the publication of this article.

Acknowledgments

The authors would like to thank MLFRL and SUST for the field work and laboratory support, respectively. They are also grateful to VVBDI, Tanzania, for molecular technique and their special thanks are due to Dr. Imna Malele, Mr. Peter Paul, and Miss Delphina.

References

[1] T. E. N. Angara, *The Socio-economic aspects of brucellosis in Khartoum dairy scheme, Khartoum State [Ph.D. thesis]*, Sudan University of Science and Technology, Khartoum, Sudan, 2005.

[2] H. Hoogstraal, *African Ixodidae Volume I, Ticks of the Sudan*, Department of Medical Zoology, U.S. Naval Medical Res. Unit (NAMRU) No. 3, Cairo, Egypt, 1956.

[3] E. J. L. Soulsby, Ed., *Helminths, Arthropods & Protozoa of Domesticated Animals*, Bailliere Tindall, London, UK, 7th edition, 1986.

[4] A. M. Ibrahim, D. Geysen, A. A. Ismail, and S. A. Mohammed, "Haemoparasites identification in two dairy cattle farms in Khartoum State with reference of *Babesia bigemina*: molecular confirmation," *The Sudan Journal of Veterinary Research*, vol. 25, pp. 37–42, 2010.

[5] B. S. Abd-Elmaleck, G. H. Abed, and A. M. Mandourt, "Some protozoan parasites infecting blood of camels (*Camelus dromedarius*) at Assiut locality, Upper Egypt," *Journal of Bacteriology & Parasitology*, vol. 5, article 184, 2014.

[6] H. J. Jasim, G. Y. Azzal, and R. M. Othman, "Conventional and molecular detection of *Babesia caballi* and *Theileria equi* parasites in infected camels in south of Iraq," *Basrah Journal of Veterinary Research*, vol. 14, no. 2, pp. 110–121, 2015.

[7] F. Khamesipour, A. Doosti, A. Koohi, M. Chehelgerdi, A. Mokhtari-Farsani, and A. A. Chengula, "Determination of the presence of Babesia DNA in blood samples of cattle, camel and sheep in Iran by PCR," *Archives of Biological Sciences*, vol. 67, no. 1, pp. 83–90, 2015.

[8] I. A. Abdelrahim, A. A. Ismail, A. M. Majid et al., "Detection of *Babesia caballi* in the one-humped Camel (*Camelius dromedarius*) using the Reverse Line Block (RLB) in Sudan," *The Sudan Journal of Veterinary Research*, vol. 24, pp. 69–72, 2009.

[9] B. Salim, M. A. Bakheit, J. Kamau, and C. Sugimoto, "Current status of equine piroplasmosis in the Sudan," *Infection, Genetics and Evolution*, vol. 16, pp. 191–199, 2013.

[10] S. R. Hosseini, T. Taktaz-Hafshejani, and F. Khamesipour, "Molecular detection of *Theileria equi* and *Babesia caballi* infections in horses by PCR method in Iran," *Kafkas Universitesi Veteriner Fakultesi Dergisi Journal*, vol. 23, no. 1, pp. 161–164, 2017.

[11] A. A. Swelum, A. B. Ismael, A. F. Khalaf, and M. A. Abouheif, "Clinical and laboratory findings associated with naturally occurring babesiosis in dromedary camels," *Bulletin of the Veterinary Institute in Pulawy*, vol. 58, no. 2, pp. 229–233, 2014.

[12] I. Kohler-Rollefson, B. E. Musa, and M. F. Achmed, "The camel pastoral system of the southern Rashaida in eastern Sudan," *Nomadic Peoples*, vol. 29, pp. 68–76, 1991.

[13] A. Shommein and A. Osman, "Diseases of camels in the Sudan," *Revue Scientifique et Technique de l'OIE*, vol. 6, no. 2, pp. 481–486, 1987.

[14] H. Hilpertshauser, P. Deplazes, M. Schnyder, L. Gern, and A. Mathis, "Babesia spp. identified by PCR in ticks collected from domestic and wild ruminants in Southern Switzerland," *Applied and Environmental Microbiology*, vol. 72, no. 10, pp. 6503–6507, 2006.

[15] M. A. Taylor, R. L. Coop, and R. L. Wall, Eds., *Veterinary Parasitology*, Blackwell Publishing, 3rd edition, 2007.

26

Brazilian Spotted Fever with an Approach in Veterinary Medicine and One Health Perspective

Sabrina Destri Emmerick Campos,[1] **Nathalie Costa da Cunha,**[2] **and Nádia Regina Pereira Almosny**[1]

[1]*Departamento de Patologia e Clínica Veterinária, Universidade Federal Fluminense, 24230-340 Niterói, RJ, Brazil*
[2]*Departamento de Saúde Coletiva Veterinária e Saúde Pública, Universidade Federal Fluminense, 24230-340 Niterói, RJ, Brazil*

Correspondence should be addressed to Sabrina Destri Emmerick Campos; s.destri@gmail.com

Academic Editor: Francesca Mancianti

There is increasing interaction between man and pathogens transmitted by arthropods, especially by ticks. It is on this background that a holistic approach stands out, for the sake of Public Health. Brazilian Spotted Fever is an endemic disease at the country's southeast, with *Amblyomma sculptum* as its major contributor, followed by *A. aureolatum* and potentially *Rhipicephalus sanguineus*. Dogs have been considered sentinels, and in some areas the disease in dogs can precede human disease. Considering the importance of this disease for human health, the serological evidence in dogs, and the transmission of ticks between dogs and their owners, this review aimed to elucidate the importance of the epidemiological investigation, the diagnosis in dogs, and the role of veterinarians in Public Health to control vector-borne zoonotic diseases. We encourage veterinarians to include this rickettsial infection in the diagnosis of febrile diseases of common occurrence in dogs.

1. Introduction

Vector-borne diseases are globally important to human and animal health, since pathogens, vectors, and animal hosts reveal interactions through pathologies and their epidemiology, which differ among geographic zones, and may change over time [1]. Ticks and wildlife are among the main reservoirs of pathogens transmitted by arthropods of veterinary importance [2].

Human beings are causing important changes in the ecosystem, such as habitat fragmentation, global warming, and exploitation of natural resources, which have allowed interaction between man and pathogens potentially transmitted by arthropods [3, 4]. The global Strategic Framework for health has been created to decrease the risk and minimize the impact of emerging infectious diseases at the animal-human-ecosystem and socioeconomic interface [3]. Shaffer [5] suggested the use of surveillance policies for animals as part of an approach in One Health Perspective, in order to contribute to more coordinated actions towards human health.

It is against this background that stands out a holistic approach for the sake of Public Health, applying the concept of One Health, which recognizes that human welfare is linked to animals and the environment and so it seeks a combined action between physicians, ecologists, and veterinarians in the control of threats to Public Health.

Rickettsia rickettsii is the major bacterium responsible for the Brazilian Spotted Fever (BSF), a highly fatal disease with challenging diagnosis due to its nonspecific signs [6, 7]. To assist the epidemiological surveillance, studies have been searching for sentinel animals, such as horses and dogs, with positive serological reaction in endemic areas [8, 9].

Based on the importance of BSF to human health, the evidence of clinical illness in dogs from areas with laboratory-confirmed BSF in humans, and the potential transmission of ticks between dogs and their owners, this review aimed to discuss the importance of epidemiological surveys and laboratory diagnosis of BSF in dogs for Public Health, inspired by the principles of One World, One Health, a Strategic Framework that has been raised jointly by specialized agencies, such as World Health Organization (WHO), United Nations (UN) Food and Agriculture Organization (FAO), International Organization for Animal Health (OIE), and UN Children's Fund (UNICEF).

2. The One Health Idea

The idea that humans, animals, and the ecosystems are closely related has been under discussion since the late nineteenth century, when the first movements to integrate activities and research in human and animal health were raised [3, 10].

It is believed that emerging infectious diseases are related to socioeconomic conditions and ecological features, which allow identifying potential hotspots of injuries of animal origin, particularly at low latitudes, at areas where the notifications are substantially weak [11], a pattern that fits the epidemiological situation of BSF.

The Strategic Framework establishes a more interdisciplinary approach with international cooperation, in order to ensure health for humans, animals, and ecosystems [3, 10, 12]. However, people are reservoir of only a small number of zoonotic pathogens, so it is understood that an effective monitoring system requires the integration of physicians, who can identify human outbreaks, and veterinarians, that can identify animal reservoirs and sentinels [5, 13].

Veterinarians can contribute to the promotion of health through their knowledge on environmental conservation, the use of domestic animals as sentinels for the circulation of pathogens in the domestic and/or wildlife arenas, and occupational risk (due to the exposure to ticks) [12, 14, 15]. A study with veterinary students revealed that animal treatment with acaricides, avoiding contact with ticks, keeping vegetation cut down, and inspecting the body every three hours for the presence of ticks were the main prevention methods cited in control of BSF [15].

We believe that interdisciplinary participation in epidemiological investigation research and dissemination of articles and reports to scientific and health care assistance communities could be a mechanism to integrate information and improve strategies to control this disease.

3. Brazilian Spotted Fever

3.1. History. A disease caused by *Rickettsia rickettsii* was first described in the USA, and since then it has been confirmed in several countries, including Canada, Mexico, Panama, Costa Rica, Colombia, Brazil, Argentina, and possibly Guatemala [16–21]. In Brazil, this disease has been called Brazilian Spotted Fever (BSF) and it was first discovered in the state of São Paulo in 1928, where it was originally treated as "Exanthematic Typhus" [22]. The return of BSF reports in the 80s has shown that the disease has never ceased to occur; however it became detected as an acute disease affecting people from the same household or labor, albeit isolated cases have been described [23, 24]. Since 2001, BSF is a nationally notifiable disease, considered endemic in southeastern Brazil [23, 25].

According to the Center of Disease Control, the gold standard serologic test for diagnosis of the disease is the indirect immunofluorescence assay (IFA) with *R. rickettsii* antigen, performed on two paired serum samples to demonstrate a significant (fourfold) rise in IgG antibody titers, since molecular diagnosis is not always routinely available to confirm cases (http://www.cdc.gov/rmsf/symptoms). In Brazil, 1141 human cases confirmed by IFA were notified between 2007 and 2015, being 61.26% (699/1141) in the southeast, especially in the states of São Paulo (43.21%, 493/1141), Minas Gerais (8.15%, 93/1141), and Rio de Janeiro (7.19%, 82/1141). The state of Santa Catarina is highlighted with 23.05% of human cases (263/1141). Amapá, Rondônia, and Amazonas contributed with a single confirmed human case each, in 2007, 2008, and 2011 (http://www.saude.gov.br/sinan).

3.2. Vectors, Reservoir, and Amplifying Hosts. Due to their capability to transmit a variety of zoonotic pathogens, ticks stand out on the concept of One Health. Brazil contains many biomes, rich and abundant fauna, and several species of arthropods, such as ticks of the *Amblyomma* genus, widely distributed in the Neotropical region [21].

Based on recent reassessment of the taxonomic and morphological status of *Amblyomma cajennense* (Fabricius, 1787), currently, the name *A. cajennense sensu lato* (*s.l.*) refers to a group of six species. According to geographical distributions, and host associations, *A. cajennense sensu stricto* (*s.s.*) applies to the tick found in the Amazonian region of South America, while *A. sculptum* applies to the tick found in the coastal states, and degraded areas of the Atlantic Forest, including all states in the southeast [26, 27].

Interestingly, the low host specificity of *A. cajennense s.l.* allows for their detection in many mammals including cattle, deer, and wild and domestic canids, besides man [7, 28, 29]. *Amblyomma cajennense s.l.* is implicated as the major species responsible for BSF, followed by *A. aureolatum* [29, 30]. In addition, the potential disease-transmission role of *Rhipicephalus sanguineus* is also increasingly studied [9, 31–35].

In the tick, transstadial and transovarian systems maintain the bacteria, which are transmitted to the vertebrate host during blood feeding, making arthropods simultaneously vector and reservoir [36–39]. However, infection rates by *R. rickettsii* in ticks under natural conditions tend to be low (<1%), evidencing that *R. rickettsii* is pathogenic to ticks, and reinforcing the need of an amplifying host to ensure the maintenance of bacteria, such as capybaras, especially in endemic areas of São Paulo [40–44].

3.3. Amblyomma sculptum. In southeastern Brazil, the area with the highest concentration of BSF reports, the ecological setting in which the disease occurs is well described, including a voluminous population of *Amblyomma* ticks [21]. Horses and capybaras are among the most important primary hosts for all parasitic stages of *A. cajennense s.l.* [38, 45]. The capybara population has greatly increased in the state of São Paulo, and at this point it raises suspicions of its relationship to the emergence of BSF [44].

Although massive infestations with adult ticks occur in horses and capybaras in southeastern Brazil, nymphs of *A. cajennense s.l.* have shown better competence as vectors of

R. rickettsii experimentally [46, 47], which is important, since these stages have less requirements regarding their hosts including dogs and people [28, 29]. In fact, most human cases of BSF seem to occur during the nymphs season of *A. cajennense s.l.*, from July to November, possibly related to the aggressive behavior of nymphs, their effective spreading through the environment, and their small size, making their removal quite difficult [48].

3.4. Amblyomma aureolatum.

Amblyomma aureolatum is yet another vector involved in BSF, with its ecological peculiarities. The "yellow dog tick" is found mainly in subtropical areas, with high humidity and mild temperatures throughout the year [49]. The population of *A. aureolatum* tends to be low and in southeastern Brazil, its distribution is restricted to Atlantic Forest, typically occurring in dogs with free access to rainforest [30, 49].

There are few reports of adults of *A. aureolatum* biting humans [50, 51]. Thus, human cases transmitted by *A. aureolatum* seem to occur when dogs get infected by adults of this tick during incursions into the rainforest and go on to carry *A. aureolatum* to their households [21]. However, experimentally, this tick was more susceptible to *R. rickettsii* infection and more efficient to maintain the pathogen by transstadial and transovarian transmission than *A. sculptum* [52]. Another study with experimental infection of *A. aureolatum* demonstrated that *R. rickettsii* was preserved between transstadial and transovarial stages in 100% of the *A. aureolatum* ticks for several consecutive generations, and larvae, nymphs, and adults transmitted *R. rickettsii* to susceptible guinea pigs [53]. Recently it was suggested that the adult *A. aureolatum* needs only approximately 10 minutes attached to the body of a vertebrate host to transmit *R. rickettsii* [35].

Note that in some areas of southeastern Brazil, particularly in areas of the state of São Paulo, *A. aureolatum* can replace *A. sculptum* as the main vector of *R. rickettsii* to humans, being even more effective in transmitting the pathogen [30, 31, 53].

3.5. Amblyomma ovale.

In the past years, *A. ovale* has been implicated as a possible vector of new rickettsiosis in Brazil, since a human case of febrile disease with eschar (*tache noire*) was observed after tick biting in an Atlantic (ATL) Rainforest region of the state of São Paulo. Phylogenetic analysis revealed a new human rickettsiosis of the Spotted Fever Group (SFG), named ATL Rainforest Rickettsiosis, distinct from that caused by *R. rickettsia* [54]. Due to its phylogenetic similarity to *R. parkeri*, this new strain was called *R. parkeri* strain ATL Rainforest, which has been detected naturally infecting *A. ovale* ticks [55, 56]. So far *A. triste* was the vector associated with infection by *R. parkeri* in South America, including Brazil [57, 58].

Experimentally, 100% of transstadial and transovarian transmission of *R. parkeri* to *A. ovale* was confirmed by PCR. Larvae and nymphs demonstrated high competence in transmission of the bacteria because all animals infested by these ticks' stages presented seroconversion when tested by IFA using *R. parkeri* antigens, but only half of the animals presented seroconversion after being infested by infected-adult ticks. Reproductive parameters of infected *A. ovale* females were low when compared to uninfected females, indicating deleterious effect of *R. parkeri* on this tick [56].

Amplifier hosts and reservoir in the ATL Rainforest Rickettsiosis have not been determined so far, but small rodents were shown to be important for *A. ovale* immature stages and high seroconversion prevalence [59]. Krawczak [56] suggested that *A. ovale* is an important vector on the epidemiology of *R. parkeri* strain ATL Rainforest, since this tick is often found in the ATL Rainforest ecosystem. Moreover, human bites by adult *A. ovale* tick are common [50]. Thus, humans can become infected if bitten by ticks detached from the dogs, suggesting the importance of dogs from the forests of endemic areas, mainly infested with *A. ovale* ticks [21, 59].

Serology studies have reported that dogs seroconvert, attaining very high titers against *R. parkeri* antigens [55, 59, 60]. Furthermore, Medeiros et al. [60] reported identical sequences to *R. parkeri* strain ATL Rainforest in dogs coinfested with *A. ovale* ticks. So far, it can be supposed that some febrile human cases diagnosed as mild BSF were in fact ATL Rainforest Rickettsiosis [59].

3.6. Rhipicephalus sanguineus.

The "brown dog tick" is possibly the tick with greater distribution, inhabiting urban and rural environments where dogs and humans live [18]. It is a three-host tick that feeds primarily on dogs and occasionally on other hosts [61]. Participation of *Rh. sanguineus* in the transmission of BSF is still a source of speculation, although this tick is already an important vector and reservoir of *R. conorii* responsible for the Mediterranean Spotted Fever in Europe, Africa, and Asia [21].

In Brazil, human parasitism by *Rh. sanguineus* has been reported [61] but is still considered a rare event, particularly considering the close proximity of these ticks with man [51, 61]. Natural infection of *Rh. sanguineus* by *R. rickettsii* in Brazil has been observed in endemic areas for BSF [30, 33, 62]. And even if the transmission to humans has not been proven yet, there is a favorable outlook in urban areas where *Rh. sanguineus* is often found in pet or stray dogs [21]. Furthermore, these dogs can often move between urban and rural farming areas, being parasitized by ticks from both environments [30].

It is noteworthy that *Rh. sanguineus* tends to be less aggressive to man, making the transmission occasional, particularly for those dealing with dogs most of the time [21].

The traditional mechanism by which the tick gets infected by *R. rickettsia* is during blood feeding of the vertebrate host or by transstadial and transovarian transmission [36, 37]. However, under natural conditions, low infection rates among tick populations suggest that these mechanisms are not enough to maintain the pathogen in the ecosystem [40, 41]. It is important to consider that *R. rickettsii* is pathogenic to the tick, causing decreased fertility and death [41]. Cofeeding transmission of *R. rickettsii* is not fully elucidated but may have an important role in the transmission of bacteria among ticks that feed in close proximity at the same host [39].

Considering that dogs can become infected by *A. aureolatum* during incursions into the rainforest and that bacteria-infected *A. aureolatum* can remain on the dog for several weeks, it is possible that tick-infested dogs carry infected ticks back to human households. The ticks may then drop off from the dog, contaminate the household environment, and accidentally bite humans. In a different scenario, *Rh. sanguineus* ticks can become infected by cofeeding on the same dog with infected *A. aureolatum* ticks [21, 49, 59].

4. *Rickettsia rickettsii* Infection in Dogs and the Role of Sentinels in Brazil

Clinical disease caused by *R. rickettsii* in dogs is not easy to diagnose and has not been well described in South America, with few cases reported in the state of São Paulo, Brazil [7, 63].

Experimentally, dogs developed clinical illness characterized by fever, lethargy, anorexia, bilateral ocular discharge, scleral congestion, conjunctival edema, thrombocytopenia, and anemia [64]. *Rickettsia rickettsii*-reactive antibodies were shown in serum samples, and rickettsial DNA was detectable in blood 3 to 13 days after infection, indicating that a Brazilian strain of *R. rickettsii* is pathogenic for dogs [64].

Dogs, which remain close to both humans and naturally infected areas, can play a role as sentinels in an epidemiological approach [34, 65]. The use of serological methods for the detection of anti-*Rickettsia* spp. antibodies in dogs has been reported in several Brazilian states, especially in the southeast [9, 32, 34, 62, 66].

According to Cunha et al. [34], the dog's habit of entering rainforest regions and living in rural environments indicated a risk factor to the presence of anti-SFG rickettsiae antibodies.

Although SFG species share antigens that might cause group reactive serological responses, IFA is a highly sensitive and specific technique, used as the method of choice in serosurvey and screening tests in Brazil [67, 68]. In addition, if serology to several SFG antigens demonstrates titers to one antigen at least fourfold higher than the others, we can assume which pathogen stimulated the immune response [9]. High titers to *R. rickettsii* in endemic areas for BSF, up to 1 : 4096, or more, reinforce this hypothesis [34].

Clinical signs in dogs and humans may be similar, in such a way that the disease in dogs can precede the disease in humans, reinforcing the role of dogs as sentinels of BSF, a hypothesis that becomes stronger in USA, where cases of *R. rickettsii* in dogs and their owners have been found [8, 69, 70].

In Brazil, canine monocytic ehrlichiosis (CME), caused by *Ehrlichia canis*, is the most common tick-transmitted canine disease [71]. As many clinical and laboratorial findings described in CME, fever, depression, petechial hemorrhage, and thrombocytopenia, are also described in dogs infected by *R. rickettsii* [72], and given that doxycycline is the treatment of choice for both diseases, it is possible that rickettsial infection in dogs is being misdiagnosed as CME [7, 9, 72].

Differential diagnosis is a great challenge, because dogs may present with subclinical infections or nonspecific clinical signs, often misdiagnosed as other diseases transmitted by arthropods like CME, Lyme's disease, babesiosis, leishmaniasis, anaplasmosis, and any febrile disease of unspecified etiology [73].

According to Labruna et al. [7], definitive diagnosis of naturally infected dogs is based on (1) serological analysis

of paired samples; (2) anti-*R. rickettsii* titers fourfold higher than other spotted-fever group antigens occurring in Brazil; (3) rickettsial DNA detection in blood; (4) both clinical and laboratorial findings compatible with the disease; (5) doxycycline responsive treatment; and (6) epidemiological history with tick infestation and exposure to endemic areas.

Besides the dog, authors have attempted to elucidate the role of other domestic animals as sentinels of the BSF. Horses, considered primary hosts of *A. cajennense s.l.*, are also an important object of study in the epidemiology of the disease.

Participation of horses as sentinels of infections caused by SFG has also been reported. One study suggested the ecological importance of cart horses as sentinels for BSF, since these horses are extensively used for transporting humans and heavy loads in urban and rural areas, being heavily infested with ticks [74]. Vianna et al. [75] believed that horses could be better sentinels to *R. rickettsii* than dogs, due to the presence of antibodies anti-*R. rickettsii* in 100% of the equine sera tested by IFA. However, Cunha et al. [34] after serosurvey in human foci of BSF observed that if the vector is not *A. sculptum*, horses present low serological reaction rate, which rules out these animals as good sentinels, while dogs can perform the role of sentinel for different vectors, since they can be parasitized by *A. sculptum*, *A. aureolatum*, *A. ovale*, and *Rh. sanguineus*. This was reinforced by other studies in the state of São Paulo, which observed a higher frequency of horses with positive serology in areas with strong evidence that the main vector was *A. cajennense s.l.* [66].

5. Conclusion and Perspectives

Ticks of domestic animals may be involved in the epidemiology of several vector-borne diseases, which also affect humans. Even though the dogs are not the main host for *R. rickettsii*, they may carry infected ticks into the human dwellings. One of the most effective ways to assess the evidence of SFG pathogens circulation in sentinel animals is through serological tests, among which the IFA has been widely employed in dogs, particularly because of the easy access to samples, their intimate relationship with man, and parasitism by the same ticks.

Due to this challenging outlook it is possible that BSF in dogs is underestimated, since the nonspecific clinical signs may get confused with EMC, which is the most prevalent tick-borne disease in dogs. As doxycycline is an effective treatment for patients with BSF or EMC, it is possible that dogs with acute febrile illness are not being routinely molecularly tested for BSF, since its cost is a limiting factor. Veterinarians should include rickettsial infections in the differential diagnosis of CME and other febrile diseases of nonspecific signs transmitted by common ticks, facilitating monitoring of BSF, since it is an important zoonosis with human fatalities when the diagnosis is delayed and treatment cannot be implemented in time.

Serology of these dogs could indicate prior exposure to rickettsial agents by the presence of IgG antibodies even before the reporting of human cases of BSF, warning about circulation of the bacteria, which added to the knowledge of the presence of ticks could help to improve BSF monitoring.

When physicians, veterinarians, and other health professionals face every challenge the same way, they will understand that the traditional mechanisms for the study of diseases are full of unresolved gaps that can be addressed with interdisciplinary actions.

Conflict of Interests

The authors declare that there is no conflict of interests regarding the publication of this paper.

Acknowledgments

The authors are thankful to CNPq, Capes, and Faperj for the financial support.

References

[1] S. Harrus and G. Baneth, "Drivers for the emergence and re-emergence of vector-borne protozoal and bacterial diseases," *International Journal for Parasitology*, vol. 35, no. 11-12, pp. 1309–1318, 2005.

[2] D. D. Colwell, F. Dantas-Torres, and D. Otranto, "Vector-borne parasitic zoonoses: emerging scenarios and new perspectives," *Veterinary Parasitology*, vol. 182, no. 1, pp. 14–21, 2011.

[3] World Organisation for Animal Health (OIE), *Contributing to One World, One Health. A Strategic Framework for Reducing Risks of Infectious Diseases at the Animal-Human-Ecosystems Interface*, World Organisation for Animal Health (OIE), Paris, France, 2008.

[4] A. K. Silveira and A. H. Fonseca, *Caracterização de Ambientes com Potencial para Ocorrência de Carrapatos Transmissores de Agentes Patogênicos para Humanos*, vol. 13 of *Boletim do Parque Nacional Do Itatiaia*, Ministério do Meio Ambiente, Instituto Chico Mendes de Conservação da Biodiversidade, ICMBio, 2011.

[5] L. E. Shaffer, "Role of surveillance in disease prevention and control: crossspecies surveillance contribution to one medicine," in *Proceedings of the 145th AVMA Annual Convention*, Schaumburg, Ill, USA, July 2008.

[6] D. H. Walker, "*Rickettsia rickettsii*: as virulent as ever," *The American Journal of Tropical Medicine and Hygiene*, vol. 66, no. 5, pp. 448–449, 2002.

[7] M. B. Labruna, O. Kamakura, J. Moraes-Filho, M. C. Horta, and R. C. Pacheco, "Rocky mountain spotted fever in dogs, Brazil," *Emerging Infectious Diseases*, vol. 15, no. 3, pp. 458–460, 2009.

[8] C. D. Paddock, O. Brenner, C. Vaid et al., "Short report: concurrent Rocky Mountain spotted fever in a dog and its owner," *The American Journal of Tropical Medicine and Hygiene*, vol. 66, no. 2, pp. 197–199, 2002.

[9] A. Pinter, M. C. Horta, R. C. Pacheco, J. Moraes-Filho, and M. B. Labruna, "Serosurvey of *Rickettsia* spp. in dogs and humans from an endemic area for Brazilian spotted fever in the State of São Paulo, Brazil," *Cadernos de Saúde Pública*, vol. 24, no. 2, pp. 247–252, 2008.

[10] P. D. Van Helden, L. S. Van Helden, and E. G. Hoal, "One world, one health: humans, animals and the environment are inextricably linked—a fact that needs to be remembered and exploited in our modern approach to health," *EMBO Reports*, vol. 14, no. 6, pp. 497–501, 2013.

[11] K. E. Jones, N. G. Patel, M. A. Levy et al., "Global trends in emerging infectious diseases," *Nature*, vol. 451, no. 7181, pp. 990–993, 2008.

[12] D. Frank, "One world, one health, one medicine," *Canadian Veterinary Journal*, vol. 49, no. 11, pp. 1063–1065, 2008.

[13] J. Childs, R. E. Shope, D. Fish et al., "Emerging zoonoses," *Emerging Infectious Diseases*, vol. 4, no. 3, pp. 453–454, 1998.

[14] D. A. Jessup, M. A. Miller, C. Kreuder-Johnson et al., "Sea otters in a dirty ocean," *Journal of the American Veterinary Medical Association*, vol. 231, no. 11, pp. 1648–1652, 2007.

[15] P. M. R. Barros-Silva, L. X. Fonseca, M. E. Carneiro, K. M. A. Vilges, S. V. Oliveira, and R. Gurgel-Gonçalves, "Occupational risk of spotted fever: an evaluation of knowledge, attitudes and prevention practices among veterinary medicine students," *Revista de Patologia Tropical*, vol. 43, no. 4, pp. 389–397, 2014.

[16] A. S. Chapman, S. M. Murphy, L. J. Demma et al., "Rocky Mountain spotted fever in the United States, 1997–2002," *Vector-Borne and Zoonotic Diseases*, vol. 6, no. 2, pp. 170–178, 2006.

[17] D. Estripeaut, M. G. Aramburú, X. Sáez-Llorens et al., "Rocky Mountain spotted fever, Panama," *Emerging Infectious Diseases*, vol. 13, no. 11, pp. 1763–1765, 2007.

[18] D. Raoult and P. Parola, *Rickettsial Diseases (Infectious Disease and Therapy)*, CRC Press, New York, NY, USA, 2007.

[19] L. Hun, X. Cortés, and L. Taylor, "Molecular characterization of Rickettsia rickettsii isolated from human clinical samples and from the rabbit tick *Haemaphysalis leporispalustris* collected at different geographic zones in Costa Rica," *American Journal of Tropical Medicine and Hygiene*, vol. 79, no. 6, pp. 899–902, 2008.

[20] M. E. Eremeeva, E. Berganza, G. Suarez et al., "Investigation of an outbreak of rickettsial febrile illness in Guatemala, 2007," *International Journal of Infectious Diseases*, vol. 17, no. 5, pp. e304–e311, 2013.

[21] M. P. J. Szabó, A. Pinter, and M. B. Labruna, "Ecology, biology and distribution of spotted-fever tick vectors in Brazil," *Frontiers in Cellular and Infection Microbiology*, vol. 3, no. 27, pp. 1–9, 2013.

[22] E. Dias and A. V. Martins, "Spotted fever in Brazil," *American Journal of Tropical Medicine*, no. 19, pp. 103–108, 1939.

[23] E. R. S. De Lemos, F. B. F. Alvarenga, M. L. Cintra et al., "Spotted fever in Brazil: a seroepidemiological study and description of clinical cases in an endemic area in the state of São Paulo," *The American Journal of Tropical Medicine and Hygiene*, vol. 65, no. 4, pp. 329–334, 2001.

[24] M. A. M. Galvão, "Diagnósticos e inquéritos sorológicos para riquetsioses do gênero rickettsia no Brasil," *Revista Brasileira de Parasitologia Veterinária*, vol. 13, no. 1, pp. 188–189, 2004.

[25] J. Brites-Neto, F. A. Nieri-Bastos, J. Brasil et al., "Environmental infestation and rickettsial infection in ticks in an area endemic for Brazilian spotted fever," *Revista Brasileira de Parasitologia Veterinaria*, vol. 22, no. 3, pp. 367–372, 2013.

[26] T. F. Martins, A. R. M. Barbieri, F. B. Costa et al., "Estudo do complexo *Amblyomma cajennense* (Acari: Ixodidae) no Brasil," *BEPA, Boletim Epidemiológico Paulista*, vol. 10, no. 117, pp. 8–13, 2013.

[27] S. Nava, L. Beati, M. B. Labruna, A. G. Cáceres, A. J. Mangold, and A. A. Guglielmone, "Reassessment of the taxonomic status of *Amblyomma cajennense* (Fabricius, 1787) with the description of three new species, *Amblyomma tonelliae* n. sp., *Amblyomma interandinum* n. sp. and *Amblyomma patinoi* n. sp., and reinstatement of *Amblyomma mixtum* Koch, 1844, and *Amblyomma sculptum* Berlese, 1888 (Ixodida: Ixodidae)," *Ticks and Tick-Borne Diseases*, vol. 5, no. 3, pp. 252–276, 2014.

[28] M. B. Labruna, C. E. Kerber, F. Ferreira, J. L. Faccini, D. T. De Waal, and S. M. Gennari, "Risk factors to tick infestations and their occurrence on horses in the state of São Paulo, Brazil," *Veterinary Parasitology*, vol. 97, no. 1, pp. 1–14, 2001.

[29] M. B. Labruna, "Ecology of *Rickettsia* in South America," *Annals of the New York Academy of Sciences*, vol. 1166, pp. 156–166, 2009.

[30] M. Ogrzewalska, D. G. Saraiva, J. Moraes-Filho et al., "Epidemiology of Brazilian spotted fever in the Atlantic Forest, state of Sao Paulo, Brazil," *Parasitology*, vol. 139, no. 10, pp. 1283–1300, 2012.

[31] A. Pinter and M. B. Labruna, "Isolation of *Rickettsia rickettsii* and *Rickettsia bellii* in cell culture from the tick *Amblyomma aureolatum* in Brazil," *Annals of the New York Academy of Sciences*, vol. 1078, pp. 523–529, 2006.

[32] J. Moraes-Filho, A. Pinter, R. C. Pacheco et al., "New epidemiological data on Brazilian spotted fever in an endemic area of the state of São Paulo, Brazil," *Vector-Borne and Zoonotic Diseases*, vol. 9, no. 1, pp. 73–78, 2009.

[33] N. C. Cunha, A. H. Fonseca, J. Rezende et al., "First identification of natural infection of *Rickettsia rickettsii* in the *Rhipicephalus sanguineus* tick, in the State of Rio de Janeiro," *Pesquisa Veterinaria Brasileira*, vol. 29, no. 2, pp. 105–108, 2009.

[34] N. C. Cunha, E. R. S. Lemos, T. Rozental et al., "Rickettsiae of the Spotted Fever group in dogs, horses and ticks: an epidemiological study in an endemic region of the State of Rio de Janeiro, Brazil," *Revista Brasileira de Medicina Veterinária*, vol. 36, no. 3, pp. 294–300, 2014.

[35] D. G. Saraiva, H. S. Soares, J. F. Soares, and M. B. Labruna, "Feeding period required by *Amblyomma aureolatum* ticks for transmission of *Rickettsia rickettsii* to vertebrate hosts," *Emerging Infectious Diseases*, vol. 20, no. 9, pp. 1504–1510, 2014.

[36] D. Raoult and V. Roux, "Rickettsioses as paradigms of new or emerging infectious diseases," *Clinical Microbiology Reviews*, vol. 10, no. 4, pp. 694–719, 1997.

[37] M. A. M. Galvão, L. J. da Silva, E. M. Mendes Nascimento, S. B. Calic, R. de Sousa, and F. Bacellar, "Riquetsioses no Brasil e Portugal: ocorrência, distribuição e diagnóstico," *Revista de Saude Publica*, vol. 39, no. 5, pp. 850–856, 2005.

[38] E. Guedes, R. C. Leite, M. C. A. Prata, R. C. Pacheco, D. H. Walker, and M. B. Labruna, "Detection of *Rickettsia rickettsii* in the tick *Amblyomma cajennense* in a new Brazilian spotted fever-endemic area in the state of Minas Gerais," *Memórias do Instituto Oswaldo Cruz*, vol. 100, no. 8, pp. 841–845, 2005.

[39] P. Parola, C. D. Paddock, and D. Raoult, "Tick-borne rickettsioses around the world: emerging diseases challenging old concepts," *Clinical Microbiology Reviews*, vol. 18, no. 4, pp. 719–756, 2005.

[40] J. E. McDade and V. F. Newhouse, "Natural history of *Rickettsia rickettsii*," *Annual Review of Microbiology*, vol. 40, pp. 287–309, 1986.

[41] M. L. Niebylski, M. G. Peacock, and T. G. Schwan, "Lethal effect of *Rickettsia rickettsii* on its tick vector (*Dermacentor andersoni*)," *Applied and Environmental Microbiology*, vol. 65, no. 2, pp. 773–778, 1999.

[42] M. B. Labruna, T. Whitworth, M. C. Horta et al., "Rickettsia species infecting *Amblyomma cooperi* ticks from an area in the state of São Paulo, Brazil, where Brazilian Spotted Fever is endemic," *Journal of Clinical Microbiology*, vol. 42, no. 1, pp. 90–98, 2004.

[43] R. C. Pacheco, M. C. Horta, J. Moraes-Filho, A. C. Ataliba, A. Pinter, and M. B. Labruna, "Rickettsial infection in capybaras (*Hydrochoerus hydrochaeris*) from São Paulo, Brazil: serological evidence for infection by *Rickettsia bellii* and *Rickettsia parkeri*," *Biomédica*, vol. 27, no. 3, pp. 364–371, 2007.

[44] C. E. Souza, J. Moraes-Filho, M. Ogrzewalska et al., "Experimental infection of capybaras *Hydrochoerus hydrochaeris* by *Rickettsia rickettsii* and evaluation of the transmission of the infection to ticks *Amblyomma cajennense*," *Veterinary Parasitology*, vol. 161, no. 1-2, pp. 116–121, 2009.

[45] A. M. L. Vieira, C. E. Souza, M. B. Labruna, R. C. Mayo, S. S. L. Souza, and V. L. F. Camargo-Neves, *Manual de Vigilância Acarológica, Estado de São Paulo*, Secretaria de Saúde, Estado da São Paulo, São Paulo, Brazil, 2004.

[46] D. M. Barros-Battesti, M. Arzua, and G. H. Bechara, *Carrapatos de Importancia Médico-Veterinaria da Regiao Neotropical: Um Guia Ilustrado Para Identificação de Espécies*, Vox/ICTTD-3/Butantan, São Paulo, Brazil, 2006.

[47] J. F. Soares, H. S. Soares, A. M. Barbieri, and M. B. Labruna, "Experimental infection of the tick *Amblyomma cajennense*, cayenne tick, with *Rickettsia rickettsii*, the agent of Rocky Mountain spotted fever," *Medical and Veterinary Entomology*, vol. 26, no. 2, pp. 139–151, 2012.

[48] A. Pinter, A. C. França, C. E. Souza et al., "Febre Maculosa Brasileira," *BEPA Suplemento*, vol. 8, no. 1, pp. 3–31, 2011.

[49] A. Pinter, R. A. Dias, S. M. Gennari, and M. B. Labruna, "Study of the seasonal dynamics, life cycle, and host specificity of *Amblyomma aureolatum* (Acari: Ixodidae)," *Journal of Medical Entomology*, vol. 41, no. 3, pp. 324–332, 2004.

[50] A. A. Guglielmone, L. Beati, D. M. Barros-Battesti et al., "Ticks (Ixodidae) on humans in South America," *Experimental and Applied Acarology*, vol. 40, no. 2, pp. 83–100, 2006.

[51] N. M. Serra-Freire, "Occurrence of ticks (Acari: Ixodidae) on human hosts, in three municipalities in the State of Pará, Brazil," *Revista Brasileira de Parasitologia Veterinaria*, vol. 19, no. 3, pp. 141–147, 2010.

[52] M. B. Labruna, M. Ogrzewalska, T. F. Martins, A. Pinter, and M. C. Horta, "Comparative susceptibility of larval stages of *Amblyomma aureolatum*, *Amblyomma cajennense*, and *Rhipicephalus sanguineus* to infection by *Rickettsia rickettsii*," *Journal of Medical Entomology*, vol. 45, no. 6, pp. 1156–1159, 2008.

[53] M. B. Labruna, M. Ogrzewalska, J. F. Soares et al., "Experimental infection of *Amblyomma aureolatum* ticks with *Rickettsia rickettsii*," *Emerging Infectious Diseases*, vol. 17, no. 5, pp. 829–834, 2011.

[54] M. G. Spolidorio, M. B. Labruna, E. Mantovani, P. E. Brandão, L. J. Richtzenhain, and N. H. Yoshinari, "Novel spotted fever group rickettsiosis, Brazil," *Emerging Infectious Diseases*, vol. 16, no. 3, pp. 521–523, 2010.

[55] G. S. Sabatini, A. Pinter, F. A. Nieri-Bastos, A. Marcili, and M. B. Labruna, "Survey of ticks (Acari: Ixodidae) and their rickettsia in an Atlantic rain forest reserve in the state of São Paulo, Brazil," *Journal of Medical Entomology*, vol. 47, no. 5, pp. 913–916, 2010.

[56] F. S. Krawczak, *Avaliação da dinâmica da infecção por Rickettsia parkeri cepa Mata Atlântica, agente etiológico de uma nova riquetsiose brasileira, em carrapatos Amblyomma ovale Koch, 1844 naturalmente infectados [M.S. dissertation]*, Universidade de São Paulo, São Paulo, Brazil, 2012, http://www.teses.usp.br/teses/disponiveis/10/10134/tde-11062013-155536/pt-br.php.

[57] Y. Romer, A. C. Seijo, F. Crudo et al., "*Rickettsia parkeri* rickettsiosis, Argentina," *Emerging Infectious Diseases*, vol. 17, no. 7, pp. 1169–1173, 2011.

[58] I. Silveira, R. C. Pacheco, M. P. J. Szabó, H. G. C. Ramos, and M. B. Labruna, "*Rickettsia parkeri* in Brazil," *Emerging Infectious Diseases*, vol. 13, no. 7, pp. 1111–1113, 2007.

[59] M. P. J. Szabó, F. A. Nieri-Bastos, M. G. Spolidorio, T. F. Martins, A. M. Barbieri, and M. B. Labruna, "*In vitro* isolation from *Amblyomma ovale* (Acari: Ixodidae) and ecological aspects of the Atlantic rainforest *Rickettsia*, the causative agent of a novel spotted fever rickettsiosis in Brazil," *Parasitology*, vol. 140, no. 6, pp. 719–728, 2013.

[60] A. P. Medeiros, A. P. de Souza, A. B. de Moura et al., "Spotted fever group *Rickettsia* infecting ticks (Acari: Ixodidae) in the state of Santa Catarina, Brazil," *Memórias do Instituto Oswaldo Cruz*, vol. 106, no. 8, pp. 926–930, 2011.

[61] F. Dantas-Torres, L. A. Figueredo, and S. P. Brandão-Filho, "*Rhipicephalus sanguineus* (Acari: Ixodidae), o carrapato vermelho do cão, parasitando humanos no Brasil," *Revista da Sociedade Brasileira de Medicina Tropical*, vol. 39, pp. 64–67, 2006.

[62] R. C. Pacheco, J. Moraes-Filho, E. Guedes et al., "Rickettsial infections of dogs, horses and ticks in Juiz de Fora, southeastern Brazil, and isolation of *Rickettsia rickettsii* from *Rhipicephalus sanguineus* ticks," *Medical and Veterinary Entomology*, vol. 25, no. 2, pp. 148–155, 2011.

[63] P. Parola, C. D. Paddock, C. Socolovschi et al., "Update on tick-borne rickettsioses around the world: a geographic approach," *Clinical Microbiology Reviews*, vol. 26, no. 4, pp. 657–702, 2013.

[64] E. M. Piranda, J. L. H. Faccini, A. Pinter et al., "Experimental infection of dogs with a Brazilian strain of *Rickettsia rickettsii*: clinical and laboratory findings," *Memorias do Instituto Oswaldo Cruz*, vol. 103, no. 7, pp. 696–701, 2008.

[65] L. D. Cardoso, R. N. Freitas, C. L. Mafra et al., "Caracterização de *Rickettsia* spp. circulante em foco silencioso de febre maculosa brasileira no município de Caratinga, Minas Gerais, Brasil," *Cadernos de Saúde Pública*, vol. 22, no. 3, pp. 495–501, 2006.

[66] M. C. Horta, M. B. Labruna, A. Pinter, P. M. Linardi, and T. T. S. Schumaker, "*Rickettsia* infection in five areas of the state of São Paulo, Brazil," *Memórias do Instituto Oswaldo Cruz*, vol. 102, no. 7, pp. 793–801, 2007.

[67] V. M. F. Del Guercio, M. M. M. Rocha, H. H. B. Melles, V. C. L. Lima, and M. G. Pignatti, "Febre maculosa no município de Pedreira, SP, Brasil. Inquérito sorológico," *Revista da Sociedade Brasileira de Medicina Tropical*, vol. 30, no. 1, pp. 47–52, 1997.

[68] H. H. Melles, S. Colombo, and E. R. S. Lemos, "Isolamento de rickettsia em cultura de célula vero," *Revista da Sociedade Brasileira de Medicina Tropical*, vol. 32, no. 5, pp. 469–473, 1999.

[69] L. Kidd, B. Hegarty, D. Sexton, and E. Breitschwerdt, "Molecular characterization of *Rickettsia rickettsii* infecting dogs and people in North Carolina," *Annals of the New York Academy of Sciences*, vol. 1078, pp. 400–409, 2006.

[70] B. N. Elchos and J. Goddard, "Implications of presumptive fatal Rocky Mountain spotted fever in two dogs and their owner," *Journal of the American Veterinary Medical Association*, vol. 223, no. 10, pp. 1450–1452, 2003.

[71] D. M. Aguiar, G. T. Cavalcante, A. Pinter, S. M. Gennari, L. M. A. Camargo, and M. B. Labruna, "Prevalence of *Ehrlichia canis* (Rickettsiales: Anaplasmataceae) in dogs and *Rhipicephalus sanguineus* (Acari: Ixodidae) ticks from Brazil," *Journal of Medical Entomology*, vol. 44, no. 1, pp. 126–132, 2007.

[72] C. B. Grindem, E. B. Breitschwerdt, P. C. Perkins, L. D. Cullins, T. J. Thomas, and B. C. Hegarty, "Platelet-associated immunoglobulin (antiplatelet antibody) in canine rocky mountain spotted fever and ehrlichiosis," *Journal of the American Animal Hospital Association*, vol. 35, no. 1, pp. 56–61, 1999.

[73] F. Dantas-Torres, "Canine vector-borne diseases in Brazil," *Parasites and Vectors*, vol. 1, no. 1, article 25, 2008.

[74] B. S. Milagres, A. F. Padilha, R. M. Barcelos et al., "*Rickettsia* in synanthropic and domestic animals and their hosts from two areas of low endemicity for Brazilian spotted fever in the Eastern Region of Minas Gerais, Brazil," *The American Journal of Tropical Medicine and Hygiene*, vol. 83, no. 6, pp. 1305–1307, 2010.

[75] M. C. B. Vianna, M. C. Horta, L. A. Sangioni et al., "Rickettsial spotted fever in Capoeirão village, Itabira, Minas Gerais, Brazil," *Revista do Instituto de Medicina Tropical de Sao Paulo*, vol. 50, no. 5, pp. 297–301, 2008.

27

Interpretation Criteria for Comparative Intradermal Tuberculin Test for Diagnosis of Bovine Tuberculosis in Cattle in Maroua Area of Cameroon

J. Awah-Ndukum,[1] J. Temwa,[1] V. Ngu Ngwa,[1] M. M. Mouiche,[1] D. Iyawa,[2] and P. A. Zoli[1]

[1]*School of Veterinary Medicine and Sciences, University of Ngaoundéré, BP 454, Ngaoundéré, Cameroon*
[2]*Regional Delegation of Livestock, Fisheries, Animal Industries, Far North Region, Cameroon*

Correspondence should be addressed to J. Awah-Ndukum; awahndukum@yahoo.co.uk

Academic Editor: Francesca Mancianti

Intradermal tuberculin test (TST) is the choice method for diagnosis of bovine tuberculosis (Tb) in live animals. This work was done to assess the performance of single intradermal comparative cervical tuberculin (SICCT) test in randomly selected cattle in Maroua, Cameroon, against detection of Tb lesions and detection of Tb lesions plus acid fast bacilli in lesions. While 22.28% of slaughtered cattle presented Tb lesions at meat inspection, detection rates of anti-bovine-Tb antibody, Tb lesions, and Tb lesions plus acid fast bacilli were 68.57%, 32.95%, and 22.35%, respectively. SICCT-bovine-Tb positive cattle were 35.29%, 29.41%, 25.88%, 24.7%, and 21.18% at ≥2 mm, ≥2.5 mm, ≥3 mm, ≥3.5 mm, and ≥4 mm cut-offs, respectively. Higher sensitivity and predictive values were obtained at severe interpretations. The best performance was at ≥3 mm and ≥3.5 mm cut-offs. Against detection of Tb lesions, ≥3 mm and ≥3.5 mm showed sensitivity of 67.8% and specificity of 94.7% and 96.5%, respectively. For detection of Tb lesions accompanied with acid fast bacilli in lesions, ≥3 mm and ≥3.5 mm showed sensitivity of 89.4% and specificity of 92.4% and 93.9%, respectively. These findings revealed that interpretations of SICCT-bovine-Tb should be at ≥3 mm and/or ≥3.5 mm cut-offs. Severe interpretation of TST is essential for optimal diagnosis of bovine Tb in cattle in Maroua, Cameroon.

1. Introduction

Bovine tuberculosis (Tb) is a major chronic bacterial disease of animals and humans caused by *Mycobacterium bovis*. Though zoonotic, bovine Tb is neglected and underinvestigated in Sub-Saharan Africa including Cameroon [1, 2]. In areas where bovine Tb is endemic and not controlled or partially controlled, human Tb due to *M. bovis* may occur resulting from ingesting contaminated fresh milk and meat products and by inhaling cough spray from infected cattle [3–8]. Widespread bovine Tb in cattle has been diagnosed in some parts of Cameroon following comparative cervical tuberculin test, detection of Tb lesions during abattoir slaughter meat inspection, acid fast staining of bacilli, and molecular analysis of cultured isolates [1, 9, 10]. Also, *M. bovis* in human has been reported in the West and Northwest Regions of Cameroon [11, 12].

Bovine Tb has significant impact on international trade of livestock and animal products [13]. Intradermal tuberculin skin test (TST) is the international choice method for field diagnosis of bovine Tb in live animals and the World Organisation for Animal Health (OIE) recommended difference between the increases in skin thickness for the test to be positive should be at least 4 mm after 72 hours [13]. However, the performance of TST is affected by environmental and host factors and the nature of the tuberculin used [14–19]. A perfect cut-off point in a specific geographic area or country may not be useful in another environment or another country [14, 17, 20] and the ability of the test to accurately predict true positive disease status depends on its sensitivity, specificity, and prevalence of the disease in the population tested [14]. The OIE recommended cut-off value was established mainly in developed countries for *Bos taurus* cattle and different cut-off values are applied according to a particular country's disease status and objective of its disease control programme [17]. Severe interpretations have been used in Chad, Ethiopia, and Tanzania [15, 17, 21–23] and in regions or herds where *M. bovis* infection had been confirmed based on the discretion of the veterinarian [17].

TST together with slaughter of positive reactors to examine for Tb lesions; culture of suspected Tb specimens; and other modern diagnostic techniques (e.g., gamma-interferon, ESAT-6 tests, and serologic and fluorescence polarization assays) have been compared and are being validated for maximum diagnosis of bovine Tb in cattle in various environmental conditions [14, 24–28]. This study was therefore carried out to estimate the prevalence of bovine Tb and assess the diagnostic performance of TST in the diagnosis of bovine Tb zebu cattle in Maroua area of Cameroon.

2. Materials and Methods

2.1. Study Area and Population. Cattle from the livestock markets in the environs of Maroua destined for slaughter at the Makabaye abattoir were sampled for the study. About twenty cattle are slaughtered daily in the Makabaye abattoir which provides beef to inhabitants of Maroua city and neighbouring areas ($10°30'–10°40'$N and $14°20'–14°30'$E). A TST bovine Tb prevalence rate of 4.67% (3.89%–5.44%) recorded by Awah-Ndukum et al. [29] in the highlands of Cameroon using OIE recommended standards was used to estimate the number of cattle required to detect at least one positive reactor with 95% confidence and a desired precision of ≥5% as previously described [30]. The selection of cattle for the study was based on haphazard arrival of animals at the abattoir and on random-number generation method of cattle owners from the daily abattoir records whose animals were judged as fit to be slaughtered. However, cattle used for the TST performance study were animals that were judged as fit to be slaughtered and were not slaughtered until at least 72-hour stay at the abattoir.

2.2. Detection of Bovine Tuberculosis. During November 2013 to March 2014, blood was collected by venopuncture of the jugular vein from 175 randomly selected cattle intended for slaughter to extract serum for lateral flow assay of anti-BTb antibody (Anti-Bovine Ab®). Single intradermal comparative cervical tuberculin (SICCT) skin test was done on 86 random cattle of the 175 selected animals [13] that were slaughtered at least 72 hours later. Following slaughter of these 175 animals, intensive meat inspections were carried out by JT assisted by veterinary staff of the abattoir based on the government's legislation regulating veterinary health inspection and notification of contagious animal diseases [31]. Evidence of pathologies was also supported by postmortem examination of carcasses as earlier described [32–34]. Briefly, the inspection procedure employed visual examination and palpation of the lungs, liver, and kidneys, lymph nodes of the thoracic and head regions, the mesenteric lymph nodes, and other lymph nodes of the body and various other parts/organs of the carcass.

The sera were extracted and stored at −20°C until analysis was carried out. Similarly, 68 tissues specimens, with suspicious TB lesions (53 thoracic and 7 abdominal lymph nodes and 8 liver tissues) from the 86 SICCT bovine Tb cattle of the 175 slaughtered zebu cattle in the study were collected into sterile plastic containers and also stored at −20°C for up to two months before analysis. Individual animal information such as age estimated by examining the incisors [35], sex, breed [31, 36], and body condition scores [37] was recorded during blood collection. Grinding of TB lesions [38] and direct smear microscopy with Ziehl-Neelsen (ZN) staining for confirmation of acid fast tubercle bacilli and lateral-flow-based rapid test for detection of antibodies in serum were done following standard procedures [13, 39–41] and as described by manufacturer (Anigen Bovine Tb Ab®, BioNote Inc., Korea). Briefly, in the ready-to-use disposable lateral flow kit, 10 μL of test serum was poured into the sample well and, after 1 minute, 3 drops of developing buffer (provided as part of the kit) were placed in the buffer well. The result was interpreted after 20 minutes. The presence of two purple coloured bands within the result window, the test area and control line, indicated antibodies positive result whereas no band in the test area in addition to a visible control purple line was negative. An invalid test was one where no coloured band was visible within the result window. The appearance of a control colour band, for positive or negative assays, indicated that the test was working properly.

Risk assessments of the project were performed by the researchers to avoid hazards to all persons and animals involved in the project. Ethical clearances were obtained from the required authorities before carrying out the study. The purpose of the study was explained to the targeted participants usually with the assistance of resident veterinarians, local leaders at the abattoir, and or trusted intermediaries. An animal was tested after an informed consent was given by the owner. Apart from minor jugular vein puncture for blood collection, intradermal injections of avian and bovine tuberculin, and procedural restraining manipulations for safety purposes, the animals were not subjected to suffering. Slaughtering and dressing of cattle carcasses were done as described by the Cameroon veterinary services [31]. All laboratory analyses including ZN staining were carried out in a laboratory equipped with a category II Biosafety cabinet.

2.3. Data Analysis. The data were entered into Microsoft Excel and then transferred to SPSS 20 and R software. Frequency distributions of bovine Tb were generated for the different diagnostic techniques. The Chi-square test was used to evaluate the sensitivity of TST and assess various associations. The ROC (*Receiving Operating Characteristic*) analysis was also used to evaluate diagnostic performance of TST at different cut-off points [30].

3. Results

3.1. Prevalence of Bovine Tuberculosis. Over 22.28% (164) of 736 cattle slaughtered at Makabaye-Maroua during the study period presented macroscopic Tb lesions at meat inspection. The cattle with Tb lesions were distributed as follows: 12 of 123

(9.76%) male animals, 152 of 613 (24.80%) female animals, 44 of 133 (33.08%) animals aged 5 to 10 years, 120 of 597 (20.10%) animals aged over 10 years, 62 of 302 (20.53%) Peulh of Sahel zebu, 86 of 242 (35.54%) Bororo/Fulani zebu, and 16 of 192 (8.33%) Toupouri-Massa zebu.

However, 68.57% (95% CI: 61.69–75.45) of 175 randomly selected cattle were positive for anti-bovine Tb antibodies with lateral flow assay. Single intradermal comparative cervical tuberculin (SICCT) skin test done on 86 of these 175 cattle showed 30 (35.29%, 95% CI: 25.1–45.4), 25 (29.41%, 95% CI: 19.7–39.1), 22 (25.88%, 95% CI: 16.6–35.2), 21 (24.7%, 95% CI: 15.5–33.8), and 18 (21.18%, 95% CI: 12.5–29.8) positive reactors at ≥ 2 mm, ≥ 2.5 mm, ≥ 3 mm, ≥ 3.5 mm, and ≥ 4 mm cut-off points, respectively. Of the 86 animals, Tb lesions and Tb lesions plus acid fast bacilli were detected in 28 animals (32.95%, 95% CI: 22.95–42.93) and 19 animals (22.35%, 95% CI: 13.5–31.2), respectively. Over 73.26% (63) of the 86 SICCT animals were positive for anti-bovine Tb antibodies corresponding to apparent rates of 3.49%, 31.40%, 29.07%, 25.58%, 24.42%, and 20.93% animals positive for SICCT bovine Tb and anti-bovine Tb antibody at < 2 mm, ≥ 2 mm, ≥ 2.5 mm, ≥ 3 mm, ≥ 3.5 mm, and ≥ 4 mm cut-off points, respectively.

3.2. Diagnostic Performance of Tuberculin Skin Test to Detect Bovine Tuberculosis in Cattle. The performances of SICCT technique at various cut-off points to diagnose bovine Tb in cattle in Maroua, Cameroon, using detection of Tb lesions and detection of Tb lesions accompanied with acid fast bacilli in the lesions as references for defining the status disease are shown in Table 1. Based on computed sensitivity and specificity values of SICCT compared to detection of Tb lesions and Tb lesions plus acid fast bacilli, severe interpretations of SICCT tests detected more diseases cases. Though highest detection of disease cases by SICCT tests was detected at ≥ 2.0 mm cut-off point, the overall performances were superior at ≥ 3 mm and ≥ 3.5 mm cut-off values. The sensitivity of SICCT at ≥ 3 mm and ≥ 3.5 mm cut-off points compared to the sensitivity at ≥ 4 mm cut-off was not significantly higher [$P > 0.05$] against detection of Tb lesions but significantly higher [$P < 0.05$] against detection of Tb lesions plus acid fast bacilli to define disease status.

It is worth mentioning that overall the predictive values were usually superior at SICCT ≥ 3 mm and ≥ 3.5 mm cut-off points compared to the OIE recommended (≥ 4 mm) cut-off point. Indeed, the performance of SICCT against detection of Tb lesions revealed positive predictive values of 73.3 (63.9–82.7); 80.0 (71.5–88.5); 86.3 (78.9–93.6); 90.4 (84.1–96.6); 88.8 (82.1–95.5) and negative predictive values of 89.0 (82.3–95.6); 86.6 (79.3–93.8); 85.7 (78.2–93.1); 85.9 (78.5–93.2); 82.0 (73.8–90.1) at reactors at ≥ 2 mm, ≥ 2.5 mm, ≥ 3 mm, ≥ 3.5 mm, and ≥ 4 mm cut-off points, respectively. Accordingly, the performance of SICCT against detection of Tb lesions plus acid fast bacilli revealed positive predictive values of 63.3 (53.05–73.54); 72 (62.45–81.54); 77.3 (68.39–86.20); 81 (72.66–89.34); 77.8 (68.96–86.63) and negative predictive values of 100; 98.3 (95.5–100); 96.8 (93–100); 96.9 (93–100); 92.5 (86.9–98.1).

Furthermore, the ROC (*Receiving Operating Characteristic*) analysis showed that the area under the curve was significantly higher at cut-off points < 4 mm, particularly at ≥ 3.5 mm cut-off point according to detection of Tb lesions [0.822 (0.711–0.932)] and detection of Tb lesions plus acid fast bacilli in the lesions [0.92 (0.83–1)] [Figure 1]. The area under the ROC curves according to detection of Tb lesions for all SICCT cut-off points was between 0.7 and 0.9 suggesting that these cut-off values are only fairly informative for the detection of bovine Tb. However, SICCT at ≥ 3.5 mm cut-off point showed significantly higher ($P < 0.001$) discriminatory power compared to SICCT at ≥ 4 mm cut-off point. For the ROC curves according to detection of detection of Tb lesions plus acid fast bacilli in the lesions, all SICCT cut-off points < 4 mm were between 0.9 and 1, particularly for ≥ 3 mm and ≥ 3.5 mm cut-off points, indicating that these cut-off values are very informative for the detection of bovine Tb. Therefore, the ROC findings also confirmed severe interpretations of SICCT bovine Tb detection [particularly at ≥ 3 mm and ≥ 3.5 mm cut-off points] as for sensitivity and specificity evaluations.

4. Discussion

The detection rates of macroscopic Tb lesions [22.28–32.95%] in cattle in this study are much higher than values, ranging from < 1 to 4.25%, reported in the littoral and western highland regions of Cameroon [29, 42], while the prevalence of anti-bovine Tb antibodies [68.57% and 73.26%] was higher than 60% recorded in the Bamenda area [42] and 37.17% recorded in the highland regions [43]. Also, significantly higher SICCT bovine Tb prevalence estimates based on tuberculin skin tests at cut-off points ≥ 4 mm, ≥ 3 mm, and ≥ 2 mm were obtained compared to 3.59%–7.48%, 8.92%–13.25%, and 11.77%–17.26% recorded by Awah-Ndukum et al. [43] in the highland regions. However, the rates of SICCT bovine Tb/anti-bovine Tb antibodies animal responses in this study agree with that of Awah-Ndukum et al. [43] who reported that the proportion of SICCT bovine Tb/anti-bovine Tb antibody reactors was significantly higher at the ≥ 2 mm followed by the ≥ 3 mm and ≥ 4 mm cut-off point groups. These findings suggest that bovine Tb is highly endemic in cattle in the Maroua area compared to other parts of Cameroon and require severe interpretations of SICCT bovine Tb results.

Postmortem examination of Tb lesions and demonstration of acid fast bacilli by direct microscopy were used in this study to define disease status of bovine Tb in cattle, to evaluate the performance of tuberculin skin test as opposed to bacteriological culture that was used elsewhere as reference diagnostic test [13]. However, detection of Tb lesions showed lower sensitivity values compared to detection of Tb lesions accompanied with demonstration of acid fast bacilli in the lesions. Macroscopic examination of Tb lesions and demonstration of acid fast bacilli have also been used by Ameni et al. [15] in Ethiopia and Ngandolo et al. [21] in Chad to evaluate the diagnostic performances of tuberculin skin tests. In this study optimal detection of bovine Tb in cattle in Maroua, Cameroon, was obtained at severe interpretations of SICCT and particularly at ≥ 3 mm and ≥ 3.5 mm. These findings are similar to those of Ameni et al. [15] who reported that

TABLE 1: Performances of single intradermal comparative cervical tuberculin (SICCT) skin test at various cut-off points to diagnose bovine tuberculosis in zebu cattle in Maroua, Cameroon, using detection of tuberculosis lesions and detection of tuberculosis lesions accompanied with acid fast bacilli in lesions to define disease status.

SICCT cut-off point	Detection of tuberculosis lesions to define disease status				Detection of tuberculosis lesions and acid fast bacilli in lesions to define disease status			
	Sensitivity		Specificity		Sensitivity		Specificity	
	Value, % (95% CI)	P value [χ^2]	Value, % (95% CI)	P value [χ^2]	Value, % (95% CI)	P value [χ^2]	Value, % (95% CI)	P value [χ^2]
≥2 mm	78.5 (69.7–87.2)	0.001* [10.49]	85.9 (78.5–93.2)	0.008* [7.0]	100	0.000* [30.41]	83.3 (75.37–91.23)	0.018* [5.56]
≥2.5 mm	71.4 (61.8–81.0)	0.034* [4.45]	91.2 (85.1–97.2)	0.118 [2.43]	94.7 (89.9–99.4)	0.000* [16.69]	89.4 (82.85–95.94)	0.250 [1.32]
≥3.0 mm	67.8 (57.8–77.7)	0.118 [2.44]	94.7 (89.9–99.4)	0.534 [0.38]	89.4 (82.8–95.9)	0.004* [8.28]	92.4 (86.76–98.03)	0.674 [0.17]
≥3.5 mm	67.8 (57.8–77.7)	0.118 [2.44]	96.5 (92.6–100)	1 [0]	89.4 (82.8–95.9)	0.004* [8.28]	93.9 (88.81–98.98)	1 [0]
≥4 mm	57.1 (46.5–67.6)	—	96.5 (92.6–100)	—	73.6 (64.2–82.9)	—	93.9 (88.81–98.98)	—

*Significantly different [$P < 0.05$] when compared to ≥4 mm cut-off point.

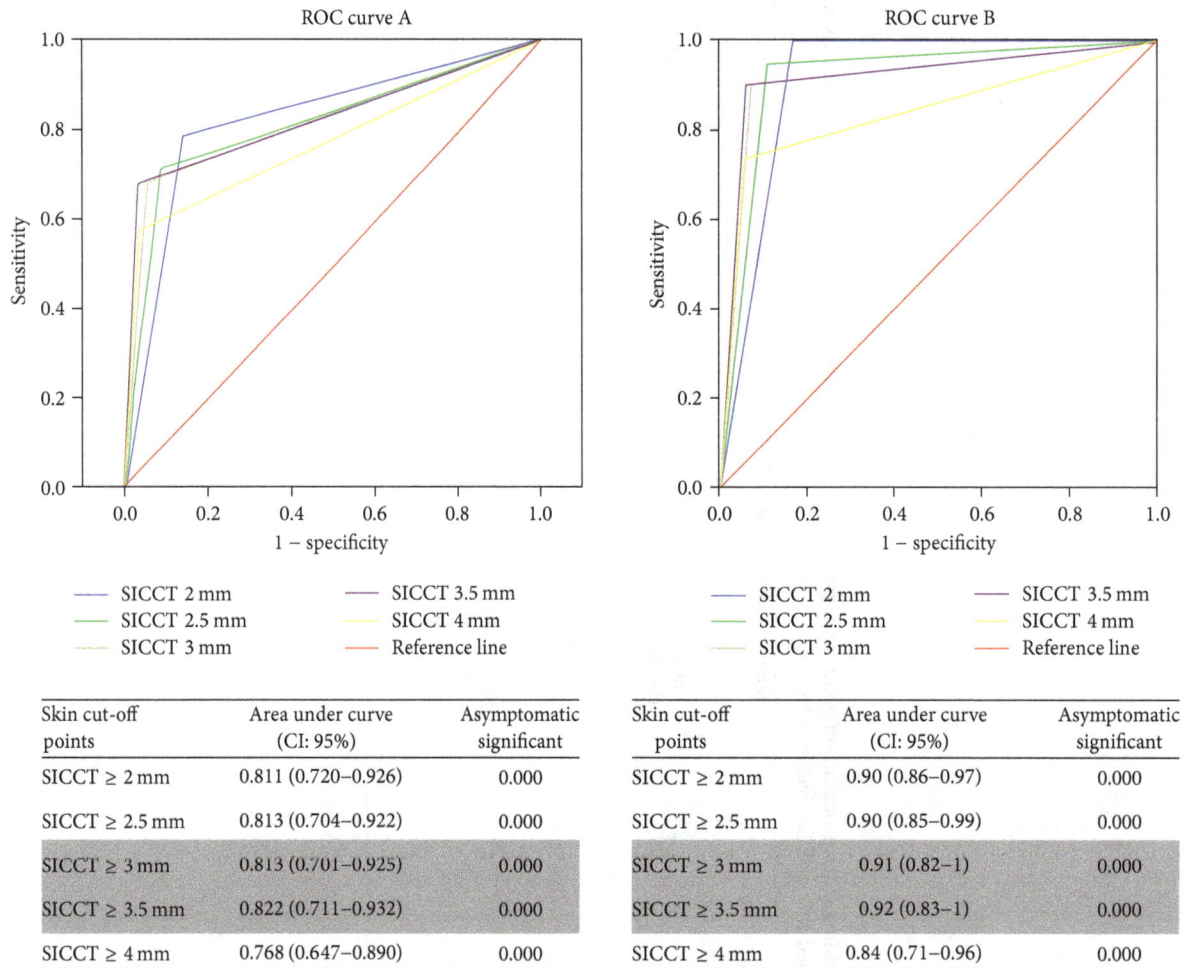

FIGURE 1: ROC (*Receiving Operating Characteristic*) analysis of the performances of SICCT to detect bovine Tb. Classification of the single intradermal comparative cervical tuberculin (SICCT) skin test cut-off point performance with detection of tuberculous lesions as reference test (curve A). Classification of the single intradermal comparative cervical tuberculin (SICCT) skin test cut-off point performance with detection of tuberculous lesions and acid fast bacilli as reference test (curve B).

improved diagnostic performances of tuberculin skin test in zebu cattle in Ethiopia were obtained at severe interpretations of >2 mm cut-off point. In Chad, Ngandolo et al. [21] also stated that optimum diagnostic performance of tuberculin skin test in Arab zebus and Bororo zebus was >2 mm cut-off point. The present results agree with those of Awah-Ndukum et al. [43] who observed that improved diagnosis of bovine Tb by tuberculin skin test was obtained at ≥3 mm cut-off when compared to anti-bovine Tb antibody detection in Goudali, Red Bororo, and White Fulani zebus and their crosses in the highlands [Adamawa and Northwest] of Cameroon.

The tuberculin skin tests are currently the best available and affordable techniques for international field diagnosis of bovine TB in live animals [14, 24]. Also, the tests are based on delayed hypersensitivity reactions [13]. The intradermal comparative cervical tuberculin (ICCT) skin test involving the intradermal injection of bovine tuberculin (BT) and avian tuberculin (AT) at separate sites in the skin of the neck gives more specific results than the simple intradermal tuberculin (SIT) skin test which uses only BT [16, 17]. The World

Organisation for Animal Health (OIE) recommended difference between the increases in skin thickness for the test to be positive should be >4 mm after 72 hours [13]. However, the OIE recommended cut-off value was established mainly in developed countries for *Bos taurus* cattle [15], in an epidemiologic context of very low prevalence of bovine Tb [≤0.1%] and the implementation of a strict test and slaughter eradication policy [24]. Indeed, different cut-off values have been applied worldwide according to a particular country's disease status and objective of its disease control programme [17]. In Africa, for example, the >2 mm, ≥3 mm, >4 mm, and ≥4 mm cut-off points have been used in Chad, Ethiopia, and Tanzania [15, 17, 22, 23, 44].

The ROC analysis and sensitivity evaluations support severe interpretation of tuberculin skin tests in this study, particularly at ≥3 mm and ≥3.5 mm cut-off points and [43] had proposed severe interpretations of tuberculin skin tests for the diagnosis of bovine Tb in *Bos indicus* cattle in Cameroon, where the prevalence of bovine Tb is high and widespread. The performance of tuberculin skin tests has also been affected by environmental factors, host factors (status of immunity, genetics, etc.), prevalence of the disease in the population tested, and the nature of the tuberculin used [14–19]. A perfect cut-off point in a specific geographic area may not be so useful at another environment [14, 17] and the ability of the test to accurately predict the true positive disease status depends on its sensitivity, specificity, and prevalence of the disease in the population tested [14]. Excessively high sensitivity of tuberculin skin tests will generate false positive reactions during interpretations of test results. However, severe interpretations for improved diagnosis have been done in regions or herds where *M. bovis* infection had been confirmed based on the discretion of the veterinarian [17].

In this study, the best individual sensitivity [67.8% (57.8–77.7) at ≥3.5 mm cut-off point] of tuberculin skin test, with detection of Tb lesions as the reference test, recorded is lower than the median individual sensitivity [80% (52.0–100)] stated by OIE [13] at the recommended >4 mm cut-off point [14]. The best individual sensitivity [89.4% (82.8–95.9) at ≥3.5 mm cut-off point] of tuberculin skin test, with detection of Tb lesions plus acid fast bacilli in lesions as the reference test, recorded is higher than the median individual sensitivity stated by OIE at the recommended cut-off point. The OIE proposed value is a median from a very wide dispersion (52.0–100%) compared to very narrower dispersions for best overall values in the present study (57.8–77.7% and 82.8–95.9%). For SICCT bovine Tb detection, the study showed higher (nonsignificant for detection of Tb lesions and significant for detection of Tb lesions accompanied with AFB in lesions as gold standards) sensitivities at severe (<4 mm cut-off) interpretation compared to interpretation at the OIE recommended (≥4 mm) cut-off value. Severe interpretation of SICCT results diagnosed more bovine Tb cases and is very essential in managing high zoonotic potential [1] as well as high socioeconomic and cultural implication [45] of bovine Tb in Cameroon. The sensitivities obtained in this study are similar to the values of Ameni et al. [15] who reported 68.8% at >2 mm cut-off point in Ethiopia and Delafosse et al. [23] who reported 94% at ≥4 mm in Chad. Various factors can influence the sensitivity of tuberculin skin test and the hypersensitivity reactions can fluctuate considerably depending on the animal. Delayed hypersensitivity reactions provoked by tuberculin injection can become established 3 to 6 weeks after exposure of the host to bacilli agents while recently infected animals may not react sufficiently to tuberculin injection [46]. The reaction is reduced in young animals [calves] and pregnant females [cow] near term [47].

Anergy has been reported to cause false negative reactions during tuberculin skin test but the reasons are still poorly understood [48]. However, recently infected cattle, cattle under stress due to malnutrition, gastrointestinal parasitoses, other concurrent infections, and cattle with generalized Tb would be anergic and fail to react to tuberculin skin test [47, 48]. Therefore, cattle presenting differential SICCT skin thickness of ≤4 mm should not be excluded that they are not affected by bovine Tb, especially animals in highly endemic areas and animals sensitized to environmental mycobacteria such as in Cameroon [29]. These animals could actually be infected but low reacting or not reacting

at all because their immune systems may not be sufficiently stimulated for a positive response to occur at the ≥4 mm OIE recommended cut-off point [47, 48]. Also, conditions such as stress may compromise their immune function [49] and animals may be sensitized to environmental mycobacteria [50]. Furthermore, in late stages or towards the end of the course of the disease, the capacities of the infected hosts may become saturated and the expected hypersensitivity reactions may not be observed [51]. Also, 1–5% of some animals may be totally anergic during their entire lifespan [24, 52]. These phenomena are responsible for the fluctuating sensitivities of tuberculin skin tests according to environments and amongst animal populations.

This study revealed that severe interpretation of tuberculin skin tests, at cut-off values less than the OIE recommended cut-off value of >4 mm, is essential for optimal diagnosis of bovine Tb in *Bos indicus* cattle in Maroua, Cameroon. The interpretations should be done at either ≥3 mm or ≥3.5 mm cut-off points given the epidemiological and environmental context of the region.

Competing Interests

The authors declare that they have no competing interests.

References

[1] J. Awah-Ndukum, A. C. Kudi, G. S. Bah, G. Bradley, V. Ngu-Ngwa, and P. L. Dickmu, "Risk factors analysis and implications for public health of bovine tuberculosis in the highlands of Cameroon," *Bulletin of Animal Health and Production in Africa*, vol. 62, no. 4, pp. 353–376, 2014.

[2] A. R. Boukary, E. Thys, S. Mamadou et al., "La tuberculose à *Mycobacterium bovis* en Afrique subsaharienne," *Annales de Médecine Vétérinaire*, vol. 155, pp. 23–37, 2011.

[3] C. H. Collins and J. M. Grange, "Zoonotic implication of *Mycobacterium bovis* infection," *Irish Veterinary Journal*, vol. 41, pp. 363–366, 1987.

[4] O. Cosivi, J. M. Grange, C. J. Daborn et al., "Zoonotic tuberculosis due to *Mycobacterium bovis* in developing countries," *Emerging Infectious Diseases*, vol. 4, no. 1, pp. 59–70, 1998.

[5] E. Etter, P. Donado, F. Jori, A. Caron, F. Goutard, and F. Roger, "Risk analysis and bovine tuberculosis, a re-emerging zoonosis," *Annals of the New York Academy of Sciences*, vol. 1081, pp. 61–73, 2006, Impact of Emerging Zoonotic Diseases on Animal Health: 8th Biennial Conference of the Society for Tropical Veterinary Medicine.

[6] G. Moda, C. J. Daborn, J. M. Grange, and O. Cosivi, "The zoonotic importance of *Mycobacterium bovis*," *Tubercle and Lung Disease*, vol. 77, no. 2, pp. 103–108, 1996.

[7] C. Thoen, P. LoBue, and I. de Kantor, "The importance of *Mycobacterium bovis* as a zoonosis," *Veterinary Microbiology*, vol. 112, no. 2-4, pp. 339–345, 2006.

[8] J. E. Shitaye, W. Tsegaye, and I. Pavlik, "Bovine tuberculosis infection in animal and human populations in Ethiopia: a review," *Veterinarni Medicina*, vol. 52, no. 8, pp. 317–332, 2007.

[9] J. Awah-Ndukum, A. C. Kudi, G. Bradley et al., "Molecular genotyping of *Mycobacterium bovis* isolated from cattle tissues in the North West Region of Cameroon," *Tropical Animal Health and Production*, vol. 45, no. 3, pp. 829–836, 2013.

[10] F. Koro-Koro, E. F. Bouba, A. F. Ngatchou, S. Eyangoh, and F.-X. Etoa, "First insight into the current prevalence of bovine tuberculosis in cattle slaughtered in Cameroon: the case of main abattoirs of Yaoundé and Douala," *British Microbiology Research Journal*, vol. 3, no. 3, pp. 272–279, 2013.

[11] S. N. Niobe-Eyangoh, C. Kuaban, P. Sorlin et al., "Genetic biodiversity of *Mycobacterium tuberculosis* complex strains from patients with pulmonary tuberculosis in Cameroon," *Journal of Clinical Microbiology*, vol. 41, no. 6, pp. 2547–2553, 2003.

[12] F. Nkongho, R. Kelly, L. Ndip et al., "Molecular epidemiology of bovine tuberculosis in Cameroon," in *Proceedings of the 6th International M. Bovis Conference*, Cardiff, UK, 2014.

[13] OIE, *Manual of Diagnostic Tests and Vaccines for Terrestrial Animals 2009*, OIE Terrestrial Manual 2008, World Organisation for Animal Health, Paris, France, 2009, http://www.oie.int/eng/normes/mmanual/A_summry.htm.

[14] R. T. Goodchild, M. Vordermeier, R. Clifton-Hadley, and R. de la Rua-Domenech, "Ante mortem diagnosis of Bovine Tuberculosis: the significance of unconfirmed test reactors," *Government Veterinary Journal*, vol. 16, no. 1, pp. 65–71, 2006.

[15] G. Ameni, G. Hewinson, A. Aseffa, D. Young, and M. Vordermeier, "Appraisal of interpretation criteria for the comparative intradermal tuberculin test for diagnosis of tuberculosis in cattle in central Ethiopia," *Clinical and Vaccine Immunology*, vol. 15, no. 8, pp. 1272–1276, 2008.

[16] J. Francis, C. L. Choi, and A. J. Frost, "The diagnosis of tuberculosis in cattle with special reference to bovine PPD tuberculin," *Australian Veterinary Journal*, vol. 49, no. 5, pp. 246–251, 1973.

[17] M. L. Monaghan, M. L. Doherty, J. D. Collins, J. F. Kazda, and P. J. Quinn, "The tuberculin test," *Veterinary Microbiology*, vol. 40, no. 1-2, pp. 111–124, 1994.

[18] T. Marcotty, F. Matthys, J. Godfroid et al., "Zoonotic tuberculosis and brucellosis in Africa: neglected zoonoses or minor public-health issues? The outcomes of a multi-disciplinary workshop," *Annals of Tropical Medicine and Parasitology*, vol. 103, no. 5, pp. 401–411, 2009.

[19] M.-F. Humblet, M. Gilbert, M. Govaerts, M. Fauville-Dufaux, K. Walravens, and C. Saegerman, "New assessment of bovine tuberculosis risk factors in Belgium based on nationwide molecular epidemiology," *Journal of Clinical Microbiology*, vol. 48, no. 8, pp. 2802–2808, 2010.

[20] S. A. J. Strain, M. James, and W. J. M. Stanley, "Bovine tuberculosis: a review of diagnostic tests for M. bovis infection in cattle," *Bacteriology Branch Veterinary Sciences Division, Agri-Food and Biosciences Institute*, vol. 45, pp. 8–23, 2011.

[21] B. N. Ngandolo, C. Diguimbaye-Djaïbé, B. Müller et al., "Diagnostics ante et post mortem de la tuberculose bovine au sud du Tchad: cas des bovins destinés à l'abattage," *Revue d'Élevage et de Médecine Vétérinaire des Pays Tropicaux*, vol. 62, no. 1, pp. 5–12, 2009.

[22] R. R. Kazwala, D. M. Kambarage, C. J. Daborn, J. Nyange, S. F. H. Jiwa, and J. M. Sharp, "Risk factors associated with the occurrence of bovine tuberculosis in cattle in the Southern Highlands of Tanzania," *Veterinary Research Communications*, vol. 25, no. 8, pp. 609–614, 2001.

[23] A. Delafosse, F. Goutard, and E. Thébaud, "Epidémiologie de la tuberculose et de la brucellose des bovins en zone périurbaine d'Abéché, Tchad," *Revue d'Élevage et de Médecine Vétérinaire des Pays Tropicaux*, vol. 55, no. 1, pp. 5–13, 2002.

[24] R. de la Rua-Domenech, A. T. Goodchild, H. M. Vordermeier, R. G. Hewinson, K. H. Christiansen, and R. S. Clifton-Hadley, "Ante mortem diagnosis of tuberculosis in cattle: a review of the tuberculin tests, γ-interferon assay and other ancillary diagnostic techniques," *Research in Veterinary Science*, vol. 81, no. 2, pp. 190–210, 2006.

[25] J. M. Pollock, J. McNair, H. Bassett et al., "Specific delayed-type hypersensitivity responses to ESAT-6 identify tuberculosis-infected cattle," *Journal of Clinical Microbiology*, vol. 41, no. 5, pp. 1856–1860, 2003.

[26] M. Amadori, S. Tameni, P. Scaccaglia, S. Cavirani, I. L. Archetti, and R. Q. Giandomenico, "Antibody tests for identification of *Mycobacterium bovis*—infected bovine herds," *Journal of Clinical Microbiology*, vol. 36, no. 2, pp. 566–568, 1998.

[27] B. M. Buddle, P. G. Livingstone, and G. W. de Lisle, "Advances in ante-mortem diagnosis of tuberculosis in cattle," *New Zealand Veterinary Journal*, vol. 57, no. 4, pp. 173–180, 2009.

[28] M. L. Thom, J. C. Hope, M. McAulay et al., "The effect of tuberculin testing on the development of cell-mediated immune responses during Mycobacterium bovis infection," *Veterinary Immunology and Immunopathology*, vol. 114, no. 1-2, pp. 25–36, 2006.

[29] J. Awah-Ndukum, A. C. Kudi, G. Bradley et al., "Prevalence of bovine tuberculosis in cattle in the highlands of Cameroon based on the detection of lesions in slaughtered cattle and tuberculin skin tests of live cattle," *Veterinarni Medicina*, vol. 57, no. 2, pp. 59–76, 2012.

[30] M. Thrusfield, *Veterinary Epidemiology*, vol. 610 of *Blackwell Publishing Company*, Blackwell Science, Oxford, UK, 3rd edition, 2007.

[31] MINEPIA, "La stratégie sectoriel de l'élevage, des peches et industries animales," in *Cabinet Management 2000 MINEPIA*, A. Doufissa, Ed., Ministry of Livestock, Fisheries and Animal Industries, Yaounde, Yaounde, Cameroon, 2002.

[32] FAO, *A Manual for the Primary Animal Health Care Worker*, Food and Agriculture Organization of the United Nations, Rome, Italy, 1994.

[33] J. F. Gracey and D. S. Collins, *Meat Hygiene*, Bailliére Tindall, London, UK, 9th edition, 1992.

[34] A. Grist, *Bovine Meat Inspection—Anatomy, Physiology and Disease Conditions*, Nottingham University Press, Nottingham, UK, 2nd edition, 2008.

[35] J. Turton, *How to Estimate the Age of Cattle*, National Department of Agriculture, ARC-Onderstepoort Veterinary Institute, Pretoria, South Africa, 1999.

[36] R. Blench, *Traditional Livestock Breeds: Geographical Distribution and Dynamics in Relation to the Ecology of West Africa*, Overseas Development Institute, London, UK, 1999.

[37] M. J. Nicholson and M. H. Butterworth, *A Guide to Condition Scoring of Zebu Cattle*, International Livestock Centre for Africa, Addis Ababa, Ethiopia, 1986.

[38] C. Diguimbaye, M. Hilty, R. Ngandolo et al., "Molecular characterization and drug resistance testing of *Mycobacterium tuberculosis* isolates from Chad," *Journal of Clinical Microbiology*, vol. 44, no. 4, pp. 1575–1577, 2006.

[39] B. E. Strong and G. P. Kubica, *Isolation and Identification of Mycobacterium Tuberculosis—A Guide for the Level II Laboratory*, Department of Health and Human Services, Public Health Service, Laboratory Improvement Program Office, Division of Laboratory Training and Consultation Atlanta, Atlanta, Ga, USA, 1985.

[40] World Health Organization (WHO), *Laboratory Services in Tuberculosis Control. Part III : Culture*, World Health Organization (WHO), Geneva, Switzerland, 1998.

[41] WHO, *Laboratory Services in Tuberculosis Control Part II: Microscopy*, World Health Organization, Geneva, Switzerland, 1998.

[42] J. Awah Ndukum, A. Caleb Kudi, G. Bradley, I. N. Ane-Anyangwe, S. Fon-Tebug, and J. Tchoumboue, "Prevalence of bovine tuberculosis in abattoirs of the littoral and western highland regions of cameroon: a cause for public health concern," *Veterinary Medicine International*, vol. 2010, Article ID 495015, 8 pages, 2010.

[43] J. Awah-Ndukum, A. C. Kudi, G. S. Bah et al., "Bovine tuberculosis in cattle in the highlands of cameroon: seroprevalence estimates and rates of tuberculin skin test reactors at modified cut-offs," *Veterinary Medicine International*, vol. 2012, Article ID 798502, 13 pages, 2012.

[44] B. N. R. Ngandolo, B. Müller, C. Diguimbaye-Djaïbe et al., "Comparative assessment of fluorescence polarization and tuberculin skin testing for the diagnosis of bovine tuberculosis in Chadian cattle," *Preventive Veterinary Medicine*, vol. 89, no. 1-2, pp. 81–89, 2009.

[45] J. Awah-Ndukum, K. J. P. Mingoas, V. Ngu Ngwa, M. G. V. Ndjaro Leng, and P. A. Zoli, "Causes and associated financial losses of carcass and organ condemnations in the SODEPA abattoir of Yaoundé, Cameroon," *Global Veterinara*, In press.

[46] J. Francis, "Susceptibility to tuberculosis and the route of infection," *Australian Veterinary Journal*, vol. 47, no. 9, p. 414, 1971.

[47] G. Ameni and G. Medhin, "Effect of gastro-intestinal parasitosis on tuberculin test for the diagnosis of bovine tuberculosis," *Journal of Applied Animal Research*, vol. 18, no. 2, pp. 221–224, 2000.

[48] F. O. Inangolet, B. Demelash, J. Oloya, J. Opuda-Asibo, and E. Skjerve, "A cross-sectional study of bovine tuberculosis in the transhumant and agro-pastoral cattle herds in the border areas of Katakwi and Moroto districts, Uganda," *Tropical Animal Health and Production*, vol. 40, no. 7, pp. 501–508, 2008.

[49] C. O. Thoen, P. A. LoBue, D. A. Enarson, J. B. Kaneene, and I. N. de Kantor, "Tuberculosis: a re-emerging disease of animals and humans," *Veterinaria Italiana*, vol. 45, no. 1, pp. 135–181, 2009.

[50] M. V. Palmer, W. R. Waters, T. C. Thacker, R. Greenwald, J. Esfandiari, and K. P. Lyashchenko, "Effects of different tuberculin skin-testing regimens on gamma interferon and antibody responses in cattle experimentally infected with *Mycobacterium bovis*," *Clinical and Vaccine Immunology*, vol. 13, no. 3, pp. 387–394, 2006.

[51] A. W. Lepper, C. W. Pearson, and L. A. Corner, "Anergy to tuberculin in beef cattle," *Australian Veterinary Journal*, vol. 53, no. 5, pp. 214–216, 1977.

[52] J. M. Pollock and S. D. Neill, "*Mycobacterium boviss* infection and tuberculosis in cattle," *The Veterinary Journal*, vol. 163, no. 2, pp. 115–127, 2002.

28

Circadian Rhythm and Stress Response in Droppings of *Serinus canaria*

Maura Turriani,[1] **Nicola Bernabò,**[1] **Barbara Barboni,**[1]
Gianluca Todisco,[2] **Luigi Montini,**[3] **and Paolo Berardinelli**[1]

[1]*Unit of Basic and Applied Bioscience, Faculty of Veterinary Medicine, University of Teramo, Via Renato Balzarini 1, 64100 Teramo, Italy*
[2]*Via per Mosciano, No. 96, Giulianova, 64021 Teramo, Italy*
[3]*Via Villafranca No. 11, 72100 Brindisi, Italy*

Correspondence should be addressed to Barbara Barboni; bbarboni@unite.it

Academic Editor: Francesca Mancianti

Serinus canaria is a widespread domestic ornamental songbird, whose limited knowledge of biology make compelling studies aimed to monitor stress. Here, a commercial enzyme immunoassay was adopted to measure immunoreactive corticosterone (CORT) in single *Serinus canaria* dropping sample, to monitor the daily fecal excretion of CORT in birds bred singly or in-group and to detect the effect promoted by aviary or small transport cage restraint. A robust daily rhythm of CORT was recorded in animals held on short-day light cycle, independent of bred conditions (single or group), which persisted when space availability was modified in single bred animal (transfer in aviary and transport cages). By contrast, a significant change in CORT excretion was recorded when group bred animals are restrained in a smaller cage. The daily rhythm in CORT excretion in response to manipulation showed the greatest response at the beginning of the light period, followed by the absence of the peak usually recorded at the end of the dark phase. These data indicated that EIA could be used as a reliable noninvasive approach to monitor the stress induced by restraint conditions in *Serinus canaria*.

1. Introduction

The *Serinus canaria* is a small domestic songbird native of Canaria Islands that is usually maintained in captivity for ornamental purposes. Despite its spread and the increasing evidences demonstrating that stress is related to several environmental and social conditions as well the human-induced disturbances, scarce information on the physiology of this bird is still available. Stress plays an important role in the maintenance of body homeostasis, conditioning health, and breeding outcomes. It is known that CORT are front-line hormones to overcome stressful situations. During short-term stress, they improve fitness by energy mobilization [1, 2] and regulate behavior and suppress metabolic processes nonessential for survival. However, severe or chronic stress may decrease individual fitness by immunosuppression and atrophy of tissues [3, 4] and the decreases of reproductive performance [5, 6] and there are also indications of stereotypies [7].

In the past, CORT have typically been quantified in blood [8–14] while, more recently, noninvasive methods are being developed and applied to several avian species, since they offer several advantages [15–25]. In particular, fecal steroid hormones assays are now being used in a variety of disciplines (e.g., animal science, behavioral ecology, conservation biology, ornithology, and primatology) to examine the reproductive and adrenocortical status of a variety of taxa [12, 16, 21, 22, 26–39]. These noninvasive methods allow easy collection of samples without disturbing the animals. Samples can be collected at regular intervals through time, thus providing an accurate assessment of stress without the bias of capture-induced increases in CORT [22, 31, 40, 41].

Differently from blood CORT, steroids in feces are cumulative thus provide a measure of circulating CORT over time [23, 31, 42, 43].

Although use of noninvasive techniques has increased for many species, several confounding factors must be considered before using them: the specie-specific modality of CORT excretion, the daily [44, 45] and seasonal patterns [11, 46, 47], the reproductive status [11, 48], the sex [21], the body condition [49, 50], and the photoperiod [51, 52]. In addition, steroids such as CORT are metabolized in the liver and excreted into the gut through bile [20, 22, 24] and are present in the feces either as metabolites [51, 52] or native hormones.

Fecal CORT assays have been validated in several species [16, 22, 53] but only fewer studies have focused on parrots [54, 55] or small (<200 g body mass) birds [15, 56]. In this context, no information regarding normal values of excreted CORT in *Serinus canaria* is now available despite the widespread diffusion of this breeding.

The possibility to enlarge the use of fecal CORT measurement for detecting the wellbeing in birds is limited by the validation of radioimmunoassay (RIA), in spotted owls [57] and in stonechats [58].

To detect minute quantities of feces commercial EIA kits can be adopted, due to their advantages in terms of costs, ease of use, and availability.

A negative relationship between fecal sample mass and fecal CORT concentration has been found previously [23, 40], leading to the suggestion of only analyzing larger fecal samples (>20 mg dried mass). This may potentially preclude the analysis of individual samples from many species of smaller birds, which typically produce a fecal sample smaller than 20 mg [16]. This problem could be overcome by combining multiple fecal samples or collecting them over a larger windows of time [31, 40, 59, 60]. Starting from these premises, the present research has been designed in order to test if a commercial EIA, previously used to assay CORT in zebra finches [61], can be adopted to detect fecal CORT at individual level.

Once assay has been adapted to record CORT in *Serinus canaria* feces and tested for its analytical performances (parallelism, intra- and interassay variation, and sensitivity) and biological reality (oral corticosterone challenge), the EIA was used to record the basal daily secretion of CORT in adult females (1-year olds) bred into conventional cages, during a short-light period, at stable 20°C of environmental temperature and feed ad libitum.

First, social effect has been evaluated by comparing fecal CORT excretion in individually *versus* group bred birds. Then, the effect of spatial availability has been determined by transfer bird bred individually or in group into smaller (conventional transport cages) or lager cages (aviary).

2. Materials and Methods

All research was approved by the ethical committee of the University of Teramo even if the experimental plan reproduces conventional animal management.

2.1. Animal Study. Adult, female bred *Serinus canaria* were housed under control conditions in cages of 55 × 60 × 90 cm individually or in group (4 birds) to detect the basal levels of excreted CORT collected during 24 h. They were given water and a commercial seed diet ad libitum and housed on short day photoperiod (a 10 hours of light/14 dark cycle). The animals were maintained under stable temperature of 20°C.

For the biological validation, 10 *Serinus canaria* bred individually were randomly divided in two experimental groups: Ctr and oral corticosterone challenged birds according to previously validated protocols [58, 62, 63].

To this aim *Serinus canaria* were fed with exogenous corticosterone suspended in peanut oil (1.0 mg/mL). Corticosterone solution was administered orally in a single morning dose of 0.1 mL while Ctr were feed with oil alone. Dropping were sampled four times after corticosterone administration performed at 7.00 am (time 0: prior to administration and times 3, 6, 9, and 24 indicated the hours after administration).

The experimental trials were performed singly ($n = 5$) or in group ($n = 5$ for 4 birds each) held birds; they were caught by hand and placed individually or in group, respectively, into smaller transport cages (15 × 60 × 30 cm) or in aviary (120 × 100 × 100 cm) and then transferred again into control cages the day after.

During the experimental periods all droppings excreted by animals were collected at 3 h intervals (from 10.00 am of the first day until 10.00 am of the following day). In order to facilitate dropping collection, the bottom of the cages was lined with plasticized sheet. Whole excreted samples deprived only of feathers/food contaminants were immediately deposited in cryotubes, identified, and stored at −20°C.

Then the birds were transferred into their original bred condition.

The dropping were stored frozen at −20°C until the last collection when the extraction procedure was performed.

2.2. Preparation of Droppings. Before assay, droppings were thawed at room temperature, placed in glass tubes, and weighed wet. Samples were dried in a forced-air oven at 90°C for 1 h to destroy bacterial enzymes [24, 25]. The samples were ground, homogenized, and weighed.

Glucocorticoids were extracted by first normalizing in each experiment the weight of dropping to extract on the minimum weight obtained amongst samples. In this way, within each experiment, a similar amount of dropping/samples were extracted with 75% methanol and 25% double distilled water normalizing the volume on the basis of sample weight (max 2 mL) followed by vigorous vortexing for 5 min, centrifugation (2.300 ×g, 15 min, 4°C), and freezing (−85°C for 15 min).

Centrifugation and freezing that resulted in the solidification of the samples at the bottom of tube are required to decant the supernatant methanol in another grass tube (12 × 75 mm). The supernatant was THEN evaporated under a stream of air at 90°C. Finally, we added 0.01 M Phosphate Buffered Saline with 0.1% gelatin to each tube and vortexed them vigorously for 5 min, and then assay was carried out.

2.3. Immunoassay Procedures and Validation. In the present study, the Enzo Enzyme Immunoassay kit (Enzo Life Science; Cat n° ADI900-097) was used. The first step was a standard analytical validation of the commercial EIA on CORT dropping extracts, collected from individual bird realized including assessment of parallelism, intra-assay and interassay precision, and assay sensitivity. To this aim, CORT dropping extracts obtained from samples containing high levels of CORT were used.

Samples were initially spiked with approximately 1 pg of tritiated corticosterone prior to steroid extraction and ~84,6% of recovery was obtained (max coefficient of variation 16,3%) according to results described by [61] by adopting the same commercial EIA on avian blood samples.

For parallelism assessment, curves of percent binding of EIA standard corticosterone ($\%B/B_0$) were analyzed *versus* serially diluted high dropping extract samples log-transformed doses 1 : 2 (dilution 1), 1 : 10 (dilution 2), 1 : 100 (dilution 3), and 1 : 200 (dilution 4).

Lastly, a biological test was performed by dosing fecal CORT dropping samples collected from oral corticosterone challenged animals.

The EIA analysis was performed according to manufacturing instructions. The antibody specificity was not internally determined. However, the manufacturers declare for corticosterone EIA antibody 100% cross reactivity, 28% for desoxycorticosterone, 0.3% for tetrahydrocorticosterone, and 0.2% for aldosterone.

2.4. Statistical Analysis. Each analytical sample (standard curve points and experimental points) was analyzed in triplicate while each experimental data was the mean of at least five different birds or group of animals. Reported hormone values are based on the average of at least closest two of the triplicate values obtained within each assay, except in cases where these had greater than 10% variation. In such instances, remaining samples was reanalyzed in an additional assay. All the calculations have been performed considering the data as not normally distributed (D'Agostino and Pearson omnibus test), by using not parametrical tests: Mann–Whitney U test for two samples or Kruskal-Wallis test for more samples (Past 3). The data are represented as median $\pm 25°$–$75°$ percentile.

3. Results

3.1. EIA Validation. The quality control of assay was obtained by evaluating the standard curves ($\%B/B_0$ versus CORT concentration and CORT concentration versus Optical Density) (see Figure 1(a)) in which the quality of fit is always >0.99, whereas the ability of EIA to actually measure the CORT concentrations was assessed by the parallelism assay (see Figure 1(b)). Based on the results of serial dilutions, fecal extracts were usually diluted to 1 : 10 prior to assay.

The EIA sensitivity was ~20 pg/mL. The intra-assay and the interassay coefficients of variation were 10.4% and 16.9%, respectively, similar to those declared by manufacturing guidelines. The reality of EIA protocol applied of individual dropping CORT collected during the interval time of 3 hours is considered for the following experiments since it allowed detection of ~81.2% of the collected samples instead of the 47.4% of samples collected at 1 hour of interval.

3.2. Fecal Excretion. Quantities of dropping varied amongst birds (from 0.046 g to 0.121 g/3 h) and they did not change during the days (early morning 0.064 ± 0.021 g/3 h; afternoon 0.096 ± 0.049 gr/3 h, $p > 0.05$: data not shown) in single animals bred under short day photoperiod.

3.3. Daily Excretion of CORT. The four time points (10.00, 13.00, 16.00, and 7.00) analyzed through repeated measures documented a daily rhythm in CORT excretion, either in individual or in group bred birds (Figure 2). On short day photoperiod, basal low levels of CORT were recorded through the light (active) period to increase significantly in dropping samples collected immediately after light came on. The pattern and the levels of CORT excretion over the 24 h interval did not differ between single and in group bred animals (Figure 2).

3.4. Oral Corticosterone Challenge Effect on Daily CORT Excretion. The profile of fecal CORT did not change in birds of control (5 animals) feed with peanut oil alone (CTR in Figure 3). Differently, the birds ($n = 5$) feed early in the morning with one dose of corticosterone suspended in 0.1 mL of peanut oil (1 mg/mL) displayed significantly higher level of CORT 3 and 6 hours later ($p < 0.01$ and $p < 0.05$, respectively, Figure 3). The CORT excretion, then, acquired a pattern and levels similar to those recorded under CTR conditions.

3.5. Effect of Different Restraint Conditions on CORT Excretion. The fecal CORT concentrations remained unchanged when *Serinus canaria* bred individually or in group were moved into aviary. Birds transfer in a larger cage never modified the daily pattern and the levels of excreted CORT (data shown).

On the contrary, the daily dropping levels of CORT measured after bird transfer in smaller cages, as summarized in Figure 4, were conditioned to preliminary bred conditions.

The levels as well the daily circadian excreted CORT remained unchanged in *Serinus canaria* bred individually and moved into small transport cages (Figure 4). Differently, the pattern of CORT excretion was modified when *Serinus canaria* had bred preliminary in group. In this experimental condition, higher levels of dropping CORT levels were recorded at 13.00 and 16.00 ($p < 0.01$ *versus* single bred animals). In addition, the early morning peaks usually recorded in samples collected immediately after light came on (7.00: $p < 0.01$ *versus* single bred birds, Figure 4) were not observed.

The birds acquired again the daily CORT rhythm the day after they were transferred in group in normal cages (data not shown).

4. Discussion

4.1. EIA Validation. The present data demonstrated, for the first time, the validity of a commercial double antibody EIA

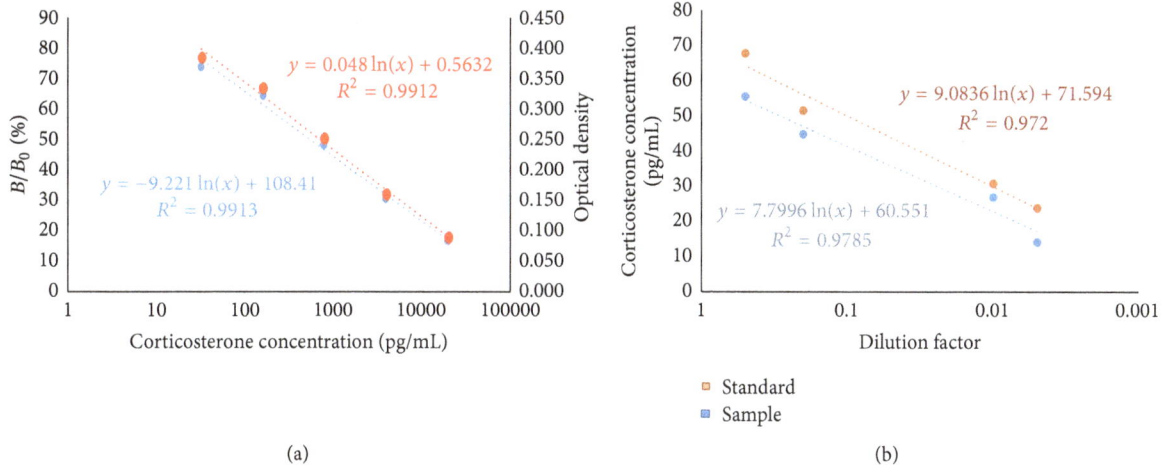

(a)

(b)

FIGURE 1: (a) Standard curves. (b) Diagram showing the curves slope at different dilutions (dilution 1 = 1:2, dilution 2 = 1:10, dilution 3 = 1/100, and dilution 4 = 1/200). X-axis in logarithmic scale.

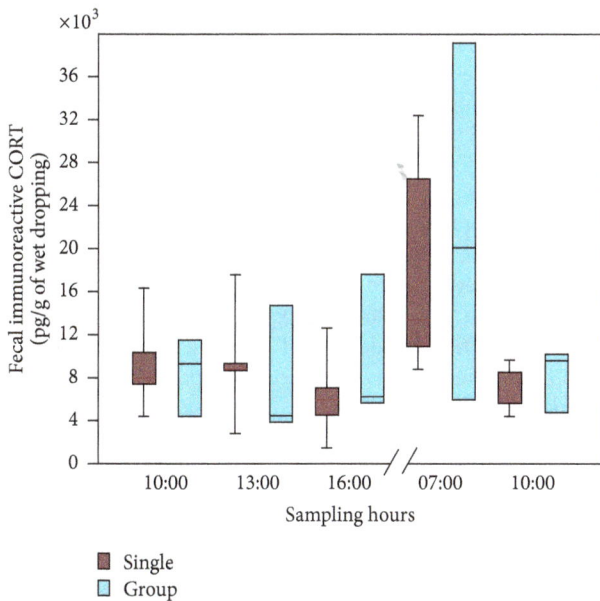

FIGURE 2: Diagram showing the daily rhythm in CORT excretion either in single (blue) or in grouped (red) bred birds. The sampling was carried out at different times, as reported on x-axis. For statistical analysis, refer to the result section of the manuscript.

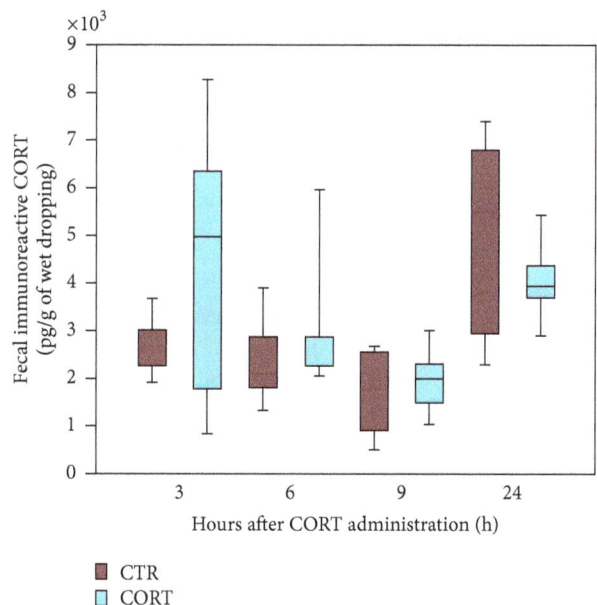

FIGURE 3: Diagram showing the daily rhythm in CORT excretion in control animals (CTR) or in birds feed with one dose of corticosterone suspended in 0.1 mL of peanut oil (1 mg/mL) (FEED). 3 h, 6 h, 9 h, and 24 h are referred to as the hours after the CORT administration. For statistical analysis, refer to the result section of the manuscript.

kit for detecting excreted CORT in *Serinus canaria*, probably the most widespread songbird domesticated avian species.

The specificity of EIA was confirmed through the parallelism experiments and by detecting increased fecal levels of CORT in birds orally treated with corticosterone. Unfortunately, the small size of *Serinus canaria* did not allow us to design, in parallel, experiments aimed to pharmacologically induce circulatory changes of CORT, as proposed by Young and Hallford [58].

Analogously, the daily rhythm recorded in single and group bred birds has represented, indirectly, a further approach to validate the use of this commercial kit for

monitoring stressful conditions on small amount of dropping collected from single bred *Serinus canaria*.

In this context, the several technical (the absence of radioactivity, minimal equipment requirement, etc.) and biological advantages of a commercial EIA cannot be underestimated when the assay can be adopted, in particular, for practical aims. The high impact of translating stress detection to clinical and breeding practices of widespread species like *Serinus canaria* could justify a qualitative use of the assay (for example, CORT values over basal daily levels)

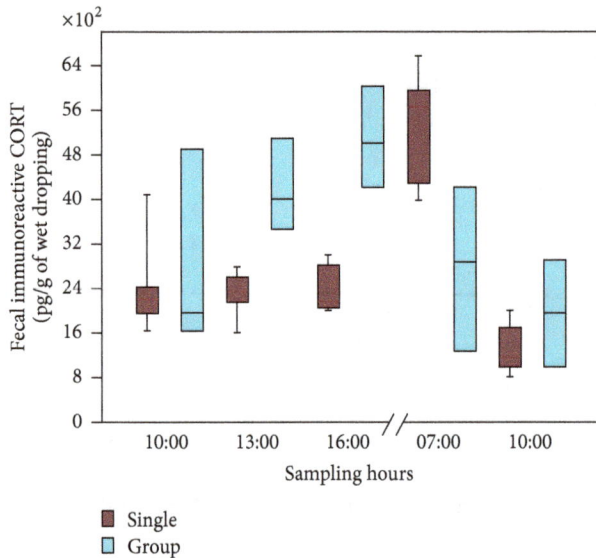

FIGURE 4: Diagram showing the daily rhythm in CORT excretion measured after bird transfer in smaller cages in single (blue) or in grouped animals (red). The sampling was carried out at different times, as reported on x-axis. For statistical analysis, refer to the result section of the manuscript.

thus underestimating limit imposed by a precise quantitative dosage.

4.2. Daily Rhythm. EIA analysis enabled us to describe, for the first time, the CORT daily rhythm of *Serinus canaria*, evaluated on single dropping sample collected from animals bred under short day photoperiod and maintained under controlled bred conditions.

The *Serinus canaria* showed, indeed, a 24-hour cyclic CORT excretion. The repetitiveness of CORT data that constitutes itself as a strong validation of EIA assay was not affected by the bred conditions considered (single *versus* group).

Under short days (10L/14D), basal levels remained low throughout the light period (one sample each 3 h from 10.00 am to 16.00) to peak in before lights came on (7.00). Considering the delay in the feces, it may be presumed that also in *Serinus canaria* the CORT peak in the plasma occurred during or at the end of the dark hours.

The CORT levels during a 3 h interval before light double, even if the birds did not eat during this inactive period. This entails that the increase in CORT rate cannot be attributed to differential food intake while lights are off but to a preactive peak of CORT that was similarly observed in other avian taxa [44, 51, 52, 64–67]. The preactive peak may be necessary to prepare an appropriate physiological state to meet energetic demands as active period begins. In mammals CORT daily rhythm is thought to regulate overall metabolism [9, 68] and, together with insulin, regulates energy acquisition, deposition, and mobilization [69, 70]. A similar assumption has been translated to some birds (e.g., pigeons and chickens) that displayed CORT rhythms

similar to that of mammals [8, 10, 71]. Relatively few studies, instead, have evaluated CORT rhythm in passerine such as white-throated sparrow, *Zonotrichia albicollis* [66], Gambel's white-crowned sparrow (*Zonotrichia leucophrys gambelii*) [44], the European stonechat (fecal CORT) (*Saxicola torquata rubicola*) [30], house sparrow (*Passer domesticus*) [45], the starling, *Sturnus vulgaris* [45], the great tit, *Parus major* [51, 52], and more recently in zebra finches [72].

On the basis of fecal CORT diel rhythm, two interesting hypothesizes may be proposed. Firstly, since under two different bred conditions CORT reached similar daily levels in dropping sample before the active period, this finding seems to suggest a potential biological relevance of the peak during the preactive period driving behavioral and physiological processes. Second, like other passerine species, the excreted CORT levels in *Serinus canaria* are very low during the active period, as a consequence of a sharp drop in CORT metabolites occurring immediately after the first hour of the day. This peculiarity has suggested avian-specific mechanisms of regulation. This hypothesis was firstly advanced from Breuner et al. [44] that recorded a rapid decrease in CORT plasma levels during most of active day in Gambel's white-crowed sparrow (differently from mammals [44]). This could not be ascribable to high mass specific metabolic rate since also in smaller mammals, like mice or rat, the blood CORT basal levels are 5–10 times higher than in sparrow [69, 73, 74]. In addition, low active CORT blood levels in avian cannot be due to a greater intestinal clearance since, as documented in the present paper, low and stable fecal CORT levels were similarly recorded at least in the *Serinus canaria*. Even if further experiments investigating the changes in CORT secretion and clearances are required to establish the cause of this rapid decline, a passerine specificity could be hypothesized.

4.3. Response to Modified Restraint Condition. As regards the relationship between stress-induced levels and rhythm, it seems that, in most of avian species, the intensity of the CORT response to stressors is dependent on the day at which the stimulus is presented. The stress response has a daily rhythm, which approximately mimics the pattern of the basal fluctuation, at least on a winter photoperiod [44, 45, 51, 52]. This was, partly, confirmed in the *Serinus canaria*. The hypothalamic-pituitary-adrenal (HPA) axis appeared to be sensitive to specific stressor just after light came on, but the daily basal rhythm was slightly impaired under persistent stressor conditions. Moreover, the perception of a stimulus as stressor seems to be strictly conditioned by the preliminary bred condition. Indeed, whereas single bred animal did not modify the CORT basal levels, when they are transferred in cages of different size (aviary and transport cages). By contrast, the transfer in transport cages applied to birds bred in group became able to increase CORT secretion in few hours early in the morning.

The explanation of this different behavior in steroids secretion cannot be easily interpreted based exclusively on fecal CORT dosages. Firstly, since several evidences demonstrated that CORT secretion plays a key role in the consolidation of memories of a stressful events, the subject can respond more effectively when the events reoccur in the future [75, 76]. If this is the case, the lower sensitivity to transport restraint, observed in single bred animal could be interpreted as their more practice to tolerate stressor conditions in comparison to group bred ones that could have experienced greater stressor live conditions (ex. hierarchy within birds). Based on this hypothesis, it is possible to explain, for example, the different levels of CORT recorded in the Bengalese finch (*Lonchura striata* var. *domestica*), a domesticated strain of the white-backed munia (Lonchura striata). The domesticated songbirds have reduced CORT levels because of reduced levels of environmental stresses (compared to wild related species) and reductions in the role of CORT, which is necessary for survival in the wild.

In addition, another mechanism regulating CORT individual can be considered. Indeed, it has recently been demonstrated in mice that the effects of stress on free CORT are stressor specific, with respect both to the magnitude and to the duration of the response and that they are mediated by circulatory corticosteroid binding globulins (CBG). CBG seems to be released from the liver at high levels only in response to stressors of moderate to strong intensity. Thus, the increase in circulating CBG levels after stress restrains the rise in free CORT concentrations in the face of mounting total hormone levels in the circulation. This highly dynamic mechanism involved in the regulation of glucocorticoid hormone physiology complicates the interpretation of CORT fecal secretion levels after acute stress.

However, even if it is quite difficult to interpret the mechanism involved in these different CORT responses, the combination of the group bred and transport restraint condition was able to evoke a significant increase in CORT over basal levels that, however, determine a transitory reduction of the daily rhythm. The day after, indeed, the preactive morning CORT peak was significantly inhibited. Interesting, the modification of space in not per se a condition sufficient to evoke stress in *Serinus canaria* since restraint in larger cages that did not modify CORT secretion. Exclusively the limitation of space may determine a CORT response when, however, it was applied to group bred birds.

The rapid reduction of fecal CORT levels can offer a protective response, able to limit the long term adverse effects that chronic elevations can have on the brain, such as hippocampal atrophy, increased feeding rate, and immune function [4].

Instead, the detrimental effects of prolonged low concentration of systemic CORT levels have not yet studied in avian species even if exhaustion of glucocorticoid response may represent a very critical situation for animals homeostasis that, however, should take place under pathological conditions (endocrine syndrome) or after more prolonged stressor exposure.

5. Conclusion

The availability of commercial EIA for the noninvasive monitoring of stress in captive widespread bird species like *Serinus canaria* has a large clinical and breeding management impact. The identification of an endogenous CORT variations over the 24 h is essential to interpret the stressor effects and to approach future focused experiments. The description of the baseline circulating CORT fluctuates on a diel basis would, indeed, allow researchers to remove that source of variation by planning experiments at appropriate time of day.

The experimental results suggested, in addition, that domesticated *Serinus canaria* bred individually does not experience stressor modified restraint conditions (aviary or transport cage transfer). On the contrary, higher attention must be addressed to the management of *Serinus canaria* bred in group in order to prevent stress response determined by the reduction of cage space.

Competing Interests

The authors declare that they have no competing interests.

Acknowledgments

The authors thank Francesca Pettinella for her technical support. This research was supported by grants from the Società Ornitologica Reggiana (SOR).

References

[1] R. Reynaert, S. Marcus, M. De Paepe, and G. Peeters, "Influences of stress, age and sex on serum growth hormone and free fatty acid levels in cattle," *Hormone and Metabolic Research*, vol. 8, no. 2, pp. 109–114, 1976.

[2] S. M. Korte, G. A. H. Bouws, and B. Bohus, "Central actions of corticotropin-releasing hormone (CRH) on behavioral, neuroendocrine, and cardiovascular regulation: brain corticoid receptor involvement," *Hormones and Behavior*, vol. 27, no. 2, pp. 167–183, 1993.

[3] A. Munck and N. J. Holbrook, "Glucocorticoid-receptor complexes in rat thymus cells. Rapid kinetic behavior and a cyclic model," *Journal of Biological Chemistry*, vol. 259, no. 2, pp. 820–831, 1984.

[4] T. B. VanItallie, "Stress: a risk factor for serious illness," *Metabolism: Clinical and Experimental*, vol. 51, no. 6, pp. 40–45, 2002.

[5] R. M. Liptrap, "Stress and reproduction in domestic animals," *Annals of the New York Academy of Sciences*, vol. 697, pp. 275–284, 1993.

[6] H. Dobson and R. F. Smith, "Stress and reproduction in farm animals," *Journal of Reproduction and Fertility. Supplement*, vol. 49, pp. 451–461, 1995.

[7] S. D. McBride and D. Cuddeford, "The putative welfare-reducing effects of preventing equine stereotypic behaviour," *Animal Welfare*, vol. 10, no. 2, pp. 173–189, 2001.

[8] M. M. Joseph and A. H. Meier, "Daily rhythms of plasma corticosterone in the common pigeon, Columba livia," *General and Comparative Endocrinology*, vol. 20, no. 2, pp. 326–330, 1973.

[9] E. P. Widmaier, T. L. Harmer, A. M. Sulak, and T. H. Kunz, "Further characterization of the pituitary-adrenocortical responses to stress in Chiroptera," *Journal of Experimental Zoology*, vol. 269, no. 5, pp. 442–449, 1994.

[10] I. Westerhof, W. E. Van den Brom, J. A. Mol, J. T. Lumeij, and A. Rijnberk, "Sensitivity of the hypothalamic-pituitary-adrenal system of pigeons (Columba livia domestica) to suppression by dexamethasone, cortisol, and prednisolone," *Avian Diseases*, vol. 38, no. 3, pp. 435–445, 1994.

[11] J. C. Wingfield, J. C. Wingfield, D. Monk, and D. Monk, "Behavioral and hormonal responses of male song sparrows to estradiol-treated females during the non-breeding season," *Hormones and Behavior*, vol. 28, no. 2, pp. 146–154, 1994.

[12] R. Palme and E. Möstl, "Measurement of cortisol metabolites in faeces of sheep as a parameter of cortisol concentration in blood," *International Journal of Mammalian Biology*, vol. 62, supplement 2, pp. 192–197, 1997.

[13] L. F. Gregory and J. R. Schmid, "Stress responses and sexing of wild Kemp's ridley sea turtles (Lepidochelys kempii) in the Northeastern Gulf of Mexico," *General and Comparative Endocrinology*, vol. 124, no. 1, pp. 66–74, 2001.

[14] T. Mathies, T. A. Felix, and V. A. Lance, "Effects of trapping and subsequent short-term confinement stress on plasma corticosterone in the brown treesnake (*Boiga irregularis*) on Guam," *General and Comparative Endocrinology*, vol. 124, no. 1, pp. 106–114, 2001.

[15] S. M. Hiebert, M. Ramenofsky, K. Salvante, J. C. Wingfield, and C. L. Gass, "Noninvasive methods for measuring and manipulating corticosterone in hummingbirds," *General and Comparative Endocrinology*, vol. 120, no. 2, pp. 235–247, 2000.

[16] S. K. Wasser, K. E. Hunt, J. L. Brown et al., "A generalized fecal glucocorticoid assay for use in a diverse array of nondomestic mammalian and avian species," *General and Comparative Endocrinology*, vol. 120, no. 3, pp. 260–275, 2000.

[17] J. W. Ludders, J. A. Langenberg, N. M. Czekala, and H. N. Erb, "Fecal corticosterone reflects serum corticosterone in Florida sandhill cranes," *Journal of Wildlife Diseases*, vol. 37, no. 3, pp. 646–652, 2001.

[18] W. Goymann, E. Möstl, T. Van't Hof, M. L. East, and H. Hofer, "Noninvasive fecal monitoring of glucocorticoids in spotted hyenas, *Crocuta crocuta*," *General and Comparative Endocrinology*, vol. 114, no. 3, pp. 340–348, 1999.

[19] E. Möstl, J. L. Maggs, G. Schrötter, U. Besenfelder, and R. Palme, "Measurement of cortisol metabolites in faeces of ruminants," *Veterinary Research Communications*, vol. 26, no. 2, pp. 127–139, 2002.

[20] E. Möstl and R. Palme, "Hormones as indicators of stress," *Domestic Animal Endocrinology*, vol. 23, no. 1-2, pp. 67–74, 2002.

[21] C. Touma, N. Sachser, E. Möstl, and R. Palme, "Effects of sex and time of day on metabolism and excretion of corticosterone in urine and feces of mice," *General and Comparative Endocrinology*, vol. 130, no. 3, pp. 267–278, 2003.

[22] C. Touma, R. Palme, and N. Sachser, "Analyzing corticosterone metabolites in fecal samples of mice: a noninvasive technique to monitor stress hormones," *Hormones and Behavior*, vol. 45, no. 1, pp. 10–22, 2004.

[23] W. Goymann, "Noninvasive monitoring of hormones in bird droppings: physiological validation, sampling, extraction, sex differences, and the influence of diet on hormone metabolite levels," *Annals of the New York Academy of Sciences*, vol. 1046, pp. 35–53, 2005.

[24] R. Palme, "Measuring fecal steroids: guidelines for practical application," *Annals of the New York Academy of Sciences*, vol. 1046, pp. 75–80, 2005.

[25] E. Möstl, S. Rettenbacher, and R. Palme, "Measurement of corticosterone metabolites in birds' droppings: an analytical approach," *Annals of the New York Academy of Sciences*, vol. 1046, pp. 17–34, 2005.

[26] M. W. Miller, N. T. Hobbs, and M. C. Sousa, "Detecting stress responses in Rocky Mountain bighorn sheep (*Ovis canadensis canadensis*): reliability of cortisol concentrations in urine and feces," *Canadian Journal of Zoology*, vol. 69, no. 1, pp. 15–24, 1991.

[27] J. F. Kirkpatrick, J. C. McCarthy, D. F. Gudermuth, S. E. Shideler, and B. L. Lasley, "An assessment of the reproductive biology of Yellowstone bison (Bison bison) subpopulations using noncapture methods," *Canadian Journal of Zoology*, vol. 74, no. 1, pp. 8–14, 1996.

[28] J. L. Brown, S. K. Wasser, D. E. Wildt, and L. H. Graham, "Comparative aspects of steroid hormone metabolism and ovarian activity in felids, measured noninvasively in feces," *Biology of Reproduction*, vol. 51, no. 4, pp. 776–786, 1994.

[29] M. H. Jurke, N. M. Czekala, D. G. Lindburg, and S. E. Millard, "Fecal corticoid metabolite measurement in the cheetah (Acinonyx jubatus)," *Zoo Biology*, vol. 16, no. 2, pp. 133–147, 1997.

[30] W. Goymann and M. Trappschuh, "Seasonal and diel variation of hormone metabolites in European stonechats: on the importance of high signal-to-noise ratios in noninvasive hormone studies," *Journal of Biological Rhythms*, vol. 26, no. 1, pp. 44–54, 2011.

[31] J. M. Harper and S. N. Austad, "Fecal glucocorticoids: a noninvasive method of measuring adrenal activity in wild and captive rodents," *Physiological and Biochemical Zoology*, vol. 73, no. 1, pp. 12–22, 2000.

[32] M. Dehnhard, M. Clauss, M. Lechner-Doll, H. H. D. Meyer, and R. Palme, "Noninvasive monitoring of adrenocortical activity in roe deer (Capreolus capreolus) by measurement of fecal cortisol metabolites," *General and Comparative Endocrinology*, vol. 123, no. 1, pp. 111–120, 2001.

[33] C. J. Morrow, E. S. Kolver, G. A. Verkerk, and L. R. Matthews, "Fecal glucocorticoid metabolites as a measure of adrenal activity in dairy cattle," *General and Comparative Endocrinology*, vol. 126, no. 2, pp. 229–241, 2002.

[34] V. Hayssen, J. M. Harper, and R. DeFina, "Fecal corticosteroids in agouti and non-agouti deer mice (*Peromyscus maniculatus*)," *Comparative Biochemistry and Physiology—A Molecular and Integrative Physiology*, vol. 132, no. 2, pp. 439–446, 2002.

[35] M. Dehnhard, A. Schreer, O. Krone, K. Jewgenow, M. Krause, and R. Grossmann, "Measurement of plasma corticosterone and fecal glucocorticoid metabolites in the chicken (*Gallus domesticus*), the great cormorant (*Phalacrocorax carbo*), and the goshawk (*Accipiter gentilis*)," *General and Comparative Endocrinology*, vol. 131, no. 3, pp. 345–352, 2003.

[36] A. Ganswindt, R. Palme, M. Heistermann, S. Borragan, and J. K. Hodges, "Non-invasive assessment of adrenocortical function in the male African elephant (*Loxodonta africana*) and its relation to musth," *General and Comparative Endocrinology*, vol. 134, no. 2, pp. 156–166, 2003.

[37] K. E. Hunt, A. W. Trites, and S. K. Wasser, "Validation of a fecal glucocorticoid assay for Steller sea lions (Eumetopias jubatus)," *Physiology and Behavior*, vol. 80, no. 5, pp. 595–601, 2004.

[38] J. W. Turner Jr., R. Nemeth, and C. Rogers, "Measurement of fecal glucocorticoids in parrotfishes to assess stress," *General and Comparative Endocrinology*, vol. 133, no. 3, pp. 341–352, 2003.

[39] W. Goymann, D. Geue, I. Schwabl et al., "Testosterone and corticosterone during the breeding cycle of equatorial and European stonechats (Saxicola torquata axillaris and S. t. rubicola)," *Hormones and Behavior*, vol. 50, no. 5, pp. 779–785, 2006.

[40] J. J. Millspaugh and B. E. Washburn, "Use of fecal glucocorticoid metabolite measures in conservation biology research: considerations for application and interpretation," *General and Comparative Endocrinology*, vol. 138, no. 3, pp. 189–199, 2004.

[41] J. J. Millspaugh, R. J. Woods, K. E. Hunt et al., "Fecal glucocorticoid assays and the physiological stress response in elk," *Wildlife Society Bulletin*, vol. 29, no. 3, pp. 899–907, 2001.

[42] K. Hirschenhauser, K. Kotrschal, and E. Möstl, "Synthesis of measuring steroid metabolites in goose feces," *Annals of the New York Academy of Sciences*, vol. 1046, no. 1, pp. 138–153, 2005.

[43] C. E. Ninnes, J. R. Waas, N. Ling et al., "Comparing plasma and faecal measures of steroid hormones in Adelie penguins *Pygoscelis adeliae*," *Journal of Comparative Physiology B*, vol. 180, no. 1, pp. 83–94, 2010.

[44] C. W. Breuner, J. C. Wingfield, and L. M. Romero, "Diel rhythms of basal and stress-induced corticosterone in a wild, seasonal vertebrate, Gambel's white-crowned sparrow," *Journal of Experimental Zoology*, vol. 284, no. 3, pp. 334–342, 1999.

[45] L. M. Romero and L. Remage-Healey, "Daily and seasonal variation in response to stress in captive starlings (Sturnus vulgaris): corticosterone," *General and Comparative Endocrinology*, vol. 119, no. 1, pp. 52–59, 2000.

[46] A. Dawson and P. D. Howe, "Plasma corticosterone in wild starlings (*Sturnus vulgaris*) immediately following capture and in relation to body weight during the annual cycle," *General and Comparative Endocrinology*, vol. 51, no. 2, pp. 303–308, 1983.

[47] J. L. F. Raminelli, M. B. C. De Sousa, M. S. Cunha, and M. F. V. Barbosa, "Morning and afternoon patterns of fecal cortisol excretion among reproductive and non-reproductive male and female common marmosets, Callithrix jacchus," *Biological Rhythm Research*, vol. 32, no. 2, pp. 159–167, 2001.

[48] J. M. Whittier, F. Corrie, and C. Limpus, "Plasma steroid profiles in nesting loggerhead turtles (Caretta caretta) in Queensland, Australia: relationship to nesting episode and season," *General and Comparative Endocrinology*, vol. 106, no. 1, pp. 39–47, 1997.

[49] J. A. Heath and A. M. Dufty Jr., "Body condition and the adrenal stress response in captive American kestrel juveniles," *Physiological Zoology*, vol. 71, no. 1, pp. 67–73, 1998.

[50] G. T. Smith, J. C. Wingfield, and R. R. Veit, "Adrenocortical response to stress in the common diving petrel, Pelecanoides urinatrix," *Physiological Zoology*, vol. 67, no. 2, pp. 526–537, 1994.

[51] C. Carere, T. G. G. Groothuis, E. Möstl, S. Daan, and J. M. Koolhaas, "Fecal corticosteroids in a territorial bird selected for different personalities: daily rhythm and the response to social stress," *Hormones and Behavior*, vol. 43, no. 5, pp. 540–548, 2003.

[52] E. Rich and L. Romero, "Daily and photoperiod variations of basal and stress-induced corticosterone concentrations in house sparrows (Passer domesticus)," *Journal of Comparative Physiology—B Biochemical, Systemic, and Environmental Physiology*, vol. 171, no. 7, pp. 543–547, 2001.

[53] S. K. Chinnadurai, J. J. Millspaugh, W. S. Matthews et al., "Validation of fecal glucocorticoid metabolite assays for South African herbivores," *Journal of Wildlife Management*, vol. 73, no. 6, pp. 1014–1020, 2009.

[54] J. F. Cockrem, D. C. Adams, E. J. Bennett et al., "Endocrinology and the conservation of New Zealand birds," in *Experimental Approaches to Conservation Biology*, M. S. Gordon and S. M. Bartol, Eds., pp. 101–121, University of California Press, Los Angeles, Calif, USA, 2004.

[55] L. G. Popp, P. P. Serafini, A. L. S. Reghelin, K. M. Spercoski, J. J. Roper, and R. N. Morais, "Annual pattern of fecal corticoid excretion in captive Red-tailed parrots (*Amazona brasiliensis*)," *Journal of Comparative Physiology B*, vol. 178, no. 4, pp. 487–493, 2008.

[56] B. E. Washburn, J. J. Millspaugh, J. H. Schulz, S. B. Jones, and T. Mong, "Using fecal glucocorticoids for stress assessment in Mourning Doves," *The Condor*, vol. 105, no. 4, pp. 696–706, 2003.

[57] L. S. Hayward, R. K. Booth, and S. K. Wasser, "Eliminating the artificial effect of sample mass on avian fecal hormone metabolite concentration," *General and Comparative Endocrinology*, vol. 169, no. 2, pp. 117–122, 2010.

[58] A. M. Young and D. M. Hallford, "Validation of a fecal glucocorticoid metabolite assay to assess stress in the budgerigar (*Melopsittacus undulatus*)," *Zoo Biology*, vol. 32, no. 1, pp. 112–116, 2013.

[59] N. E. Cyr and L. M. Romero, "Fecal glucocorticoid metabolites of experimentally stressed captive and free-living starlings: implications for conservation research," *General and Comparative Endocrinology*, vol. 158, no. 1, pp. 20–28, 2008.

[60] R. J. G. Pereira, M. A. M. Granzinolli, and J. M. B. Duarte, "Annual profile of fecal androgen and glucocorticoid levels in free-living male American kestrels from southern mid-latitude areas," *General and Comparative Endocrinology*, vol. 166, no. 1, pp. 94–103, 2010.

[61] V. Careau, W. A. Buttemer, and K. L. Buchanan, "Early-developmental stress, repeatability, and canalization in a suite of physiological and behavioral traits in female zebra finches," *Integrative and Comparative Biology*, vol. 54, no. 4, pp. 539–554, 2014.

[62] K. A. Spencer, K. L. Buchanan, A. R. Goldsmith, and C. K. Catchpole, "Song as an honest signal of developmental stress in the zebra finch (*Taeniopygia guttata*)," *Hormones and Behavior*, vol. 44, no. 2, pp. 132–139, 2003.

[63] K. A. Spencer and S. Verhulst, "Delayed behavioral effects of postnatal exposure to corticosterone in the zebra finch (Taeniopygia guttata)," *Hormones and Behavior*, vol. 51, no. 2, pp. 273–280, 2007.

[64] P. Marra, K. Lampe, and B. Tedford, "Plasma corticosterone levels in two species of Zonotrichia sparrows under captive and free-living conditions," *Wilson Bulletin*, vol. 107, no. 2, pp. 296–305, 1995.

[65] J. D. Baylé, J. Boissin, J. Y. Daniel, and I. Assenmacher, "Hypothalamic-hypophysial control of adrenal cortical function in birds," *Neuroendocrinology*, vol. 7, no. 5-6, pp. 308–321, 1971.

[66] J. W. Dusseau and A. H. Meier, "Diurnal and seasonal variations of plasma adrenal steroid hormone in the white-throated sparrow, Zonotrichia albicollis," *General and Comparative Endocrinology*, vol. 16, no. 3, pp. 399–408, 1971.

[67] A. M. Dufty Jr. and J. R. Belthoff, "Corticosterone and the stress response in young western screech-owls: effects of captivity, gender, and activity period," *Physiological Zoology*, vol. 70, no. 2, pp. 143–149, 1997.

[68] H. C. Atkinson and B. J. Waddell, "The hypothalamic-pituitary-adrenal axis in rat pregnancy and lactation: circadian variation and interrelationship of plasma adrenocorticotropin and corticosterone," *Endocrinology*, vol. 136, no. 2, pp. 512–520, 1995.

[69] M. F. Dallman, "Stress update: adaptation of the hypothalamic-pituitary-adrenal axis to chronic stress," *Trends in Endocrinology and Metabolism*, vol. 4, no. 2, pp. 62–69, 1993.

[70] P. Santana, S. F. Akana, E. S. Hanson, A. M. Strack, R. J. Sebastian, and M. F. Dallman, "Aldosterone and dexamethasone both

stimulate energy acquisition whereas only the glucocorticoid alters energy storage," *Endocrinology*, vol. 136, no. 5, pp. 2214–2222, 1995.

[71] M. Lauber, S. Sugano, T. Ohnishi, M. Okamoto, and J. Müller, "Aldosterone biosynthesis and cytochrome P-45011β: evidence for two different forms of the enzyme in rats," *Journal of Steroid Biochemistry*, vol. 26, no. 6, pp. 693–698, 1987.

[72] M. A. Rensel, D. Comito, S. Kosarussavadi, and B. A. Schlinger, "Region-specific neural corticosterone patterns differ from plasma in a male songbird," *Endocrinology*, vol. 155, no. 9, pp. 3572–3581, 2014.

[73] D. J. Nichols and P. F. D. Chevins, "Effects of housing on corticosterone rhythm and stress responses in female mice," *Physiology and Behavior*, vol. 27, no. 1, pp. 1–5, 1981.

[74] D. Weinert, H. Eimert, H. G. Erkert, and U. Schneyer, "Resynchronization of the circadian corticosterone rhythm after a light/dark shift in juvenile and adult mice," *Chronobiology International*, vol. 11, no. 4, pp. 222–231, 1994.

[75] J. M. H. M. Reul and Y. Chandramohan, "Epigenetic mechanisms in stress-related memory formation," *Psychoneuroendocrinology*, vol. 32, no. 1, pp. S21–S25, 2007.

[76] B. Roozendaal, J. R. McReynolds, E. A. Van der Zee, S. Lee, J. L. McGaugh, and C. K. McIntyre, "Glucocorticoid effects on memory consolidation depend on functional interactions between the medial prefrontal cortex and basolateral amygdala," *The Journal of Neuroscience*, vol. 29, no. 45, pp. 14299–14308, 2009.

29

Protozoan Parasites of Rodents and Their Zoonotic Significance in Boyer-Ahmad District, Southwestern Iran

Zeinab Seifollahi, Bahador Sarkari, Mohammad Hossein Motazedian, Qasem Asgari, Mohammad Javad Ranjbar, and Samaneh Abdolahi Khabisi

Department of Parasitology and Mycology, School of Medicine, Shiraz University of Medical Sciences, Shiraz, Iran

Correspondence should be addressed to Bahador Sarkari; sarkarib@sums.ac.ir

Academic Editor: Remo Lobetti

Backgrounds. Wild rodents are reservoirs of various zoonotic diseases, such as toxoplasmosis, babesiosis, and leishmaniasis. The current study aimed to assess the protozoan infection of rodents in Boyer-Ahmad district, southwestern Iran. *Materials and Methods.* A total of 52 rodents were collected from different parts of Boyer-Ahmad district, in Kohgiluyeh and Boyer-Ahmad province, using Sherman live traps. Each rodent was anesthetized with ether, according to the ethics of working with animals, and was dissected. Samples were taken from various tissues and stool samples were collected from the contents of the colon and small intestines. Moreover, 2 to 5 mL of blood was taken from each of the rodents and the sera were examined for anti-*Leishmania* antibodies, by ELISA, or anti-*T. gondii* antibodies, by modified agglutination test (MAT). DNA was extracted from brain tissue samples of each rodent and PCR was used to identify the DNA of *T. gondii*. *Results.* Of the 52 stool samples of rodents studied by parasitological methods, intestinal protozoa infection was seen in 28 cases (53.8%). From 52 rodents, 19 (36.5%) were infected with *Trichomonas*, 10 (19.2%) with *Giardia muris*, and 11 (21.2%) with *Entamoeba* spp. Also, 10 cases (19.2%) were infected with *Blastocystis*, 3 (5.8%) were infected with *Chilomastix*, 7 (13.5%) were infected with *Endolimax*, 1 (1.9%) was infected with *Retortamonas*, 3 (5.77%) were infected with *T. gondii*, and 6 (11.54%) were infected with *Trypanosoma lewisi*. Antibodies to *T. gondii* were detected in the sera of 5 (9.61%) cases. Results of the molecular study showed *T. gondii* infection in 3 (5.77%) of the rodents. Findings of this study showed that rodents in Kohgiluyeh and Boyer-Ahmad province, southwestern Iran, are infected with several blood and intestinal parasites; some of them might be potential risks to residents and domestic animals in the region.

1. Introduction

Rodents are the most frequent and important mammals on the Earth, because they can adapt themselves to the different locations and environmental changes. These animals live on almost every continent except Antarctica [1]. Rodents are considered as reservoirs of various zoonotic diseases including toxoplasmosis, babesiosis, and leishmaniasis [1–4]. Nevertheless, rodents cannot directly cause disease in humans and disease is mainly transmitted to humans if human is in contact with rodents' feces and secretory materials. Transmission of the zoonotic pathogens to humans can occur via rodent's urine, feces, hair, and saliva [2]. Human activities which change the ecosystem of rodents' living place have an important role in the epidemiology of zoonotic diseases. Given the damage of rodents to humans and economic loss

and due to their health importance, parasitological studies on rodents seem necessary [2]. Several studies have been done on parasitic infections of wild rodent in Iran [5–10]. However, due to ecological differences in different areas of the country, the parasitic fauna of the rodents in each ecological setting might be different. This notion justifies new studies on parasitic infection of the rodents in other areas of the country. The current study aimed to assess the parasitic protozoan infections of rodents in Boyer-Ahmad district, southwest Iran.

2. Materials and Methods

2.1. The Study Area. Boyer-Ahmad district is located in Kohgiluyeh and Boyer-Ahmad province. The province is located in southwest of Iran with geographical coordinates of 30° 40′ 12″ N, 51° 36′ 0″ E. The province has two types of tropical and cold climate and Boyer-Ahmad district is located in the cold area. The mean of long-term rain and snow amount is above 600 mm in this area and a wide area of the county is covered with forests of oak, wild pistachio, and mountain almond. The main professions of the people are agricultural practice and breeding and raising livestock.

2.2. Rodents' Collection and Identification. Considering the map of the study area, 52 rodents were collected from different parts of Boyer-Ahmad County, using Sherman live traps with roasted almonds, as bait, in the summer and autumn of 2014. Different areas of the district, including villages of Kakan, Madvan, Tange Sorkh, Kal Morgah, Mansourabad, and Dehno, were selected for sampling. After transferring to the laboratory, the genus and species of rodents were identified based on morphological characteristics. This was done to subsequently find out the rate of protozoan parasites in each rodent's species.

2.3. Evaluation of Rodents' Protozoan Infection. After transferring the rodents to the laboratory, they were anesthetized with ether and blood samples were taken from their heart. Different rodent parts were carefully examined and necessary samples were prepared. Smears were prepared from rodent liver, spleen, and peripheral blood on glass slides, fixed with methanol, and stained with Giemsa. Then smears were studied by an optical microscope with 100x magnification.

Temporary staining of rodent's stool samples, with Lugol's solution, was done for detection of any protozoan cysts or trophozoites. The samples were also examined with formalin-ethyl acetate sedimentation and zinc sulfate floatation techniques and the obtained materials were observed by conventional light microscope. Smears were also prepared from the rodent stool samples and stained with trichrome. Moreover, smears were prepared from the stool sediments or floated materials, obtained by concentration methods, fixed with methanol, and stained with acid-fast staining to detect coccidia parasites in fecal samples.

2.4. Serological Assessment of Rodents' Sera Samples. Rodents' sera were examined by indirect ELISA for anti-*Leishmania* antibodies. Moreover, MAT was performed on rodent sera samples, as previously described, to assess anti-*T. gondii* antibodies [11]. Sera were studied in two dilutions of 1 : 20 and 1 : 40 and samples with MAT titer of 1 : 40 or higher were considered as positive.

2.5. Molecular Analysis of Rodents' Tissue Samples. DNA was extracted from brain tissue samples of each rodent, using DNA extraction kit, based on the manufacturer's (Yekta-Tajhiz Azma, Tehran, Iran) instructions. PCR was performed to amplify a 529 bp gene of *T. gondii*, as described by Edvinsson et al. [12]. The two primers used were TOXOF CAG GGA GGA AGA CGA AAGTTG and TOXOR CAG ACA CAG TGC ATC TGG ATT. PCR products were separated in 1.5% agarose gel and stained with ethidium bromide.

2.6. Statistical Analysis. The statistical analysis was performed with SPSS software (version 16). Chi-square test was

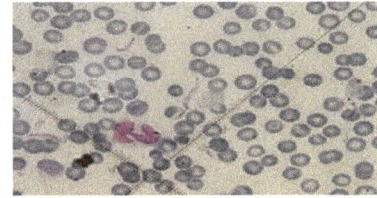

FIGURE 1: *Trypanosoma lewisi* in blood smear of the studied rodents, stained with Giemsa (100x).

used to examine the association between rodent's parasitic infections and related studied factors, such as rodent's species, gender, place of collection, and weight.

3. Results

A total of 52 rodents were captured during the course of this study, including 25 (48.1%) *Meriones*, 15 (28.8%) *Rattus*, 10 (19.2%) *Apodemus*, 1 (1.9%) *Calomyscus*, and 1 (1.9%) *Arvicola*. Among the captured rodents, 28 (53.8%) were males and 24 (46.2%) were females.

Of the 52 feces samples of rodents, examined by parasitological methods, 37 (71.1%) were infected with at least one protozoan parasite, whereas 15 (28.8%) of the rodents were not infected with any intestinal protozoan parasites. From 52 rodents, 19 (36.5%) were infected with *Trichomonas*, 10 (19.2%) with *G. muris*, 11 (21.2%) with *Entamoeba*, 10 (19.2%) with *Blastocystis*, 3 (5.8%) with *Chilomastix*, 7 (13.5%) with *Endolimax*, and 1 (1.9%) was infected with *Retortamonas*. Regarding the rodents' infection with blood and tissue protozoa, 3 (5.77%) were infected with *T. gondii* and 6 (11.54%) with *Trypanosoma lewisi* (Figure 1). Anti-*Leishmania* antibodies were detected in the sera of 8 (15.34%) of the rodents; among them were 6 rodents which were also infected with *Trypanosoma lewisi*. No *Leishmania* parasites were observed in the impression smears of liver or spleen of the seropositive rodents. Figure 2 shows a few of intestinal protozoa detected in trichrome-stained samples of rodents' feces.

Multiple infections were seen in 19 out of 52 (36.5%) rodents. Simultaneous infection with *Trichomonas* and *Entamoeba* was seen in 5.8%, *Trichomonas* and *G. muris* in 1.9%, *G. muris* and *Trypanosoma* in 1.9%, *Blastocystis* and *G. muris* in 1.9%, *Trichomonas* and *Blastocystis* in 1.9%, and *Entamoeba* and *Blastocystis* in 1.9% of the rodents. Also, simultaneous infection with *Blastocystis*, *Trypanosoma*, and *Endolimax* was observed in 1.9% of the rodents.

In this study, 54.2% of rodents, infected with intestinal protozoa, were female and 45.8% were male. Statistical analysis showed no significant correlation between various protozoa and gender of the rodents ($P > 0.05$).

The highest rates of infection with *G. muris* (70%), *Trichomonas* (36.8%), *Endolimax* (71.4%), *Trypanosoma* (100%), and *Blastocystis* (60%) were seen in *Rattus* genus and the highest infection with *Entamoeba* (54.5%) was seen in the genus *Meriones*. Statistical analysis showed significant correlation between protozoa infection and the rodent's genus ($P < 0.05$). Table 1 shows the distribution of protozoan infections according to the rodent genus.

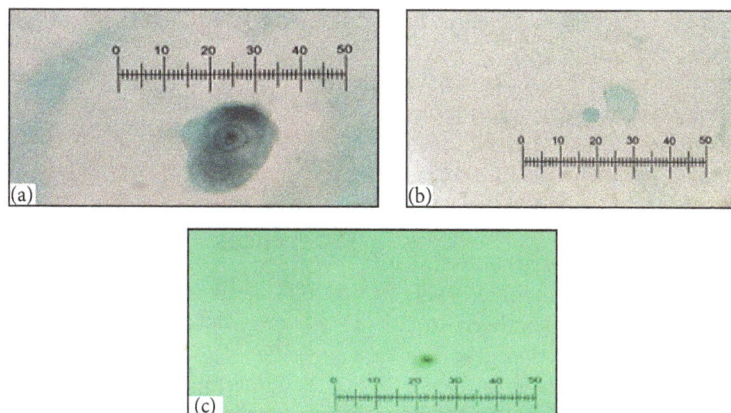

FIGURE 2: Protozoa in stool samples of the rodents, stained with trichrome. (a) *Entamoeba* trophozoite, (b) *Trichomonas* trophozoite, and (c) *Endolimax* trophozoite (100x).

TABLE 1: Distribution of protozoan infection according to genus of the studied rodents.

	Rattus		Meriones		Calomyscus		Apodemus		Arvicola		Total	
	Number	%	Number	%	Number	%	Number	%	Number	%	Number	%
G. muris	7	70	2	20	0	0	1	10	0	0	10	19.23
Trichomonas	7	36.8	4	21.1	1	5.3	7	36.8	0	0	19	36.5
Blastocystis	6	60	2	20	1	10	1	10	0	0	10	19.23
Entamoeba	4	36.4	6	54.5	0	0	1	1.9	0	0	11	21.1
Chilomastix	1	33.3	1	33.3	0	0	1	33.3	0	0	3	5.8
Endolimax	5	71.4	1	14.3	0	0	1	33.3	0	0	7	13.46
Retortamonas	0	0	0	0	0	0	1	100	0	0	1	1.92
Trypanosoma	6	100	0	0	0	0	0	0	0	0	6	11.53
T. gondii	0	0	1	33.3	1	33.3	1	33.3	0	0	3	508

Findings of the molecular study showed *T. gondii* infection in 3 (5.77%) rodents; two male and one female. Rodents infected with *T. gondii* were from *Apodemus*, *Meriones*, and *Calomyscus* genus. Figure 3 shows PCR products of DNA, isolated from rodents' brain tissue.

No cases of coccidial infection were seen in any of the fecal samples when the samples were evaluated by modified acid-fast staining method.

4. Discussion

Rodents are considered as reservoirs for a few of helminthic and protozoan parasites [1, 2]. Among the protozoa parasites of rodents is *T. gondii* which is common in rodents and these animals can behave as natural reservoir for this protozoa. Evaluation of *T. gondii* infection in rodents, as the main pray for cat, with regards to the role of cat in spreading of *T. gondii* oocyst in the environment, is important [13]. Rate of *Toxoplasma* infection in rodents is different based on ecological status of a given area. In the current study, *T. gondii* infection was common protozoa of the studied rodents. Saki and Khademvatan reported a prevalence rate of 6% for *T. gondii* in rodents of Ahvaz district, south of Iran [14]. Study of Mercier et al. in 2013, assessing 766 rodents in Niamey district of Niger, revealed *Toxoplasma* infection in 1.96%

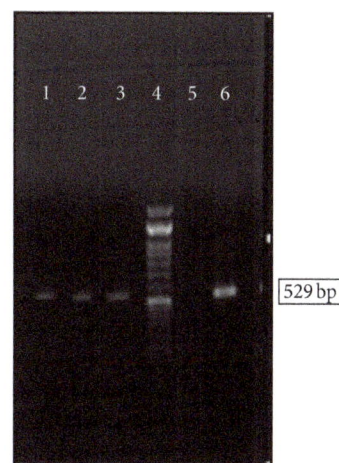

FIGURE 3: The PCR product of the DNA of *T. gondii* isolated from the rodents brain tissues. Lanes 1–3, samples isolated from rodents' brain tissue; lane 4, 50 bp DNA Ladder; lane 5, negative control; lane 6, positive control (tachyzoite prepared from mice peritonea).

of the studied rodents [15]. In the current study, *T. gondii* infection was found in *Apodemus*, *Meriones*, and *Calomyscus* genus and, to the best of our knowledge, this is the first report of molecular detection of *T. gondii* infection in *Calomyscus* from Iran.

Another important parasitic infection that rodents have an important role in its transmission, as reservoirs, is leishmaniasis. A large number of species of rodents have been identified as reservoir of cutaneous leishmaniasis in Iran [3–5]. Mohebali et al. reported the infection of different species of the rodents, including *Rhombomys opimus*, *Meriones libycus*, *Tatera indica*, and *Meriones hurrianae* with *L. major* [16]. Rassi et al. reported that *Meriones libycus* is the main reservoir of cutaneous leishmaniasis in Fars province, southern Iran [17]. In the present study, *Leishmania* infection was not detected in any of the studied rodents. The reason for this is that leishmaniasis is mainly seen in tropical and subtropical areas of Iran, while Boyer-Ahmad district is located in cold and mountainous region of the country and is not considered as an endemic focus of cutaneous leishmaniasis. Although visceral leishmaniasis is not uncommon in this district, its reservoirs are dogs, carnivores, or properly cats, rather than rodents [18–20].

Rodents are frequently infected with intestinal protozoa and may act as reservoir for a few of them. In the current study, intestinal protozoa including *Trichomonas*, *Entamoeba*, and *G. muris* were detected in the studied rodents. Rate of *Giardia* infection, as the main intestinal protozoa, in rodents was found to be 14.6% in Al Hindi and Abu-Haddaf study in 2013 in Palestine, 96.3% in *Microtus* and 48.3% in *Apodemus* species in Poland, 2.5% in the study by Rasti and colleagues in 2000 in Kashan, Iran, and 2.7% in the study by Kia and colleagues in 2001 in Ahvaz, south of Iran [7, 21–23]. In the current study, rate of *G. muris* infection in the rodents was relatively high. Further study is needed to compare the genotype of these protozoa, isolated from the rodents with the human isolates.

Infection with blood protozoa, *Trypanosoma*, was common in the studied rodents in our study. Lower rate of infection (10%) with this parasite has been reported in Kia et al. study in Ahvaz, south of Iran [7], whereas higher rates of infection have been reported from Brazil (21.7%) and India (82.3%) [24, 25].

In this study, infection with intestinal coccidia was not found in the rodents, while other studies have reported coccidia infection in these animals [21]. This difference could be due to the differences in climatic conditions in the studied areas, and also nutritional or habitat preferences of the rodents.

Taken together, findings of the current study revealed that rodents in Kohgiluyeh and Boyer-Ahmad province, in southwest of Iran, are infected with many intestinal and blood protozoa. Some of these protozoa may be potential risks to the residents and domestic animals in the region. High prevalence of intestinal protozoan infections in the rodents might be linked to the unsafe disposal of human waste and also use of human and animal fertilizers in the area.

Conflict of Interests

The authors declare that there is no conflict of interests regarding the publication of this paper.

Acknowledgments

The results described in this paper were part of MSc thesis of Zeinab Seifollahi. The study was financially supported by the office of vice-chancellor for research of Shiraz University of Medical Sciences (Grant No. 7322-93).

References

[1] B. G. Meerburg, G. R. Singleton, and A. Kijlstra, "Rodent-borne diseases and their risks for public health," *Critical Reviews in Microbiology*, vol. 35, no. 3, pp. 221–270, 2009.

[2] B. G. Meerburg, "Rodents are a risk factor for the spreading of pathogens on farms," *Veterinary Microbiology*, vol. 142, no. 3-4, pp. 464–465, 2010.

[3] M. H. Davami, M. H. Motazedian, M. Kalantari et al., "Molecular survey on detection of Leishmania infection in rodent reservoirs in Jahrom District, Southern Iran," *Journal of Arthropod-Borne Diseases*, vol. 8, no. 2, pp. 139–146, 2014.

[4] B. Pourmohammadi, M. H. Motazedian, and M. Kalantari, "Rodent infection with *Leishmania* in a new focus of human cutaneous leishmaniasis, in northern Iran," *Annals of Tropical Medicine and Parasitology*, vol. 102, no. 2, pp. 127–133, 2008.

[5] D. Mehrabani, M. H. Motazedian, A. Oryan, Q. Asgari, G. R. Hatam, and M. Karamian, "A search for the rodent hosts of *Leishmania major* in the Larestan region of southern Iran: demonstration of the parasite in *Tatera indica* and *Gerbillus* sp., by microscopy, culture and PCR," *Annals of Tropical Medicine and Parasitology*, vol. 101, no. 4, pp. 315–322, 2007.

[6] S. Gholami, H. F. Motevali, E. Moabedi, and S. Shahabi, "Study of helmintic intestinal parasites in the rodents from the rural and central regions of Mazandaran province in the years 1997 to 1999," *Journal of Mazandaran University of Medical Sciences*, vol. 12, no. 35, pp. 67–75, 2002.

[7] E. Kia, M. Homayouni, A. Farahnak, M. Mohebali, and S. Shojai, "Study of endoparasites of rodents and their zoonotic importance in Ahvaz, South West Iran," *Iranian Journal of Public Health*, vol. 30, pp. 49–52, 2001.

[8] E. B. Kia, E. Shahryary-Rad, M. Mohebali et al., "Endoparasites of rodents and their zoonotic importance in Germi, Dashte-Mogan, Ardabil Province, Iran," *Iranian Journal of Parasitology*, vol. 5, no. 4, pp. 15–20, 2010.

[9] S. M. Sadjjadi and J. Massoud, "Helminth parasites of wild rodents in Khuzestan province, south west of Iran," *Journal of Veterinary Parasitology*, vol. 13, no. 1, pp. 55–56, 1999.

[10] A. Salehabadi, G. Mowlavi, and S. M. Sadjjadi, "Human infection with *Moniliformis moniliformis* (Bremser 1811) (Travassos 1915) in Iran: another case report after three decades," *Vector-Borne and Zoonotic Diseases*, vol. 8, pp. 101–104, 2008.

[11] B. Sarkari, Q. Asgari, N. Bagherian et al., "Molecular and Serological evaluation of *Toxoplasma gondii* infection in reared turkeys in Fars Province, Iran," *Jundishapur Journal of Microbiology*, vol. 7, no. 7, Article ID e11598, 2014.

[12] B. Edvinsson, S. Jalal, C. E. Nord, B. S. Pedersen, and B. Evengård, "DNA extraction and PCR assays for detection of *Toxoplasma gondii*," *APMIS*, vol. 112, no. 6, pp. 342–348, 2004.

[13] C. Gotteland, Y. Chaval, I. Villena et al., "Species or local environment, what determines the infection of rodents by *Toxoplasma gondii*?" *Parasitology*, vol. 141, no. 2, pp. 259–268, 2014.

[14] J. Saki and S. Khademvatan, "Detection of *Toxoplasma gondii* by PCR and mouse bioassay in rodents of Ahvaz District, Southwestern Iran," *BioMed Research International*, vol. 2014, Article ID 383859, 5 pages, 2014.

[15] A. Mercier, M. Garba, H. Bonnabau et al., "Toxoplasmosis seroprevalence in urban rodents: a survey in Niamey, Niger," *Memorias do Instituto Oswaldo Cruz*, vol. 108, no. 4, pp. 399–407, 2013.

[16] M. Mohebali, E. Javadian, M. R. Yaghoobi-Ershadi, A. A. Akhavan, H. Hajjaran, and M. R. Abaei, "Characterization of Leishmania infection in rodents from endemic areas of the Islamic Republic of Iran," *Eastern Mediterranean Health Journal*, vol. 10, no. 4-5, pp. 591–599, 2004.

[17] Y. Rassi, M. Jalali, E. Javadian, and M. Moatazedian, "Confirmation of *Meriones libycus* (Rodentia; Gerbillidae) as the main reservoir host of zoonotic cutaneous leishmaniasis in arsanjan, fars province, South of Iran (1999-2000)," *Iranian Journal of Public Health*, vol. 30, no. 3-4, pp. 143–144, 2001.

[18] B. Sarkari, N. Pedram, M. Mohebali et al., "Seroepidemiological study of visceral leishmaniasis in Booyerahmad district, southwest Islamic Republic of Iran," *Eastern Mediterranean Health Journal*, vol. 16, no. 11, pp. 1133–1136, 2010.

[19] G. R. Hatam, S. J. Adnani, Q. Asgari et al., "First report of natural infection in cats with *Leishmania infantum* in Iran," *Vector-Borne and Zoonotic Diseases*, vol. 10, no. 3, pp. 313–316, 2010.

[20] B. Sarkari, G. R. Hatam, S. J. Adnani, and Q. Asgari, "Seroprevalence of feline leishmaniasis in areas of Iran where *Leishmania infantum* is endemic," *Annals of Tropical Medicine and Parasitology*, vol. 103, no. 3, pp. 275–277, 2009.

[21] A. I. Al Hindi and E. Abu-Haddaf, "Gastrointestinal parasites and ectoparasites biodiversity of *Rattus rattus* trapped from Khan Younis and Jabalia in Gaza strip, Palestine," *Journal of the Egyptian Society of Parasitology*, vol. 43, no. 1, pp. 259–268, 2013.

[22] S. Rasti, I. Moubedi, R. Dehghani, and A. Drodgar, "The survey of gastrointestinal helminths of mice in Kashan," *Journal of the Faculty of Veterinary Medicine, University of Tehran*, vol. 55, no. 4, pp. 57–59, 2000.

[23] A. Bajer, M. Bednarska, A. Pawełczyk, J. M. Behnke, F. S. Gilbert, and E. Sinski, "Prevalence and abundance of *Cryptosporidium parvum* and *Giardia* spp. in wild rural rodents from the Mazury Lake District region of Poland," *Parasitology*, vol. 125, no. 1, pp. 21–34, 2002.

[24] R. Laha, H. Hemaprasanth, and D. Bhatta-Charya, "Observations on prevalence of *Trypanosoma lewisi* infection in wild rats and a trial on its adaptation in unnatural host," *Journal of Parasitology and Applied Animal Biology*, vol. 6, pp. 5–8, 1997.

[25] P. M. Linardi and J. R. Botelho, "Prevalence of *Trypanosoma lewisi* in Rattus norvegicus from Belo Horizonte, State of Minas Gerais, Brazil," *Memórias do Instituto Oswaldo Cruz*, vol. 97, no. 3, pp. 411–414, 2002.

Permissions

List of Contributors

Amin Tamadon
Transgenic Technology Research Center, Shiraz University of Medical Sciences, Shiraz, Iran

Alireza Raayat Jahromi and Mohammad Ayaseh
Department of Clinical Sciences, School of Veterinary Medicine, Shiraz University, P.O. Box 1731-71345, Shiraz, Iran

Farhad Rahmanifar
Department of Basic Sciences, School of Veterinary Medicine, Shiraz University, P.O. Box 1731-71345, Shiraz, Iran

Omid Koohi-Hosseinabadi
Laboratory Animal Center, Shiraz University of Medical Sciences, Shiraz, Iran

Reza Moghiminasr
Department of Stem Cells and Developmental Biology, Cell Science Research Center, Royan Institute for Stem Cell Biology and Technology, ACECR, Tehran, Iran

Justin Shmalberg
Small Animal Clinical Sciences, College of Veterinary Medicine, University of Florida, Gainesville, FL 32608, USA

Mushtaq A. Memon
Department of Veterinary Clinical Sciences, College of Veterinary Medicine, Washington State University, Pullman, WA 99164, USA

Patrícia F. Castro, Denise T. Fantoni, Bruna C. Miranda and Julia M. Matera
Department of Surgery, School of Veterinary Medicine and Animal Science, University of São Paulo, Avenida Prof. Orlando Marques de Paiva 87, Cidade Universitária, 05508-270 São Paulo, SP, Brazil

T. Getachew, G. Getachew, G. Sintayehu, M. Getenet and A. Fasil
National Animal Health Diagnostic and Investigation Center (NAHDIC), EthiopianMinistry of Livestock and Fisheries Development, P.O. Box 04, Sebeta, Ethiopia

Carolina Gallego
Laboratory of Veterinary Pathology, Universidad de Ciencias Aplicadas y Ambientales, Calle 222 No. 55-37, Bogotá, Colombia
Faculty of Science, Pontificia Universidad Javeriana, Carrera 7 No. 43-82, Bogotá, Colombia

Stefany Romero
Academic Assistant, Veterinary Medicine Program, Universidad de La Salle, Cra. 7 No. 179-03, Bogotá, Colombia

Paula Esquinas
Laboratory of Cytogenetics and Genotyping of Domestic Animal UGA, Faculty of Veterinary Medicine, National University of Colombia, Bogotá, Colombia

Pilar Patiño, Nhora Martínez and Carlos Iregui
Laboratory of Veterinary Pathology, Faculty of Veterinary Medicine, National University of Colombia, Bogotá, Colombia

Yu'e Wu, Fangui Min, Jinchun Pan, Jing Wang, Wen Yuan, Yu Zhang and Ren Huang
Guangdong Laboratory Animals Monitoring Institute, Guangdong Provincial Key Laboratory of Laboratory Animals, Guangzhou 510663, China

Lixin Zhang
Institute of Microbiology, Chinese Academy of Sciences, Beijing 100080, China

Eva Spada, Daniela Proverbio, Luciana Baggiani and Roberta Perego
Veterinary Transfusion Unit (REV), Department of Health, Animal Science and Food Safety (VESPA), University ofMilan, Via G. Celoria 10, 20133Milan, Italy

Luis Miguel Viñals Flórez
Centro de Transfusión Veterinario (CTV), Arturo Soria 267, 28033 Madrid, Spain

Blanca Serra Gómez de la Serna
Clinical Veterinary Hospital, CEU Cardenal Herrera University, Alfara del Patriarca, 46115 Valencia, Spain

Maria del Rosario Perlado Chamizo
Laboratorio de Análisis Clínico, Hospital Clínico Veterinario, Universidad Alfonso X el Sabio, Avenida de la Universidad, Villanueva de la Cañada, 28691Madrid, Spain

Mauro José Lahm Cardoso, Marcelo de Souza Zanutto and Eduardo Yudi Hashizume
Department of Veterinary Clinics, State University of Londrina, Londrina, PR, Brazil

Rafael Fagnani
Northern Paraňa State University, Londrina, PR, Brazil

Carolina Zaghi Cavalcante
Pontifical Catholic University of Paraná, Curitiba, PR, Brazil

Ademir Zacarias Júnior, Luciane Holsback da Silveira Fertonani and Helena Pinheiro Costa
Northern Paraná University, Bandeirantes, PR, Brazil

Jéssica Ragazzi Calesso and Maíra Melussi
Veterinary Space Life, Londrina, PR, Brazil

C. G. Donnelly
Cornell University College of Veterinary Medicine, Ithaca, NY 14850, USA

C. T. Quinn and S. L. Raidal
School of Animal and Veterinary Sciences, Charles Sturt University, Wagga Wagga, NSW2650, Australia

S. G. Nielsen
3Quantitative Consulting Unit, Research Office, Charles Sturt University,WaggaWagga, NSW2650, Australia

Gbemisola Magaret Olabanji, Beatty VivMaikai and Gbeminiyi Richard Otolorin
Department of Veterinary Public Health and Preventive Medicine, Faculty of Veterinary Medicine, Ahmadu Bello University, Zaria, Kaduna State, Nigeria

T. K. W. Sikombe
Department of Disease Control, School of Veterinary Medicine, University of Zambia, P.O. Box 32379, Lusaka, Zambia
Central Veterinary Research Institute, P.O. Box 33980, Lusaka, Zambia

A. S. Mweene, JohnMuma and M. Simuunza
Department of Disease Control, School of Veterinary Medicine, University of Zambia, P.O. Box 32379, Lusaka, Zambia

C. Kasanga
Faculty of Veterinary Medicine, Sokoine University of Agriculture, P.O. Box 3021, Morogoro, Tanzania

Y. Sinkala
Department of Disease Control, School of Veterinary Medicine, University of Zambia, P.O. Box 32379, Lusaka, Zambia
National Livestock Epidemiology and Information Centre, P.O. Box 30041, Lusaka, Zambia

F. Banda
Central Veterinary Research Institute, P.O. Box 33980, Lusaka, Zambia

M. Mulumba
Southern African Development Community Secretariat, SADC House, Plot No. 54385, Central Business District, Private Bag 0095, Gaborone, Botswana

E. M. Fana
Botswana Vaccine Institute, Private Bag 0031, Gaborone, Botswana

C. Mundia
Department of Veterinary Services, Southern African Development Community, Trans-Boundary Animal Disease Section, Ministry of Agriculture and Livestock, P.O. Box 50060, Lusaka, Zambia

Divya Gupta, Varinder Uppal, Neelam Bansal and Anuradha Gupta
Department of Veterinary Anatomy, College of Veterinary Sciences, Guru Angad Dev Veterinary and Animal Sciences University, Ludhiana, Punjab 141004, India

Chiara Starita, Alessandra Gavazza and George Lubas
Department of Veterinary Sciences, University of Pisa, Via Livornese LatoMonte, San Piero a Grado, 56122 Pisa, Italy

Zita Talamonti, Chiara Cassis, Paola G. Brambilla, Paola Scarpa, Damiano Stefanello, Simona Cannas, Michela Minero and Clara Palestrini
Università degli Studi di Milano, Dipartimento di Scienze Veterinarie e Sanità Pubblica (DIVET), Via Celoria 10, 20133Milan, Italy

Md. Arifur Rahman, Md. Mahbub Alam, Md. Aminul Islam and A. K. M. Anisur Rahman
Department of Medicine, Faculty of Veterinary Science, Bangladesh Agricultural University (BAU), Mymensingh 2202, Bangladesh

A. K. Fazlul Haque Bhuiyan
Department of Animal Breeding and Genetics, Faculty of Animal Husbandry, BAU, Mymensingh 2202, Bangladesh

Tongku N. Siregar, Juli Melia, Rohaya, Cut Nila Thasmi, DianMasyitha, Sri Wahyuni, Juliana Rosa, Nurhafni, Budianto Panjaitan and Herrialfian
Faculty of Veterinary Medicine, Syiah Kuala University, Banda Aceh 23111, Indonesia

Silvia Mazzola, Clara Palestrini, Simona Cannas, Eleonora Fè,
Gaia Lisa Bagnato, Daniele Vigo and Michela Minero
Dipartimento di Medicina Veterinaria, Universit`a degli Studi di Milano, Via Celoria 10, 20133 Milan, Italy

Diane Frank
Faculté de Médecine Vétérinaire, Département de Sciences Cliniques, Université de Montréal, No. 3200, rue Sicotte, Saint-Hyacinthe, QC, Canada J2S 2M2

Tamer A. Sharafeldin
Department of Veterinary Population Medicine and Minnesota Veterinary Diagnostic Laboratory, Saint Paul, MN 55108, USA
Department of Pathology, Faculty of Veterinary Medicine, Zagazig University, Zagazig 44519, Egypt

Qingshan Chen
Excelen, Center for Bone & Joint Research and Education, Minneapolis, MN 55415, USA

Sunil K. Mor, Sagar M. Goyal and Robert E. Porter
Department of Veterinary Population Medicine and Minnesota Veterinary Diagnostic Laboratory, Saint Paul, MN 55108, USA

Thomas R. Tucker III and Janet E. Foley
Departments of Medicine and Epidemiology, School of Veterinary Medicine, University of California, Davis, Davis, CA 95616, USA

Sharif S. Aly
Department of Population Health and Reproduction, School of Veterinary Medicine, University of California, Davis, Davis, CA 95616, USA
Veterinary Medicine Teaching and Research Center, School of Veterinary Medicine, University of California, Davis, Tulare, CA 95616, USA

JohnMaas
Department of Population Health and Reproduction,University of California, Davis, Davis, CA 95616, USA

Josh S. Davy
Division of Agriculture and Natural Resources, University of California, Davis, Red Bluff, CA 96080, USA

Gabriela Silva-Hidalgo, Martin López-Valenzuela, Nora Cárcamo-Aréchiga,
Silvia Cota-Guajardo and Mayra López-Salazar Pathology Laboratory, Faculty of Veterinary Medicine and Animal Husbandry, Autonomous University of Sinaloa, Boulevard San Ángel s/n, Fraccionamiento San Benito, 80246 Culiacán, SIN, Mexico

Edith Montiel-Vázquez
Enteric Bacteriology Laboratory, Institute of Epidemiological Diagnosis and Reference, Francisco de P. Miranda 177, Lomas de Plateros, Álvaro Obregón, 01480 Mexico City, DF, Mexico

Philip Paul Mshelbwala, J. Scott Weese and Jibrin Manu Idris
Department of Veterinary Medicine, Faculty of Veterinary Medicine, University of Abuja, Abuja, Nigeria
Department of Pathobiology, Ontario Veterinary College, University of Guelph, Guelph, ON, Canada
African Field Epidemiology Network, Abuja, Nigeria

Ana Margarida Alho, Miguel Landum JoséMeireles and Luís Madeira de Carvalho
CIISA, Faculty of Veterinary Medicine, ULisboa, Avenida da Universidade Técnica, 1300-477 Lisboa, Portugal

António Fiarresga
Cardiology Unit, Hospital de Santa Marta, Centro Hospitalar de Lisboa Central, EPE, Rua de Santa Marta 50, 1169-024 Lisboa, Portugal

Clara Lima and Óscar Gamboa
Small Animal Teaching Hospital, Faculty of Veterinary Medicine, ULisboa, Avenida da Universidade Técnica, 1300-477 Lisboa, Portugal

José Sales Luís
CIISA, Faculty of Veterinary Medicine, ULisboa, Avenida da Universidade Técnica, 1300-477 Lisboa, Portugal
Small Animal Teaching Hospital, Faculty of Veterinary Medicine, ULisboa, Avenida da Universidade Técnica, 1300-477 Lisboa, Portugal

A. S. Aban
Department of Surgery and Gynecology, Faculty of Veterinary Medicine, Upper Nile University, Malakal, South Sudan

R. M. Abdelghafar, M. E. Badawi and A.M. Almubarak
Department of Veterinary Medicine and Surgery, College of Veterinary Medicine, Sudan University of Science and Technology, Khartoum, Sudan

Nigatu Disassa
Assosa University, P.O. Box 18, Assosa, Ethiopia

Berhanu Sibhat, Shimelis Mengistu, YimerMuktar and Dinaol Belina
Haramaya University College of Veterinary Medicine, P.O. Box 138, Dire Dawa, Ethiopia

Abdalla Mohamed Ibrahim
Abrar Research and Training Centre, Abrar University, Mogadishu, Somalia
College of Veterinary Medicine, University of Bahri, Khartoum, Sudan

Ahmed A. H. Kadle
ICRC, Mogadishu, Somalia

Hamisi Said Nyingilili
Vector and Vector Borne Diseases Institute, Tanga, Tanzania

Sabrina Destri Emmerick Campos and Nádia Regina Pereira Almosny
Departamento de Patologia e Clínica Veterinária, Universidade Federal Fluminense, 24230-340 Niterói, RJ, Brazil

Nathalie Costa da Cunha
Departamento de Saúde Coletiva Veterinária e Saúde Pública, Universidade Federal Fluminense, 24230-340 Niterói, RJ, Brazil

J. Awah-Ndukum, J. Temwa, V. Ngu Ngwa, M. M. Mouiche and P. A. Zoli
School of Veterinary Medicine and Sciences, University of Ngaoundéré, BP 454, Ngaoundéré, Cameroon

D. Iyawa
Regional Delegation of Livestock, Fisheries, Animal Industries, Far North Region, Cameroon

Maura Turriani, Nicola Bernabò, Barbara Barboni and Paolo Berardinelli
Unit of Basic and Applied Bioscience, Faculty of Veterinary Medicine, University of Teramo, Via Renato Balzarini 1, 64100 Teramo, Italy

Gianluca Todisco
Via per Mosciano, No. 96, Giulianova, 64021 Teramo, Italy

Luigi Montini
Via Villafranca No. 11, 72100 Brindisi, Italy

Zeinab Seifollahi, Bahador Sarkari,Mohammad Hossein Motazedian, Qasem Asgari, Mohammad Javad Ranjbar and Samaneh Abdolahi Khabisi
Department of Parasitology and Mycology, School of Medicine, Shiraz University of Medical Sciences, Shiraz, Iran

Index